Personalized Medicine in Oncology

Priya Hays

Personalized Medicine in Oncology

Precision Oncology and Transformative Technologies

Springer

Priya Hays
Hays Documentation Specialists, LLC
San Mateo, CA, USA

ISBN 978-3-032-14436-2 ISBN 978-3-032-14437-9 (eBook)
https://doi.org/10.1007/978-3-032-14437-9

This Springer imprint is published by the registered company Springer Nature Switzerland AG
The registered company address is: Gewerbestrasse 11, 6330 Cham, Switzerland

Hummingbirds in blue blurs whir
Necklaced around the nectar feeder,
Each creature gleaming, bright,
A piece of polished apatite
Through whose facets sunlight
Shatters into flashing gaslight
Shards that fall into the larkspur
& blaze up, igniting every flower,
Each glowing petal blue proclaims
The feast by bluer glowing
Bluer than a Day-Glo wing—
& yet, though they in flames
Are wrapped from stem to bloom,
It is the fire the flowers consume.

"The Church Gardens: A Walk,"
by Jay Hopler

For the cancer patients

for the brilliant and dedicated physician-scientists and oncologists who have made the gains of precision oncology possible

Preface

Personalized medicine for oncology had an interesting path for its development by the precision oncology community, and public perceptions remain varied. Terms such as *biomarkers*, *personalized*, *targeted therapies*, *big data*, and *electronic health records* took on a life of their own. President Barack Obama was one of the first advocates of precision medicine, and his 2015 State of the Union speech specifically addressed a cure for cancer as its main goal, which was reiterated by President Joe Biden in the Cancer Moonshot Program. Precision oncology has become a field in its own right, with journals, conferences, and courses of study having emerged and with further development of its technologies devoted to its advancement.

When I was writing the second edition of *Advancing Healthcare Through Personalized Medicine* and the collaborative edited collection "Cancer Immunotherapies" on the subject of precision oncology, the excitement in the field was palpable, and I was consequently engaged. The responses to these books were mainly positive, with a few being overwhelmingly positive, which I was greatly appreciative of.

However, a personal complacency set in when writing this edition, which had to be overcome. The contract arrived in 2022, and as of the end of 2024, I still did not have a manuscript to submit. I started to attend conferences again after having achieved professional milestones in the field, such as being ranked in ScholarGPS and having written a series of articles (including an ebook on personalized medicine) in the policy publication Open Access Government United Kingdom on personalized cancer medicines and the emergence of precision oncology, which I affectionately refer to as "the British Articles." I wrote and published an article on artificial intelligence in pathology that appeared in the *European Journal of Medical Research* and on chronic lymphocytic leukemia in *Discover Oncology*, among other significant milestones.

The field has advanced considerably, with a thriving community of cancer centers supporting it. This is shown by the increasing number of US Federal Drug Administration (FDA) approvals for precision oncology drugs. In 2023, there were 28 precision medicine approvals, whereas in 2024, there were 48 drugs, 35 being biomarker indicated and eight being autologous cell therapies, which represented a

70% increase. Cancer immunotherapies represent remarkable gains, including immune checkpoint inhibitors, bispecific antibodies, adoptive cellular therapies, and antibody drug conjugates.

The audiences for this book are varied and include oncologists, cancer patients, physicians, scientists, dedicated healthcare professionals, and the community of scholars who have helped make personalized medicine for cancer a reality.

San Mateo, CA, USA
September 2025

Priya Hays

Acknowledgments

In writing this book, I thank my mentors at the University of California, namely Sanjay Nigam and Alain Cohen of UCSD and Christopher H. Lowrey of the Geisel School of Medicine, whose spirit and generosity made this book possible. My thanks also extend to Steven Rosen of City of Hope, the series editor of Cancer Treatment Research; James Roach and Emma Frost of Open Access Government UK; Arnold Berk of UCLA; Beatles podcaster Ken Womack; Jeremy Richards of Harvard Medical School; the MD Anderson Cancer Center; ASCO, the *ASCO Post*, and SITC; and the numerous editors, conference chairs, and program managers I have had the distinct honor and privilege of interacting with.

A special thanks extends to Melanie Zerah, acquisitions editor; Michelle Tam, clinical editor; Dhanapal Palanisamy; and the wonderful and supportive team at Springer Nature.

And for Ezra Hays, who is the love of my life and I will always cherish.

Contents

Chapter 1
The Emergence of Precision Oncology

A leading cause of mortality, cancer in the year 2020 led to 10 million deaths, and 19.3 million new cases are reported each year. One in every six deaths is stipulated to be attributed to cancer, and detecting aggressive cancer early can enable more-effective treatment and improve quality of life and survival rates. Contained cancer is known as localized disease and refers to contained cancer before it spreads or stages I–II. Regional disease, or stages II–III, represents cancer that has spread to nearby organs, lymph nodes, and tissues. Metastatic cancer is distant disease and has spread to other areas of the body (stage IV). With the progression through stages, growth rates increase and the time periods between stages decrease. The impact of late-stage disease is high, which is also impacted by the tumor site, organ of location, and number of other metastatic lesions, with a general trend of increasing the cancer stages associated with a decreasing survival rate [1] (Figs. 1.1, 1.2, and 1.3).

The treatment of cancer—or, as the field is known, oncology—has certainly evolved over the past decades, from programmatic approaches, as used in a recent review, or standardized approaches to personalized ones. Oncology has undergone a transformative shift as a result of the gains in personalized medicine. Targeted approaches for diseases once thought uncurable, such as melanoma, lung cancer, and chronic lymphocytic leukemia, have led to improved and tolerable outcomes. Targeted therapies are used in combination with chemotherapy and radiation therapy. Targeted therapies paved the way for the discovery and implementation of immunotherapies, adoptive cellular therapies, bispecific antibodies, and antibody drug conjugates and combination strategies. As one observer put it, "[t]he ability to analyze and target tumor mutations has significantly altered the oncology treatment landscape over the last few decades" [2].

Oncology has undergone massive transformational changes in its management and therapy in the twenty-first century. Advances in precision medicine, immunology, and gene therapy have led to the development of targeted therapies and immuno-oncology drugs, which together constituted a major paradigm shift in the

P. Hays, *Personalized Medicine in Oncology*,
https://doi.org/10.1007/978-3-032-14437-9_1

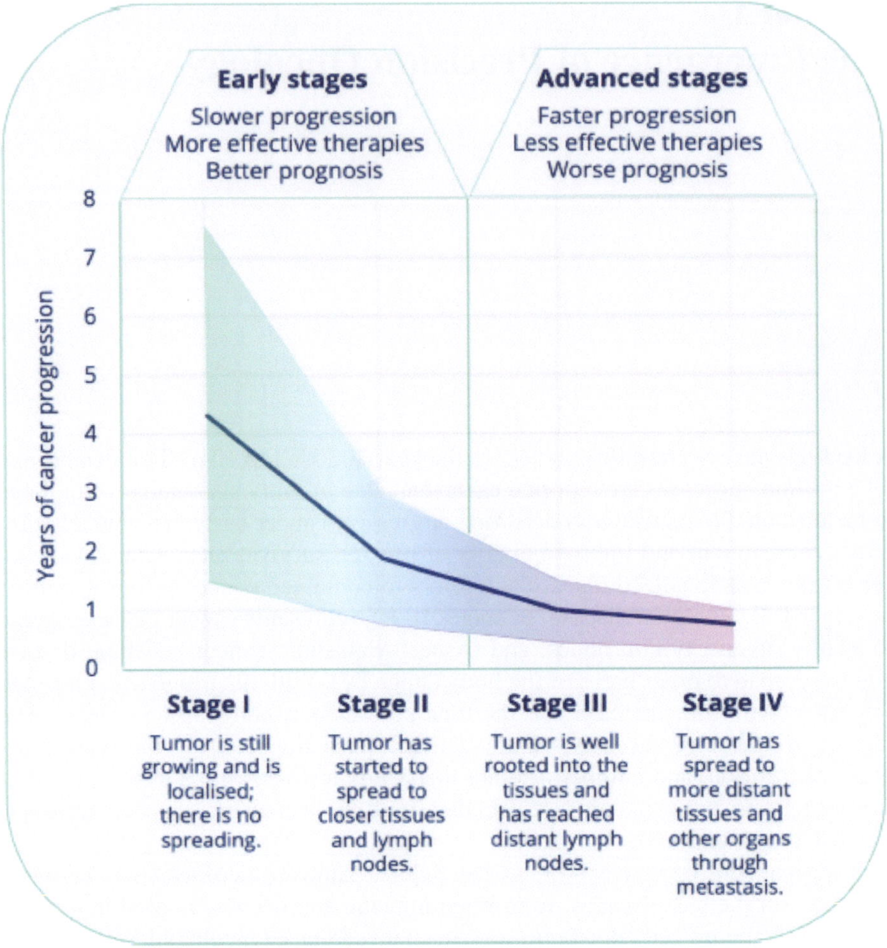

Fig. 1.1 Cancer progression over time. (Adapted from Connal [1])

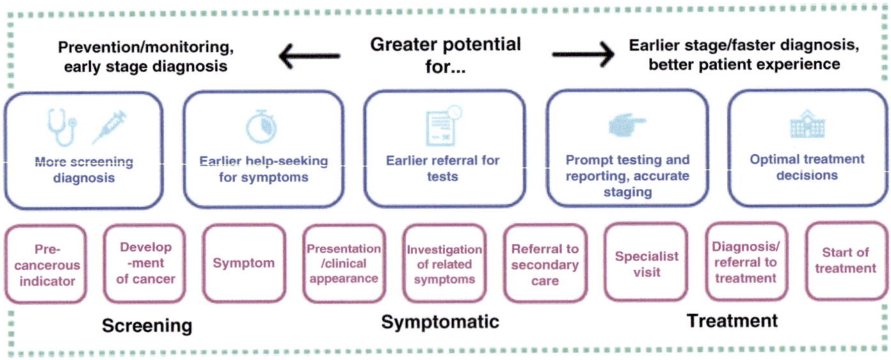

Fig. 1.2 Tumor stages with potential for prevention and early diagnosis. (Adapted from Connal [1])

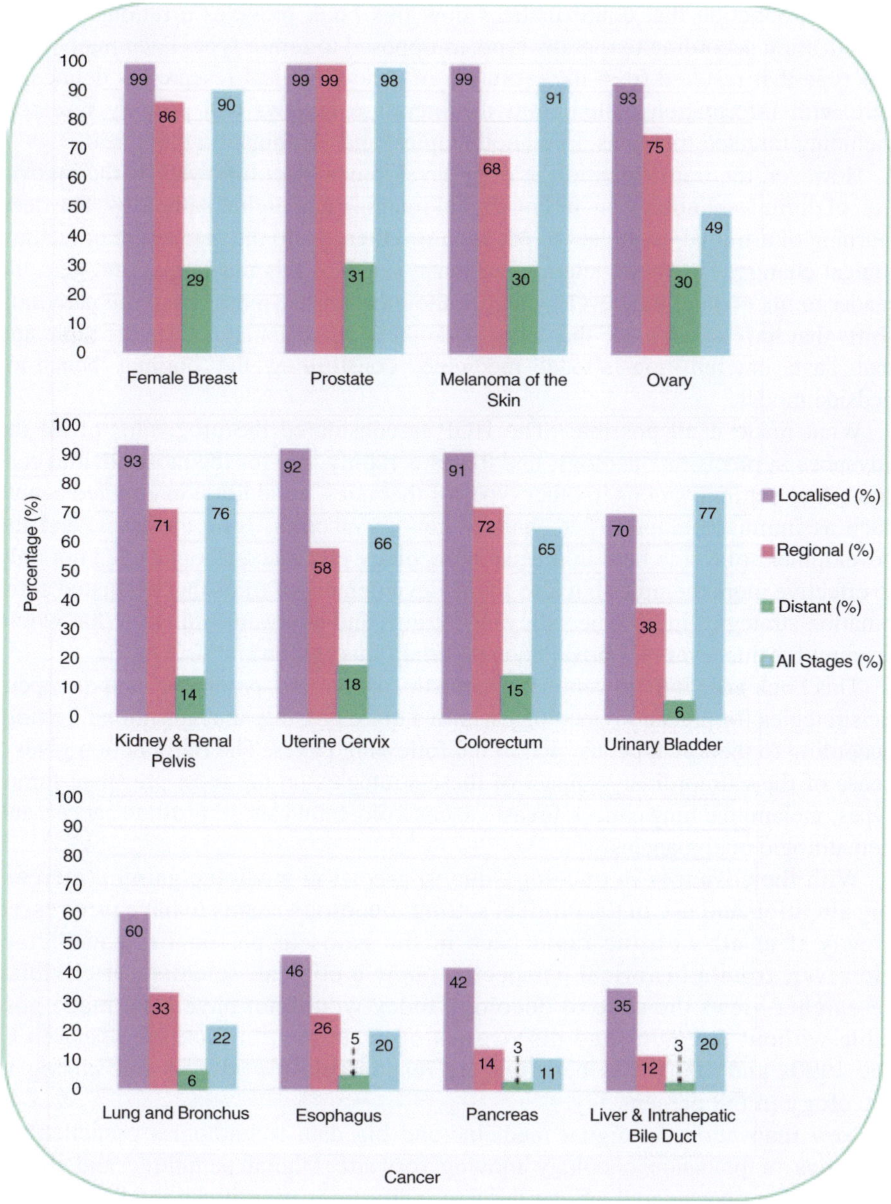

Fig. 1.3 5-year survival for cancers by stage at diagnosis. (Adapted from Connal [1])

treatment of solid tumors and hematologic malignancies. The completion of the Human Genome Project (HGP) brought about advances in genomic medicine, and our understanding of molecular variation and its diagnostic and therapeutic implications and oncology became one of its undeniable beneficiaries. This chapter serves as an introduction that contextualizes how this book provides a rationale for its organization according to therapy type, as opposed to tumor type. Each major therapy type that resulted from the evolution of cancer clinical research is delineated here with information culled from the literature reviews and primary research, including targeted therapies, immunotherapies, and combination therapies.

However, the transformation in drug development was followed by the innovation of digital technology, including digital imaging and digital pathology. The deep learning of artificial intelligence (AI)has now entered into the maelstrom of technological change. This book attempts to make sense of this maelstrom and help the reader to understand the development of the mechanistic models and the paradigm shifts that have taken place that have made these advancements even probable and that have entered translational medicine, constituting the optimal bench-to-bedside model.

What made it all possible? The HGP is considered the progenitor of all the advances in precision oncology, and this is certainly true for the most obvious reasons. And yet innovations in other types of therapies, in addition to targeted agents such as immunotherapies, personalized cancer vaccines, gene therapies, and the development of a side field in precision oncology pharmacogenomics, led not only to effective monotherapies but also to the development of trials that evaluated combination strategies in both neoadjuvant settings and adjuvant settings. What would account for this level of innovation and perhaps disruption?

This book goes into preventive, diagnostic, prognostic, predictive, and therapeutic strategies for precision oncology within a quite possibly unconventional setting: according to therapy type, as seen in the following pages. The introduction gives a sense of the extraordinary impact of these strategies on the most prevalent tumor types, melanoma, lung cancer, breast cancer, colorectal cancer, prostate cancer, and hematologic malignancies.

With the advances in oncology due to precision medicine gaining increasing attention and use in the clinical setting, oncology seems to have progressed slowly if at all with the rapid pace in the gains in personalized medicine. However, from a historical perspective, how a clinical, scientist, or clinician researcher views the state of oncology today would not have been made possible without the gains and discoveries of yesterday. In fact, the research of the 1990s and 2000s has been largely responsible for what is transpiring in oncology in the present day.

New innovations in digital medicine and big data technologies propelled the activities of precision oncology moving forward. Digital pathology and digital imaging were considered among the first innovations of artificial intelligence that challenged the diagnostic accuracies of older clinical strategies.

Personalized medicine has made significant advances in oncology since the sequencing of the human genome and the newfound understandings of the tumor microenvironment. Surgery, chemotherapy, and radiation remained the standard of care (SOC) with allogeneic hematopoietic stem cell transplantation for hematologic malignancies. A novel set of therapies has recently emerged, including targeted therapies, monoclonal antibodies, and cancer immunotherapies that are inclusive of monoclonal antibodies. A new field of precision oncology has emerged and manifested as the standard of care in neoadjuvant and adjuvant, first-line and second-line settings in both treatment naive and relapse/refractory patients with cancer.

However, this trajectory is evolving, which is the subject of this book. How—and why—did this sudden transformation take place, and why is the pace of discovery and clinical implementation so rapid that even most well-intentioned oncologists may find keeping abreast of it difficult? Sudden innovations in mobile health, machine learning, and artificial intelligence have been integrated into cancer care, and the rise of electronic health records are serving as new clinical data sources for understanding patterns in patient health. Overall, the key question remains: How clinically actionable are the results of this paradigm shift of precision oncology? This is where the main disputes may lie and will rely on a cogent synthesis and analysis of all the material and data that have been emanating from industry, National Cancer Institute (NCI)–designated cancer centers, and community hospitals and clinics. This a central focus of this book.

This book serves as a continuum of prior collections on cancer immunotherapies. The classes of cancer therapies listed in the title constitute one of the three main forms of immunotherapies that have been developed over the past 20 years as result of investigative work in cancer immunology. Trial data have emerged supporting the clinical utility of these therapies for solid tumors and hematologic malignancies. The following are the unique features of this book:

1. How each of these therapies has emerged and their clinical safety and efficacy will be discussed in detail in terms of their development for various tumor types.
2. A comparative analysis will be conducted to compare and contrast the benefits and limitations of each class of therapy and how malignancies develop resistance to them.
3. Each therapy type will have a separate chapter devoted to it describing how it is effectively (or not effectively) managed by each class of immunotherapy.

The manuscript is situated in the field of precision oncology and is aligned with the paradigm of targeted therapy drug development. The overall intention and plan of this book are to present the relevance of immunotherapies as important and pivotal treatment strategies for cancer and to appreciate how immune checkpoint inhibitors, chimeric antigen receptor (CAR) T cell therapies, and bispecific antibodies evolved through the conduct of clinical trials and resulting data to become critical components of an oncologist's armamentarium. The mechanism of each class, both textually and visually, and how each had advantages and limitations with respect to the existing standard of care and to one another will be described in detail, demonstrating that they complement and contrast with one another. Resistance mechanisms will also be discussed.

A number of biomarkers, such as tumor mutational burden and minimal residual disease, became established as clinically actionable data points in the treatment of cancer that became possible with the development of liquid biopsy, a novel, less invasive way of measuring solid tumor mutagenicity in temporal fashion. What proved pivotal in the development of immune checkpoint inhibitors is the discovery of checkpoints PD-1 and CTLA-4, becoming the foundations for the widely prescribed nivolumab and ipilimumab. The Cancer Genome Atlas, or TCGA, is the cataloging of mutations in tumors, or somatic mutations, that would lead to novel understandings of gene pair–disease associations and the further development of precision oncology drugs and their increasing use in quantifying gene expression, or transcriptomics.

One of the models underlying the immune system's relation to tumors is based on the immunosurveillance hypothesis proposed over a century ago that posits the biological phenomena of immunoediting: tumor elimination followed by the immune system existing in an equilibrium state with the cancer cells (the tumor does not grow) followed by the escape phase, whereby the cancer cells escape elimination by the immune system (the tumor grows).

The emergence of precision oncology and personalized cancer medicines has been chronicled in a series of articles that I wrote for Open Access Government United Kingdom over the course of 2 years (2023–2025). The rapid development in the implementation of personalized medicine for oncology led to profound impacts advancing both treatment options and clinical outcomes for cancer patients. The multi-institutional effort to sequence the entire human genome, the Human Genome Project, revealed the DNA base pair sequences underlying genomic variation and could be utilized to differentiate diagnosis and stratify treatment on the basis of this variation among individual genomes [2].

The application of the HGP to oncology led to the development of targeted therapies that were developed to attack tumor cells by affecting cellular signaling pathways that served as viable treatment options that eventually became defined by the personalized medicine paradigm, which led to the new and emerging field of precision oncology first constituted by small molecule inhibitor and biological therapies. Imatinib was one of the first small molecular inhibitors that were classified as tyrosine kinase inhibitors and was approved for chronic myeloid leukemia. Targeted therapies began to be developed for solid tumors such as melanoma through the BRAF mutation, breast cancer through genomic or somatic BRCA 1/2 mutations, lung cancer through ALK mutations, colorectal cancer through microsatellite instability, and prostate cancer through PARP pathways and for blood cell disorders such as chronic lymphocytic leukemia and acute lymphocytic leukemia [2] (Figs. 1.1, 1.2, and 1.3).

The major histologic subtype for lung cancer and its most prominent category, non–small cell lung cancer, was focused on in several biomarker studies to reveal a range of targetable mutations, including the targeted therapies Osimertinib for EFGR mutants, adagrasib for resistant KRAS mutants, and lorlatinib for ALK-positive mutations. BRAF mutations in melanoma also demonstrated that this tumor type would serve as a prototype for precision oncology approaches, and a class of therapies known as immune checkpoint inhibitors emerged, where two of the main examples were nivolumab and ipilimumab, also known as anti-CTLA-4 and anti-PD-1 immune checkpoint inhibitors, showing clinical efficacy by removing the brakes on cytotoxic T cells that destroy tumor cells that express foreign antigens. In gene therapy, among the best-understood advancements are chimeric antigen receptor T cell therapies, which involve genetically engineering a patient's T cells in a process known as ex vivo expansion. These personalized cytotoxic T cells are then readministered into the patient to eliminate abnormally expanding tumor cells. CAR T cell therapy was first approved for pediatric lymphomas and leukemias due to an urgent unmet need and with poor prognosis and for adult mantle cell lymphoma [2].

However, accompanying these mechanistic studies in the laboratory, clinical studies on these the small molecular inhibitors, biologics, and cellular therapies revealed a number of side effects, or adverse events, including hematologic malignancies, fatigue, gastrointestinal toxicities, cytokine release syndrome, and neurotoxicity, ranging from mild to moderate to severe and clinically known as grades 1–4; many responders to these agents "exhibited robust long-term positive clinical outcomes." Nevertheless, the toxicity profiles were overall favorable when compared to harsh chemotherapy regimens [2].

1.1 Improving Prognostic and Predictive Indicators in Cancer Care

Personalized medicine's impact on oncology was in the field of diagnostics and in cancer treatment, one of the main examples being in the development of liquid biopsy, a noninvasive way of obtaining a patient's tumor samples for the prognosis of treatment and predicting outcomes. Companion diagnostics for quantifying biomarkers were also developed, with one of the first ones to be US Food and Drug Administration (FDA) approved for detecting HER2 antibodies to detect the presence of HER2 amplification and determine which patients would respond to Herceptin. Diagnostic tools such as OncotypeDx and MammaPrint for breast cancer were widely adopted and improved the predictability of treatments [3].

Tumor biopsy is traditionally used in the diagnosis and prognosis of malignancies and determines the characteristics of a tumor in an invasive manner. Liquid biopsy involves a much less invasive approach, and it is derived from blood and consists of samples of cell-free DNA or tumor DNA. Being able to characterize minimal residual disease and a tumor's spatial and temporal heterogeneity, it is now considered a viable and valuable tool to provide measured prognostic and predictive indicators [3].

1.2 Liquid Biopsy

A novel tool for the diagnosis, prognosis and monitoring of tumors arose in the form of liquid biopsy, discussed in Chap. 3, which is considered an alternative to tissue biopsy, the gold standard for tumor profiling and are needed to determine the cancer type in the majority of cases. Surgical treatment plan and tumor location are factors that determine how a tissue biopsy is obtained. Some of the limitations of tumor biopsy are that misdiagnosis can be caused by a small sample and open surgical biopsies carry risk of infection or bleeding. Tissue biopsy is known for its "inability to capture tumor heterogeneity and clonal evolution." Liquid biopsy on the other hand, is obtaineds through blood or another bodily fluid sample, and as Connal et al. describe, "cancer is a systemic disease and not all biomarkers relate directly to the cancer. As a cancerous lesion evolves and grows, the biological signals change. In the early stages, non-tumor-derived sources—such as the immune response—dominate." However, accurate detection remains a challenge since, in the early stage, tumors are of small size and the level of tumor-derived biomarkers shed into the circulation is low. "A combination of both tumor and non-tumor-derived signals that are likely to be more prevalent in a pan-omics approach could lead to early detection of the cancer" [1].

The advantages of liquid biopsy are that it is repeatable, is more reliable, has lower procedural costs, and accounts for sample heterogeneity. Although tissue sections are preserved for immunohistochemistry (IHC), liquid biopsies offer new sources of "reliable tumor-derived components," and when carried out rapidly, they provide crucial omics information in a less invasive manner. However, liquid biopsy is currently not the standard method for the diagnosis and confirmation of disease and is considered a complement to tissue biopsy, being less sensitive and less specific and having an increased risk of false positives and false negatives; however, it is still promising in terms of increasing sensitivity [1].

1.3 New Clinical Data

As personalized medicine implementation took place, new types of clinical trials were developed that resulted from this discovery of molecular variation in patient populations that complemented randomized clinical trials. They are now being incorporated into the medical realm. Known as adaptive trials, they fall into the category of personalized medicine studies. They have the potential to reduce overall healthcare costs and accelerate the clinical trial and drug development process. These trials stratify populations through biomarkers that divide populations according to the molecular profile of the tumor. Umbrella trials lead to the distinct possibility of treatments based on these biomarker results, whereas basket trials involve the molecular profiling of tumors.

Statistical measures of clinical oncology trials known as primary and secondary endpoints give good indications of a drug's treatment potential. In precision oncology, "enormous streams of clinical data emerged for analysis and interpretation." Well-known examples of precision oncology drugs are the KEYNOTE, IMpower, and CheckMate trials that evaluated key personalized cancer medicines known as immunotherapies. These drugs, namely pembrolizumab, atezolizumab, and nivolumab, have become the standard of care for several tumor types through these studies, which have determined the clinical meaningfulness of precision medicine therapies [3].

1.4 Personalized Cancer Medicines [3]

Personalized cancer medicines have emerged with the implementation of precision medicine in oncology, a paradigm shift that had its basis in the Human Genome Project and novel discoveries in cancer biology, along with newfound understandings of the tumor microenvironment. Novel therapies targeting mutations in solid tumors, such as bevacizumab for colorectal cancer, olaparib for prostate cancer, and abemaciclib for breast cancer, are categorized according to their distinct ability to intricately affect cellular processes that lead to selective cancer cell death. Immunotherapies have emerged as a class of drugs that are now administered in front-line settings before and after surgical resection. Evolving from Coley's toxins to personalized cancer vaccines, cancer immunotherapies form a broad spectrum of therapies with a formidable armamentarium.

The emerging role for cancer immunotherapies arose from the classification of tumors as immune-desert regions ("cold tumors"), immune-excluded regions, and immune-infiltrated regions ("hot tumors"). Cold tumors are characterized by the exclusion of cytotoxic CD8+ T cells and natural killer cells and have a high degree of immunosuppressive immune cells such as Tregs. T cells cannot infiltrate the boundaries of a tumor in immune-excluded tumors.

Hot tumors have a high degree of responsiveness to therapies such as immune checkpoint inhibitors with active CD8+ T cells and natural killer cells in the tumor microenvironment. This set of tumors is responsive to immune checkpoint inhibitors. Immune checkpoint inhibitors are monoclonal antibodies that remove the inhibition on cytotoxic T cells formed by PD-1 and PD-L1 on the surfaces of cancer cells, namely solid tumors. Bispecific antibodies and chimeric antigen T cell receptor therapies have been developed to treat hematologic malignancies like acute lymphoblastic leukemia (ALL) and diffuse large B cell lymphoma (DLBCL), respectively, and an emerging class of therapies, antibody drug conjugates (ADCs), is being developed for breast cancer. CAR T cell therapies that have been FDA approved are idecabtagene vicleucel for relapsed/refractory multiple myeloma and axicabtagene ciloleucel (axi cel) and tisagenlecleucel (tisa cel) for relapsed/refractory diffuse large B cell lymphoma. Secondary malignancies have been reported as an adverse event in the treatment of CAR T cell therapies, and the US Food and Drug Administration has placed an advisory warning on these therapies. The mechanistic model underlying the efficacy of bispecific antibodies (BsAbs) is displayed by bispecific T cell engagers, or BiTEs. Bispecific antibodies have been developed to target tumor cells by redirecting T cells to distinct antigens on the surface of tumor cells. The antigens, also known as surface epitopes, were first designed with a cluster of differentiation markers, specifically CD19 and CD3 epitopes. They comprise a therapeutic class of agents that have remarkable efficacy against hematologic malignances. One of the first FDA-approved agents for BiTEs was blinatumomab, which has the canonical CD3 and CD19 epitopes. Antibody drug conjugates have a similar mechanism to that of bispecific antibodies in that they engage in immune lysis.

They bind to a receptor on a target cell, and cytotoxic agents are released after being internalized through receptor-mediated endocytosis and after being separated from the antibody in lysozyme, where a linker is cleaved, effecting tumor cell lysis. The recent DESTINY clinical trials established the antibody drug conjugate trastuzumab deruxtecan as a new standard of care for the HER2-low molecular subtype for metastatic breast cancer.

Oncolytic viral and immunotherapy combination strategies are also being developed. Oncolytic viruses replicate in cancer cells and cause cell lysis. Through a "cascade of viral transference between neoplasm and [immune activation]," oncolytic viruses lead to antigen release and recognition. Through this proinflammatory environment, the lytic virus leads to "tumor evasion by malignant cells." Recent studies have shown that these viruses can be harnessed to combine them with adoptive cellular therapies, immune checkpoint inhibitors, and bispecific antibodies to form combination strategies for developing cancer therapies. Artificial intelligence (AI), including machine learning, deep learning, and convolutional neural networks, is making sweeping changes in diagnostic pathology and automating the analysis and processing of histopathological samples from cancer patients. AI may be able "to increase accuracy and analytic validity while decreasing inter- and intra-variability among samples" [3].

1.5 Renal Cell Carcinoma or Kidney Cancer Case Study

Renal cell carcinoma, or kidney cancer, offers a case study suggesting how targeted therapies were first developed to treat with safety and efficacy, and cancer immunotherapies were later demonstrated to have superior clinical outcomes. Sunitinib was the standard of care for patients who had just been diagnosed with renal cell carcinoma. Bevacizumab (a VEFG-A targeted biologic), sunitinib, paxopanib, and axitinib (the latter three being oral small molecule tyrosine kinase inhibitors) have antiangiogenic effects and were studied in a series of clinical trials that proved it to have robust clinical outcomes and favorable safety profiles and initiated a paradigm shift in the treatment of renal cell carcinoma from cytokines to targeted therapies. A recent clinical trial later evaluated the combination of the immune checkpoint inhibitors ipilimumab and nivolumab, and this combination demonstrated better clinical efficacy over the targeted therapy sunitinib, with later trials evaluating the immune checkpoint inhibitor pembrolizumab [3].

1.6 Personalized Medicine in Oncology [4]

Advancements in cancer research have led to changes in the treatment of patients with cancer, resulting in novel personalized cancer therapies. The three major classes include small molecule inhibitors, biologics, and cancer immunotherapies. Standard first-line immunotherapies include anti-CTLA-4 inhibitor ipilimumab and anti-PD-1 inhibitor nivolumab. These are considered immune checkpoint inhibitors that remove the breaks in cytotoxic T cells from killing cancer cells. Due to the incidence of nonresponders to these first-line immunotherapies, other immunotherapies also belonging to the same immune checkpoint inhibitor class of treatments have been developed and evaluated in clinical trials, and novel therapeutic agents have been developed that could serve as the next-generation immune checkpoint inhibitors, which include anti-LAG-3 and anti-TIGIT (T cell immunoreceptor with Ig and ITIM domains) antibodies and the inhibitory receptor TIM-3. LAG-3 has been named "the third checkpoint inhibitor." Clinical trials have been conducted to study and evaluate these three agents. "These inhibitory receptors have heralded the next wave of co-inhibitory receptor targets that are being explored in clinical trials," as stated in prior reports. In vitro testing in activated T cells led to the discovery of LAG-3 as an inhibitory receptor, similar to PD-1/PD-L1 and CTLA-4. Like PD-1/PD-L1, LAG-3 inhibits T cell function and thereby its cytotoxic activity, and it inhibits CD4 T cell activation. The phase III RELATIVITY-047 trial was recently conducted and led to the FDA approval of the LAG-3 antibody relatlimab for advanced melanoma patients.

One report noted the following: "Following the approval of relatlimab, the FDA approved an agent that combines anti-LAG-3 mAB relatlimib with nivolumab for first-line treatment of metastatic melanoma in a phase 2–3, global, double-blind, randomized trial evaluating fixed-dose combination as compared with nivolumab alone when administered intravenously every four weeks to patients with previously untreated metastatic or unresectable melanoma. The primary endpoint was progression-free survival."

Other inhibitory receptors are the TIGIT antibody and the Tim-3 antibody. The TIGIT inhibitory receptor and PD-1 are "mechanistically convergent checkpoints that regulate T cell differentiation," and blockade through anti-TIGIT and PD-1 antibodies leads to the reversal of a tumor microenvironment phenomenon known as T cell exhaustion and the expansion of the cytotoxic T cell compartment.

> T cell immunoglobulin-3, or Tim-3, is expressed on interferon gamma-producing CD4+ helper and CD8+ cytotoxic T cells and serves as a cell surface marker. One monoclonal anti-TIM-3 antibody has been developed, showing clinical activity in non–small cell lung cancer and melanoma patients through a unique mechanism of action that blocks the TIM-3 interaction with a phosphatidylserine ligand. This agent, known as sabatolimab, has been evaluated with an anti-PD-1 antibody known as spartaliuzmab in a phase 1 trial for determining safety profiles and tolerability [4].

1.7 Breast Cancer Case Study [4]

Poly (adenosine diphosphate (ADP)-ribose) polymerase (PARP) inhibitors and CDK4/6 inhibitors (cyclin-dependent kinase 4 and 6 inhibitors) treat advanced and metastatic breast cancer. PARP inhibitors olaparib, talazoparib, and veliparib and CDK4/6 inhibitors abemaciclib, palbociclib, and ribociclib are considered the first-line standard of care for the treatment of advanced breast cancer, where each agent has different mechanisms of action and clinical efficacies. PARP inhibitors inhibit the enzyme PARP1, which repairs DNA double-stranded breaks, preventing cancer cell growth. CDK4/6 inhibit the cell cycle by preventing progression into the mitotic phase, and also prevent cancer cell growth, and they are usually administered with aromatase inhibitors [3, 4].

Conceptually, the management of advanced breast cancer patients could be potentially complex and involve a lengthy decision-making process of choosing between these agents. However, most of the literature on this topic is sparse. Several recent clinical trials have evaluated the various agents in both classes, and the data revealed robust clinical outcomes and manageable safety profiles for both.

The BROCADE trial showed that the PARP inhibitor veliparib in combination with chemotherapy was effective for locally advanced breast cancer patients with germline (inherited) BRCA1/2 mutations (gBRCA1/2) with increased median progression-free survival (PFS), a statistical indicator of clinical success, by nearly 3 months (7.0 months vs. 4.2 months). The EMBRACA trial likewise showed clinical effectivity for tumors harboring the gBRCA1/2 mutation for talazoparib, another PARP inhibitor, compared to the standard of care (8.6 months vs. 5.6 months). The OlympiAD trial showed clinical effectiveness for olaparib.

The MONARCH trial showed that abemaciclib, a CDK4/6 inhibitor, had a significantly longer duration of PFS when compared to the placebo (median not reached in the abemaciclib arm and 14.7 months in the placebo arm). The MONALEESA trial showed that ribociclib, also a CDK4/6 inhibitor, had significantly longer median progression-free survival (mPRS) when compared to placebo. Adverse clinical outcomes for CDK4/6 inhibitors were shown in two phase III trials, the SONIA and PALMIRA trials, suggesting the use of PARP inhibitors for breast cancer patients after testing positive for the gBRCA1/2 mutation.

The BREAKOUT study conducted in 2020 had an intriguing result that implied that advanced breast cancer patients undergo gBRCA1/2 testing after receiving CDK4/6 inhibitors when they are not effective in this population. This stemmed from data that showed that 5–10% of advanced breast cancer patients were positive for the gBRCA1/2 mutation.

> Much of this innovation and much of this progress in developing and evaluating personalized cancer medicines demonstrate the unique nature of precision oncology: Personalized cancer care is based on the instances of nonresponders in immune checkpoint inhibitors. Small molecule inhibitor drug development results from mutations in oncogenes that lead to drug resistance.. The development of the Cancer Genome Atlas; new biomarkers, such as tumor mutational burden (TMB) and PD-L1; and a novel measure of minimal residual disease (MRD) took place within the context of a rapid pace in research, development, and innovation in cancer genomics and precision oncology.

1.8 The Cancer-Immunity Cycle and the Process of Immune Evasion

Cancer immunotherapies have developed as points of intervention in the cancer-immunity cycle that was conceived of and developed by Chen and Mellman (Fig. 1.4) [5]. Immune checkpoint inhibitors in particular have been harnessed

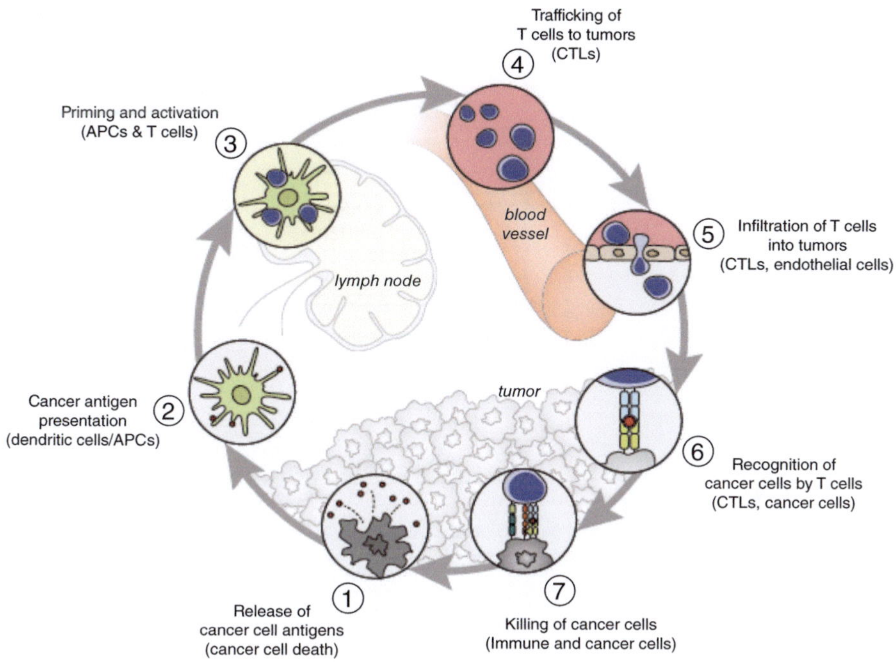

Fig. 1.4 The cancer-immunity cycle. (Adapted from Chen and Mellman [5])

for their ability to enhance the recognition of T cells by cancer cells; the trafficking of T cells has been manipulated by cellular and gene therapies; and cancer antigen presentation has been mobilized by bispecific antibodies and antibody drug conjugates. The cancer-immunity cycle describes the series of steps through which both the immune system effects the destruction of cancer cells and the immunological principles through which cancer immunotherapies carry out their therapeutic functions. In step 1, dendritic cells (DCs) release and capture the neoantigens created through oncogenesis; immunity might be induced over peripheral tolerance. In step 2, through antigen presentation on MHCI and MHCII molecules (step 2), the priming and activation of T cells occurs (step 3). The ratio of cytotoxic T cells to regulatory T cells becomes relevant at this stage. In step 4, T cells are trafficked to tumors and infiltrate them (step 5) through recognition and binding to cancer cells through MHC1 antigen binding and the binding of cancer cells to T cell receptors (step 6), and the T cells kill the cancer cells. More specifiically, its cytotoxic CD8+ T cells that kill the cancer cells (step 7). The cycle returns to step 1 with the release of additional tumor-associated antigens [5].

Mellman and colleagues in 2023 expanded on the cancer-immunity cycle (Fig. 1.5) by explaining the role of the tumor microenvironment and the concept of primary immunotypes—namely immune-desert, immune-excluded, and immune-inflamed tumor immunotypes, examples being prostate cancer, colon

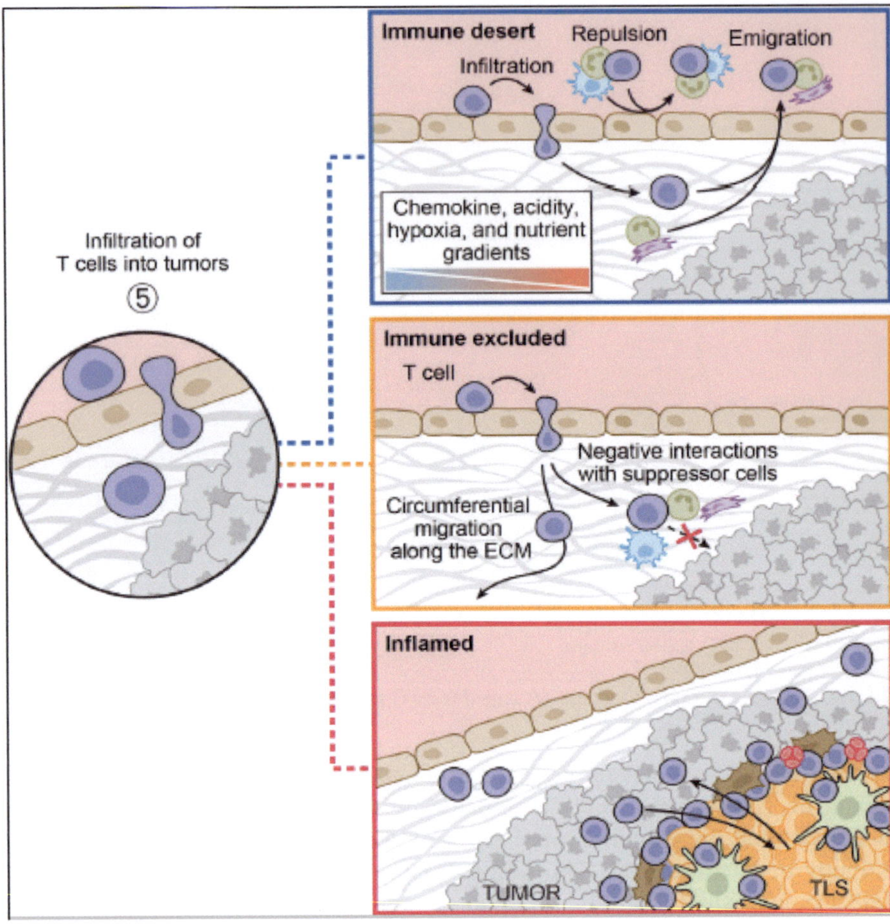

Fig. 1.5 Immune-desert, immune-excluded, and immune-inflamed tumors. (Adapted from Mellman et al. [6])

cancer, and melanoma, respectively—that are central to understanding tumor evolution and the mechanisms through which immune cells interact with tumor cells. The tumor microenvironment is considered harsh or immunosuppressive through a tumor stroma that determines immunotypes and the "trajectory and fate" of tumors, and it consists not just of T cells but also of natural killer cells and the very immunosuppressive cancer-associated fibroblasts, along with the novel discovery of exhausted T cells (Tex cells), cells that are alive but that have reduced effector activity. In addition to the PD-1/PD-L1 axis and the CTLA-4 immune checkpoint, new receptors emerged, including LAG3, TIM3, and TIGIT, that led to the development of next-generation immune checkpoint inhibitors relatllimab and sabatolimab [6].

1.9 Personalized Medicine Led to New Understandings of Medicine and Oncology

Some of the extant literature on personalized medicine—or precision medicine, as it has become to be more widely and officially known—has delved into this phenomenon in less-empirical but equally valid ways. One account is a deep dive into what this newfound understanding of medicine means for patients and healthcare: Precision medicine is based on a rewriting of the conventional cause-and-effect relationship of disease and symptoms and into one in which pathogenesis underlies disease. In other words, according to Berman in a nicely written account, trying to understand events by attributing to them a specific singular cause is considered part of the human condition. This paradigm becomes complicated in the case of cancer, in which the disease evolves via histological category: A adenocarcinoma does not transform into a squamous carcinoma, or a hepatocellular carcinoma does not morph into a renal cell carcinoma, even though many cases of oligometastasis exist [7]. By revealing the distinct sequence of events and steps, whether it be cellular signaling, cell cycle regulation, DNA repair mechanisms, or chromosomal translocations, the precise mechanistic models behind carcinogenesis could be understood and analyzed and pose as targets for the development of drugs and therapies. Hence, to understand precision medicine (and precision oncology) the nature of pathogenesis—or the cancer type, being tumor agnostic—must be understood: Tumors become identified and treated through mutations, which serve as drug targets rather

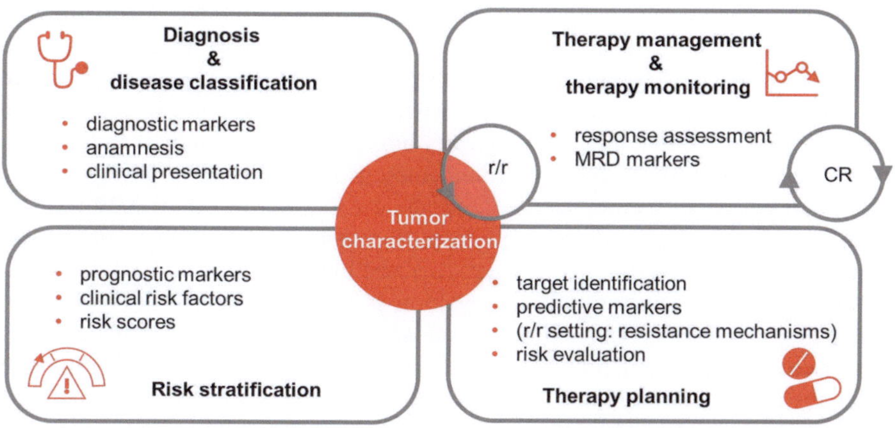

Fig. 1.6 In precision medicine, a comprehensive tumor characterization provides the basis for diagnosis, risk evaluation, therapy planning, and monitoring. (Adapted from Schmidts et al. [11])

than histological types. In turn, somatic mutations are distinct entities from germline mutations, which form the distinguishing category of hereditary cancers (Fig. 1.6).

A 2024 issue of *Nature Reviews Oncology* highlighted research advances over the past 20 years of oncology, and many of the new drugs could presumably fall into the category of personalized cancer medicines: a bispecific antibody for acute lymphoblastic leukemia, an antibody drug conjugate for cervical cancer, and a chimeric antigen receptor T cell therapy for multiple myeloma, which are therapy types discussed in this volume, specifically Chaps. 6, 7, and 8, respectively. One of the first reports on blinatumomab as an investigational agent showed how the drug improved outcomes in MRD-negative BCP-ALL. Prognosis was shown to depend on MRD status, with MRD-negative disease having superior prognosis. The CD19XCD3 bispecific antibody was added to consolidation chemotherapy and improved overall survival (OS). Patients in MRD- complete remission (CR) (0.01% leukemic cells in bone) received SOC chemotherapy and were randomly allocated in a 1:1 ratio with or without blinatumomab. + 3-year OS at a median follow-up of 43 months was 85% in patients in the blinatumomab cohort versus 68% in the chemotherapy cohort (hazard ratio (HR) 0.41, 95% CI 0.23–0.73; $p = 0.002$), with patients under 44 years old having the greatest clinical outcome (HR.016, 95% CI 0.05–0.47). Hematologic adverse events greater than grade 3 were the most common (59% vs. 52%). The FDA approved the agent in R/R BCP-ALL in 2014; expanded such approval to include MRD+ BCP-ALL in 2018; and expanded it again to include MRD- BCP-ALL in 2024 [8].

Treatment options for recurrent and advanced/metastatic cervical cancer, typically a cancer with poor prognosis, emerged with the development of the antibody drug conjugate tisotumab vedotin. As described in the anniversary issue, phase III InnovTV 301 showed that the therapeutic has a 62.8% clinical efficacy in patients who received one line of therapy and 36.8% in patients who received two lines of therapy after randomization (1:1) versus the investigator's choice of chemotherapy. OS served as the primary endpoint: 11.5 months versus 9.5 months (HR 0.70, 95% CI 0.54–0.82). A significant improvement in PFS was also observed (median 4.2 months versus 2.9 months; HR 0.67, 95% CI 0.54–0.082). The study also noted that there was no significant correlation between tumors and clinical response and tissue factor expression. Grade 3 or greater adverse events were 52% in the treatment group versus 62.3% in the chemotherapy group, with ocular adverse events (AEs) and peripheral neuropathy being notable AEs (52.8% versus 6.3%; 38.4% versus 4.2%). The data supported the use of tisotumab vedotin in recurrent and metastatic cervical cancer, and the agent received FDA approval in April 2024 [9].

The standard of care for multiple myeloma is considered the triplet regimen of CD38 targeting antibodies (daratumumab and isatuximab), immunomodulatory drugs (lenalidomide), and proteasome inhibitors (bortezomib), the therapy through which the disease is considered triple-class exposed. Patients develop recurrent and refractory disease after receiving these therapies, and therapeutic options emerged with the development of B-cell maturation antigen (BCMA)–directed therapy in the form of chimeric antigen receptor T cell therapies idecabtagene vicleucel (ide-cel) and ciltacabtagene autoleucel (cilta-cel), which became FDA approved through findings in the phase 3 KarMMa-3 and CARTITUDE-4 trials, which are discussed in detail in Chap. 9. (Other agents in the bispecific antibody and antibody drug conjugate categories that are BCMA directed were developed as well.) The CAR T cell therapy led to improved quality of life in these heavily pretreated populations; however, these therapies lead to cytokine release syndrome and neurotoxicity, which has also extensively been discussed in the literature. Objective response rate (ORR) was reported at 85% with a CR rate of 73%; PFS did not reach the 12-month PFS for cilta-cel was 76% for cilta-cel. ORR was reported at 71%, and the CR rate was 39% with a median PFS of 13.3 months for ide-cel [10].

The case studies on renal cell carcinoma and chronic lymphocytic leukemia evince the different etiological and evolutionary nature of personalized cancer medicines. Renal cell carcinoma demonstrated clear outcomes on targeted therapies, such as sunitinib and everolimus, though evidence increasingly showed that cancer immunotherapies such as pembrolizumab and nivolumab had better clinical outcomes, as shown in the KEYNOTE and CheckMate clinical trials. The Bruton tyrosine kinase inhibitor ibrutinib and the BCL2 inhibitor venetoclax constituted one of the standard treatments for chronic lymphocytic leukemia; immunotherapies such as blinatumomab (for acute lymphoblastic leukemia) were less effective; and CAR T cell therapies showed less effectivity for the malignancy. However, studies being conducted for further evaluation are ongoing.

1.10 The Structure of This Book

This book will be structured into chapters focusing on distinct therapy types and the clinical trials evaluating their efficacy and safety. The primary therapy type to be considered features targeted therapies and immune checkpoint inhibitors, which have become front-line agents. Using CAR T cells is an example of an adoptive cellular therapy that utilizes gene therapy to meet an urgent need (because they were FDA approved for hematologic cancers). Bispecific antibodies were developed as therapies for acute lymphoblastic leukemia and multiple myeloma. Antibody drug conjugates constitute one of the cutting-edge developments in this field, which are indicated for the use of both solid tumors and hematologic malignancies. Tumor infiltrating lymphocytes are nonengineered ways of transforming T cells into cancer-killing cells. These developments have been reviewed in the literature, and this work attempts to sufficiently fill a gap by coalescing these studies into a thorough yet clear compendium of these therapies. This book will describe the prognostic and predictive significance of each drug, biomarkers for determining their therapeutic potential, and the assays (e.g., NGS, IHC) that evaluate them. The innovations of liquid biopsy; clinically actionable alterations, including HER2, EGFR, KRAS, and BRAF; and the implications for oncology in pharmacogenomics are also highlighted.

Artificial intelligence and multi-omics and their impact on precision oncology and the role of big data have influenced screening, the monitoring of treatment outcomes, and the development of cancer therapies and their relevance to digital pathology. In conclusion, the scientific and medical narrative of personalized medicine's transformation of cancer and its attendant consequences on the fields of oncology, immunology, cancer immunotherapy, genomics, cellular therapy, and big data are underscored and summarized.

References

1. Connal S, Cameron JM, Sala A, Brennan PM, Palmer DS, et al. Liquid biopsies: the future of early cancer detection. J Transl Med. 2023;21:118.
2. Hays P. The emergence of precision medicine for oncology, Open Access Government July 2023, pp 98–9. Available at https://www.openaccessgovernment.org/article/emergence-precision-medicine-oncology-cancer/161135/. Accessed 25 Apr 2025.
3. Hays P. Personalized cancer medicines, Open Access Government July 2024, pp 86–7. Available at https://www.openaccessgovernment.org/article/personalized-cancer-medicines/177940/. Accessed 25 Apr 2025.
4. Hays P. Personalized medicine in oncology: Small molecule inhibitors, biologics and immunotherapies, Open Access Government April 2025, pp 120–121. Available at https://www.openaccessgovernment.org/article/personalized-medicine-in-oncology-small-molecule-inhibitors-biologics/188248/. Accessed 25 Apr 2025.
5. Chen DS, Mellman I. Oncology meets immunology: the cancer-immunity cycle. Immunity. 2013;39(1):1–10.
6. Mellman I, Chen DS, Powles T, Turley SJ. The cancer-immunity cycle: Indication, genotype, and immunotype. Immunity. 2023;56(10):2188–205.
7. Berman JJ. Precision medicine and the reinvention of human disease. London: Elsevier; 2018.
8. Romero D. Blinatumomab improves outcomes in adult MRD-negative BCP-ALL. Nat Rev Clin Oncol. 2024;21:703.
9. Sidaway P. Tisotumab vedotin effective in cervical cancer. Nat Rev Clin Oncol. 2024;21:703.
10. Van de Donk NWCJ, Zweegman S. BCMA-directed therapy for early relapased and/or refractory multiple myeloma. Nat Rev Clin Oncol. 2024;21:707–8.
11. Schmidts I, Haferlach T, Hoermann G. Precision medicine in therapy of non-solid cancer. In: Cascorbi I, Schwab M, editors. Precision medicine. Handbook of experimental pharmacology, vol. 280. Cham: Springer; 2022.

Chapter 2
The Discovery of Clinically Actionable Alterations and Pharmacogenomics

As personalized medicine for cancer may have begun to enter mainstream medicine, a significant rise in the literature that centered on the relevant themes of the field took place, and precision oncology has now become an established area of research and investigation. Journals such as *Nature Precision Oncology* and the *Journal of Clinical Oncology Precision Oncology* and journals associated with the American Association for Cancer Research, including *Clinical Cancer Research* and *Cancer Discovery*, now devote many of its studies and reports to the main topics of personalized cancer medicines, including targeted therapies for solid tumors and hematologic malignancies, cancer immunotherapies, genomic alterations, companion diagnostics, liquid biopsy, and the evaluation of precision cancer medicines, cancer genomics, multi-omics, and computational methods in artificial intelligence.

A community of physician-scientists, oncologists, academics, industry stakeholders, medical societies, scholars, and regulatory professionals coalesced around the concepts and ideas of personalized medicine and precision oncology, with the integration of targeted therapy and immunotherapy approaches in medicine and scientific laboratories, leading to improved patient outcomes and the streamlining of clinical trials for more-efficient and more-effective care. An argument could be made that healthcare was considerably enhanced by personalized medicine. Publishers and journals are now devoting their efforts to the implementation of precision medicine (PM), and a significant body of literature has emerged. The molecular diagnostic industry and the pharmaceutical industry made significant inroads into personalized and precision medicine and developed a pipeline that led to the approval of a large number of precision medicine drugs approved by the US Food and Drug Administration (FDA).

P. Hays, *Personalized Medicine in Oncology*,
https://doi.org/10.1007/978-3-032-14437-9_2

Personalized medicine in oncology was partly the result of the discovery of clinically actionable alterations and advancements in biomarker testing through applications of genomics, transcriptomics, proteomics, and metabolomics and through tumor-agnostic drug approvals. Novel innovations in the form of next-generation sequencing methods and gene panels for diagnosing these alterations led to precision oncology treatment strategies in the clinical setting. Tumor-agnostic biomarkers include the use of pembrolizumab in MSI-H/dMMR status for solid tumors and the use of entrectinib for NTRK fusions in rare cancers, such as infantile fibrosarcoma and secretory breast carcinoma [1, 2]. A category of predictive biomarkers was developed for immune checkpoint inhibitors (Chap. 6), including PD-L1 for solid tumors; mismatch repair deficiency and high microsatellite instability for solid tumors; and tumor mutational burden for melanoma and lung cancer. Prognostic biomarkers in the form of circulating tumor DNA and circulating tumor cells detected via liquid biopsy showed analytic and clinical validity for accurately determining the clinical outcomes of therapy (Chap. 3). The precision oncology paradigm comprises collecting the unique comprehensive biomarker (detected molecular alterations) profile of an individual patient to determine the most accurate diagnosis for personalized treatment strategies. The paradigm strongly suggests an improvement over the so-called one-size-fits-all approach of the traditional standard of care, such as chemotherapy and/or radiation with its attendant adverse side effects. Some of the most prominent early examples were the small molecule inhibitor imatinib for chronic myeloid leukemia targeting the BCR-ABL translocation and the Herceptin antibody targeting abnormal HER2 gene expression. Other examples include the clinical development of vemurafenib targeting the BRAFV600E mutation in melanoma and gefitinib for the treatment of EGFR-mutated non–small cell lung cancer (NSCLC). Efforts in sequencing the genome through the Cancer Genome Atlas (TCGA) also led to the identification of other clinically actionable alterations in tumors. Precision oncology workflows are illustrated in Figs. 2.1, 2.2, and 2.3.

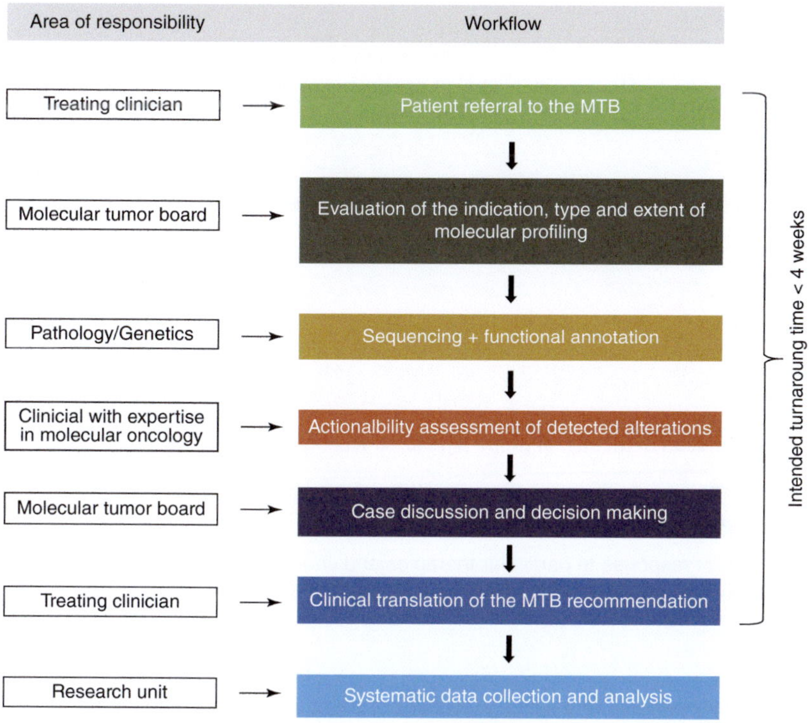

Fig. 2.1 Precision oncology clinical workflow according to area of responsibility. (Adapted from Reidl et al. [1]. Permission to reuse by Creative Commons CC BY 4.0)

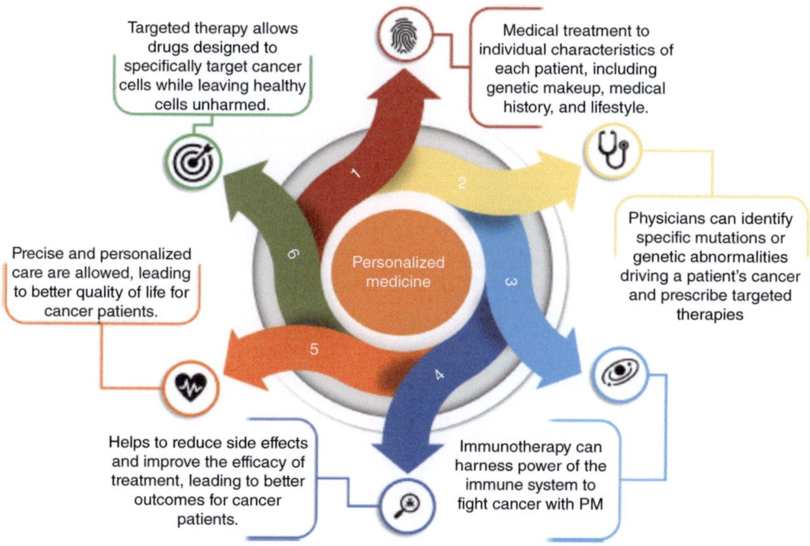

Fig. 2.2 The various aspects of personalized medicine, including treatment (targeted and immunotherapies) and the role of personalized care. (Adapted from Gadade et al. [3]. Permission to reuse by Creative Commons CC BY 4.0)

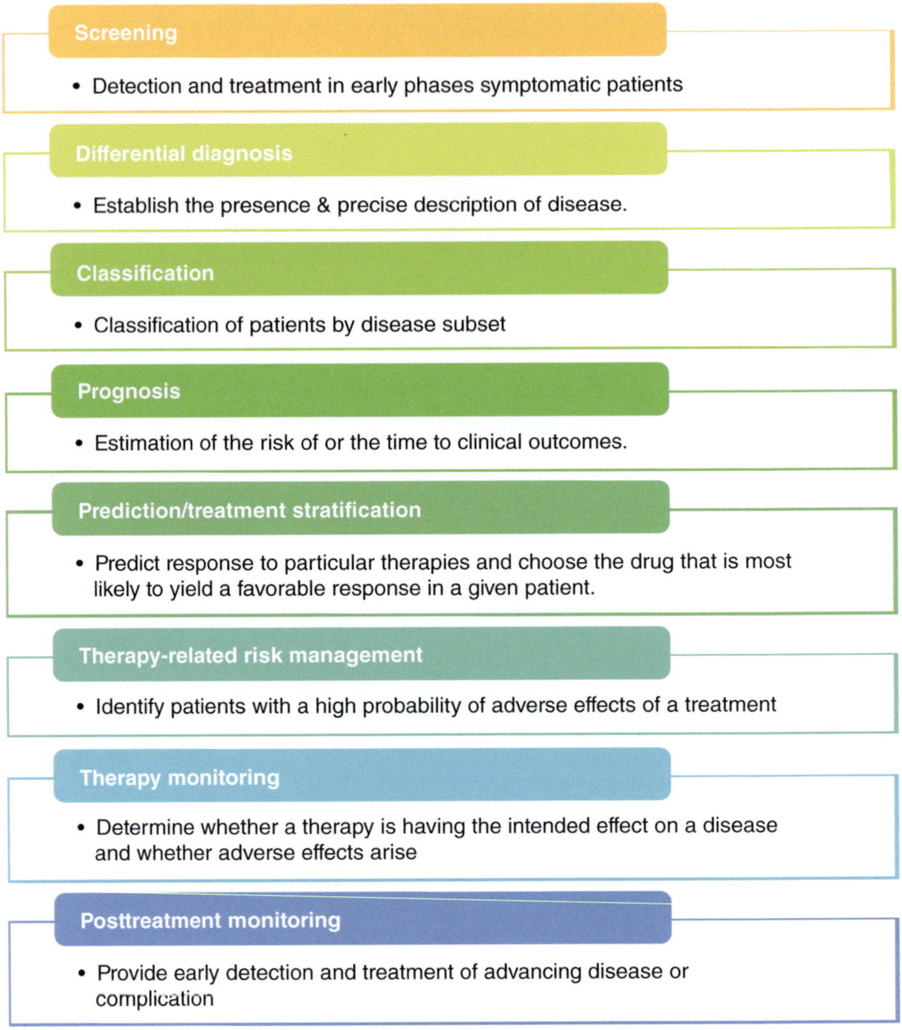

Fig. 2.3 Personalized medicine's role in reducing risk through its prognostic and predictive value, monitoring of treatments, and early detection of cancer. (Adapted from Gadade et al. [3]. Permission to reuse by Creative Commons CC BY 4.0)

2.1 Cancer Genomics

Cancer genomics, an integral component of personalized cancer medicines, emerged as a field when researchers discovered that a number of proto-oncogenes and tumor suppressor genes led to the formation of tumors as a result of genetic aberrations that led to excessive growth factor production. Uncontrolled cell division that resulted led to certain signal transduction programs going awry. When proto-oncogenes are converted into oncogenes, cellular apoptosis may be prevented and growth factor requirement is reduced, leading to continuous cellular proliferation. Accordingly, when tumor suppressor genes lose function, tumor initiation also occurs [4].

Any discussion of precision oncology would begin with the delineation of the development of targeted therapies. The activation of proto-oncogenes is the result of point mutations, chromosomal translocations, and gene amplifications. Cyclin D1, a proto-oncogene amplified in breast, bladder, and lung cancers, contributes to uncontrolled entry into the S phase of the cell cycle.

An important event in cancer cell initiation and progression is the increase in oncogenic proteins as a result of gene amplification that leads to the replication of a specific region in a chromosome several times. One of the main examples is the ERBB gene family, which includes EGFR and HER2, belonging to the tyrosine kinase receptor superfamily that is structured as transmembrane receptor proteins that are involved in the differentiation and proliferation of wild-type cells. The Ras-MAPK pathway is implicated in cell-cycle regulation. Overexpressed in 25–30% of breast cancer, 80% of lung squamous cell carcinoma, and head and neck epithelial tumors, ERBB1, ERBB2 (HER2: "human epidermal growth factor receptor"), ERBB3, and ERBB4 constitute the four members of the receptor gene family. HER2 (ERBB2) receptors are increased in 25–30% in breast, lung, and ovarian cancers. Gene amplification activates the Her2 oncoprotein with the activated tyrosine kinase, continually leading to signal cleavage in the nucleus. The ERBB2 oncogene is targeted by Herceptin for breast cancer that has ERBB2 overexpression and is preferred over standard chemotherapy [4].

Other mechanisms of proto-oncogene activation are point mutations, a well-known example being the Ras family of GTPase proteins that develop as a result proto-oncogenes whose structures have a base either leaving or entering. The c-ras oncogene leads to GTPase activity as a result of a base sequence difference in its DNA leading to its chronic stimulation due to an increase in adenylate cyclase activity. The Ras protein has GTPase activity, binds to either guanosine triphosphate (GTP) or guanosine diphosphate (GDP) , and oscillates between the active stage and the inactive stage through the oscillation of its cyclical structure (Fig. 2.4). Kras, Hras, and Nras are Ras proteins that permit signals to stimulate cell division and exist in these three homologous forms. Also, the BRAF gene is activated through point mutations and encodes tyrosine kinases known as mitogen-activated extracellular signal-regulated kinases (MEKs). After an activation chain ensues, transcription factor expression changes.

Chromosomal translocation has been well documented in the literature by implicating the c-MYC gene and the c-ABL proto-oncogene. Burkitt's lymphoma is a malignancy of antibody-producing B lymphocytes that results from the translocation of the c-MYC gene, resulting in its excessive expression and a tumorigenic phenotypic with oncogenic characteristics. Moreover, c-ABL is involved with chronic myeloid leukemia in the translocation of the Philadelphia chromosome. One of the causative phenomena resulting in chronic myeloid leukemia (CML) is the separation of the c-ABL proto-oncogene, located on chromosome 9, to

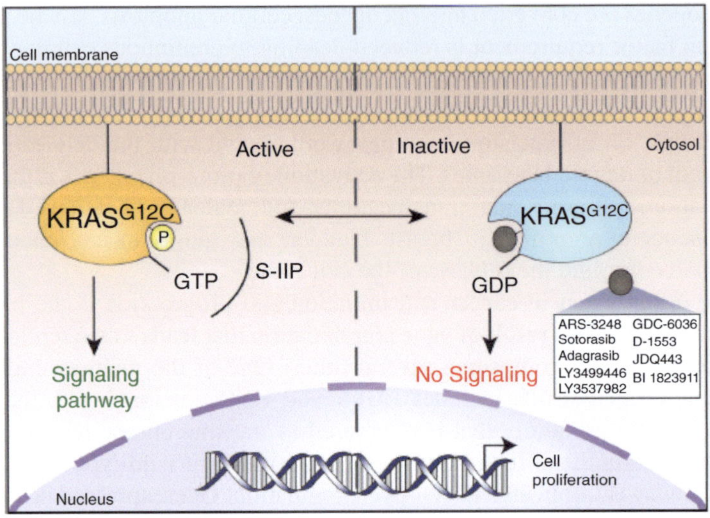

Fig. 2.4 The area of targetable alteration focus: the KRAS mutation. (Adapted from Kwan et al. [5]. Permission to reuse by Creative Commons CC BY 4.0)

chromosome 22, which contains the BCR gene region containing a very strong promoter. Tyrosine kinase activity results because the resulting BCR/ABL fusion leads to the overexpression of the synthesis of an oncogenic protein [4].

2.1.1 The Area of Targetable Alteration Focus: Clinical Workflows

Tumor suppressor genes such as p53, Rb, and PTEN prevent uncontrolled cellular proliferation. Uncontrolled proliferation and apoptotic resistance lead to neoplastic differentiation that occurs through a loss of function as a result of mutation and the chromosomal deletion of tumor suppressor genes. BRCA 1 and BRCA 2 are tumor suppressor genes integrated into genomic and somatic genetic tests. Microsatellite instability is the result of mutation in DNA repair genes MLH1 and MSH2, and it is a tumor-agnostic biomarker for pembrolizumab and a targeted mutation in colorectal cancer, notably Lynch syndrome (Fig. 2.5) [4].

A personalized cancer therapy approach was reported from an oncologist's perspective by Riedl et al. (Table 2.1). Biological understandings of the pathophysiology of cancer led to the identification of oncogenic drivers of cancer progression by identifying specific genetic alterations and led to the development of targeted therapies. The paradigm shift to tumor-agnostic, molecular-driven therapy played a prominent role in the implementation of personalized cancer medicines. The authors point out the hurdles and challenges as well, which include the complexity of the tumor microenvironment in the form of tumor heterogeneity that is based on the

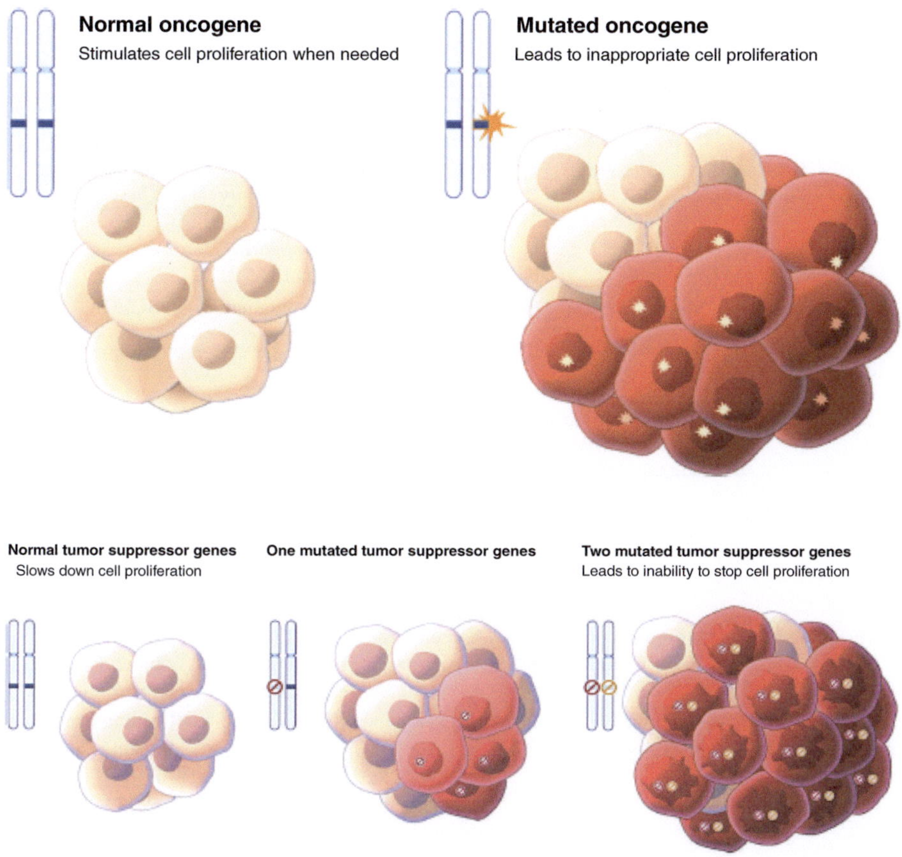

Fig. 2.5 Oncogenes and tumor suppressor genes. (Adapted from Gadade et al. [3]. Permission to reuse by Creative Commons CC BY 4.0)

Table 2.1 Approved drugs as of 2024, categorized according to their biomarker

Target	Alteration type	Testing method	Approved drugs	Clinical indication*
ALK	Gene fusion	RNA sequencing IHC screening	Alectinib Brigatinib Ceritinib Crizotinib Lorlatinib	NSCLC
BRAF	Mutation	DNA sequencing	Dabrafenib Encorafenib Vemurakenib	Anaplastic thyroid carcinoma Colorectal cancer Malignant melanoma NSCLC

(continued)

Table 2.1 (continued)

Target	Alteration type	Testing method	Approved drugs	Clinical indication*
BRCA	Mutation	DNA sequencing	Niraparib Olaparib Platinum chemotherapy Rucaparib Talamoparib Veliparib	Breast cancer Ovarian cancer Prostate cancer (PCa)
EGFR	Mutation	DNA sequencing	Amivantamab Erlotinib Gefitinib Osimertinib	NSCLC
ERBB2	Overexpression Amplification Mutation	IHC FISH DNA sequencing	Lapatinib Neratinib Pertuzumab Trastuzumab Trasturumab-emitansine Trasturumab-druxtecan	Breast cancer Colorectal cancer esophageal cancer Gastric cancer NSCLC
FGF(R)	Mutation Gerre fusion	DNA sequencing RNA sequencing	Erdafitinib Futibatinib Pemigatinib	Biliary tract cancer Urothelial cancer
Homologous recombination deficiency	Genomic instability	DNA sequencing	Niraparib Olaparib Platinum chemotherapy Rucaparib Talawoparib Veliparib	Ovarian cancer Prostate cancer
KIT	Mutation	DNA sequencing	Imatinib	Gastrointestinal stromal tumors (GIST)
MET	Amplification mutation	Flourescent in situ hybridization (FISH) DNA sequencing	Cabmatinib Tepotinib	NSCLC
Microsatellite instability/ mismatch pair deficiency	Genomic instability	DNA sequencing IHC	Pembrolizumab	Turnor agnostic
NTRK	Gene fusion	RNA sequencing IHC screening	Entrectinib Larotrectimib	Turnor agnostic
PDGF(R) A	Mutation	DNA sequencing	Avapritinib	GIST

(continued)

Table 2.1 (continued)

Target	Alteration type	Testing method	Approved drugs	Clinical indication*
PD-L1	Overexpression	IHC	Atzonlizumab Cemiplimab Durvalumab Nivolumab Pembrolizumab	Breast cancer (triple negative) Cervical canoer Esophageal canoer Gastric cancer Head and neck cancer NSCLC Urothelial cancer
PIK3CA	Mutation	DNA sequencing	Alpelisib	Breast cancer
RET	Fusion	RNA sequencing	Pralsetinib Selpercatinib	Thyroid cancer NSCLC
ROS	Fusion	RNA sequencing	Crizotinib Entrectinib Lorlatinib	NSCLC
Turnor mutational burden	Genomic instability	DNA sequencing	Pembrolizumab	Turnor agnostic

Adapted from Riedl et al. [1]
Note: *NSCLC* non–small cell lung cancer, *GIST* gastrointestinal stromal tumor, and *IHC* immunohistochemistry

temporal and spatial evaluation of tumor growth, which has the potential to be facilitated through liquid biopsy analysis (see Chap. 3). As the authors note, "precision oncology is currently revolutionizing" cancer treatment and care through next-generation sequencing (NGS)—including whole-genome sequencing (WGS) and whole-exome sequencing (WES)—and the development of molecular diagnostics, with distinct oncogenic pathways being characterized, including the elucidation of the mechanisms of key proto-oncogenes and tumors suppressors as a result of ongoing, intensive preclinical and other types of experimental studies, which also impact the cell-signaling pathways, leading to tumor abeyance as a result of small molecular inhibitors such as tyrosine kinase inhibitors (TKIs) and biologics such as monoclonal antibodies. A tumor-agnostic therapeutic decision-making process has emerged on the basis of molecular profiling, accompanied by oncology becoming the exemplar of the personalized medicine paradigm. NGS has led to decreased costs and rapid turn-around times in the process of driver alteration identification, and using NGS with comprehensive gene panels makes possible the analysis of varied genes with high accuracy, including the construction of the Cancer Genome Atlas (TCGA). Novel gene alterations such as mutations, amplifications, and rearrangements have emerged and are continually being discovered, and they are incorporated into the clinical setting for tailored molecularly stratified cancer treatment decisions on tumor-agnostic therapeutic agents for melanoma, NSCLC, and breast cancer regardless of histology. This phenomenon is situated in the context of a complex clinical workflow, according to the authors, which involves a patient journey of whether to perform a tissue biopsy or liquid biopsy, bioinformatic data processing, and the determination of the significance of the newly discovered variants, including whether they are pathogenic or likely pathogenic or benign, and which is coordinated by geneticists and pathologists, where the oncologist's role in clinical actionability assessment is crucial. Precision medicine clinical trials, as discussed in detail later, emanate from these discoveries and facilitate this workflow. Because the efficacy of the molecular process currently remains low, medical societies such as the European Society for Medical Oncology (ESMO) have taken the helm in providing guidance to the key players in the precision oncology workflow for the clinical application of NGS testing in identifying multigenes for cholangiocarcinoma, NSCLC, ovarian cancer, and prostate cancer (PCa), which involves primarily whether this genetic testing is indicated. The recommendation is that because performing molecular profile tests for every early-stage cancer is unreasonable, including late-stage cancers in patients with comorbidities, low performance status, and considerations of patient preference and patient autonomy, the implementation of molecular profiling with the most robust clinical efficacy is recommended for patients who have very limited treatment options, patients who may have undergone extensive prior therapies, and patients with rare cancers. The use of targeted gene panels versus comprehensive genomic profiling is also at issue; however, according to the authors, the data for identifying alterations remain inconclusive. My Cancer Genome is an example of a knowledge precision oncology database that has been developed to provide data on cancer-associated mutations and their potential clinical actionability for further scrutiny and the assessment of clinical annotation [1].

The ESMO score for the clinical actionability of molecular targets (ESCAT) has been put forth, and it defines six levels of evidence for molecular targets. Tier I features the strongest evidence level, which consists of genetic alterations that have been shown to be clinically efficacious to Tier Ia (randomized), Tib (nonrandomized), and Ic (basket). Tier II consists of investigational targets that are associated with clinical activity and have an undetermined benefit. Tier III drugs should be considered for N-of-1 trials as a result of their categorization in "hypothetical alteration drug matches" that show benefit as a result of prospective trial data on the same target but on a different malignancy. Tier IV constitutes agents supported by preclinical data. Finally, Tier V includes alterations that match with drugs that have antitumor activity but no observed clinical benefit. The authors also consider the financial burden of personalized cancer medicines as a major obstacle because some of the costs are associated with comprehensive genomic profiling and integrating adaptive trials into the clinical workflow, and therefore, access may be available only for a minority of patients. As the authors conclude, "with an improved understanding of complex molecular mechanisms" that integrate genetic analysis into the personalized decision-making process, with the ability to spatially and temporally monitor tumors with liquid biopsy, and with improved tools for assessing tumor heterogeneity and the microenvironment, the precision oncology paradigm shift is underway [1].

A comprehensive study by Gibbs et al. on the clinical utility of NGS showed that next-generation sequencing could lead to a meaningful improvement in overall survival (OS) and progression-free survival (PFS) when implemented in the clinical setting, demonstrating that the impact on OS and PFS rates across tumor types can be achieved through NGS-informed treatment through whole-genome, whole-exome, and targeted gene panels. A comprehensive literature review was performed on patients who received "NGS-informed cancer management" and were matched with targeted therapies. In total, 6475 publications were identified, 31 of which were evaluated for PFS and OS among patient subgroups [6].

Genomic alterations have also shown to be prognostic. The detection of genomic alterations in the PTEN gene and TP53 gene have been shown to be prognostic and predictive biomarkers. One study investigated whether the PTEN biomarker added independent prognostic value to determine prognosis in GIST patients. PTEN expression and gene loss have also been reported to be associated with the clinical significance of a localized gastrointestinal stromal tumor (GIST), and PTEN serves as a biomarker to improve the prognosis of the localized tumor. PTEN expression was shown to be associated with recurrence as compared with no recurrence ($p = 0.004$). According to the study authors, the low expression of the PTEN gene was associated with poor disease-free survival (DFS) compared with tumors with high PTEN expression (43.73 vs. 119.5 months). A loss of PTEN heterozygosity was seen in 10% of patients and was associated with poor DFS when compared with the PTEN wild type (27.56 months vs. not reached) [7].

Genomic tumor profiling has also been shown to be a putative prognostic biomarker for administering adjuvant imatinib to high-risk GIST patients, which fulfills an unmet need given that surgery cures only 50% of patients. The results found complex karyotype chromosomal aberrations in 76 of 206 tumors with losses in 14q (76%), 22q (39%), 1p (33%), and 15q (26%). Simple and complex karyotypes correlated with estimated 5-year recurrence-free survival (RFS) in high-risk patients: Simple karyotypes had an RFS of 94%, whereas complex karyotypes had an RFS of 51%. In terms of the association between genomic complexity and outcome, 23 (40%) of tumors had more than 10 chromosomal alterations, 38 (66%) had more than five alterations, and 41 tumors (71%) had more than three alterations. The authors concluded that these genomic profiles were prognostic for recurrence rates in high-risk GIST with chromosomal aberrations and that adjuvant imatinib should be de-escalated in simple karyotype GIST [8].

The genomic features and characteristics of bladder cancer and metastatic hormone-sensitive prostate cancer have led to better understandings of the need to stratify patients according to mutational alternations. According to one study, colorectal adenocarcinoma genomic profiles with frequent KRAS, PIK3CA, and TP53 mutations more closely resembled the genomic profiles of urachal and bladder adenocarcinoma. On the other hand, the genomic profile of urothelial carcinoma with glandular differentiation shared more resemblance with urothelial carcinoma not otherwise specified (UCNOS). TP53, KRAS, and PIK3CA oncogenic alterations have high incidence in primary adenocarcinoma of the bladder, comparable to observed frequences in colorectal adenocarcinoma. The urachal adenocarcinoma subtype uniquely displayed a high frequency of SMAD4 alterations (24%), detectable in 12% of colorectal adenocarcinomas and not in any primary bladder adenocarcinomas [9].

Studies continue to demonstrate how cancer genomics may lead to the discovery of actionable alterations and the stratification of patients according to these mutations designed to lead to effective therapies. Mutations in the TERT promoter differentiated urachal adenocarcinoma from primary bladder adenocarcinoma, having relative percentages of 15% and 0%, respectively, according to prior reports. Frequent alterations in chromatin-modifying regions were seen in urothelial carcinoma (UC), UC with glandular features, and regions not otherwise specified (NOS) and yet were rarely observed in urachal adenocarcinoma and primary bladder adenocarcinoma, leading to the conclusion that close resemblance existed between the genomic profiles of bladder adenocarcinoma and colorectal adenocarcinomas, whereas UC and NOS more resembled UC with glandular differentiation. Actionable alterations guiding treatment may be identified from the genomic sequencing of urachal adenocarcinoma and bladder carcinoma [9].

An interesting study found that the PTEN, SPOP, and chromosomal 8p alterations genomically characterized lung-recurrent hormone-sensitive prostate by analyzing 46 primary and 32 metastatic foci that underwent WES and targeted sequencing. These mutations characterize aggressive prostate cancer; prostate cancer that was curable was associated with the genomic landscape of lung-recurrent metastatic hormone-sensitive prostate cancer (mHSPC). TP53 and DNA damage repair genes were not found, and the study authors concluded that prospective efforts for stratifying lung-recurrent mHSPC through genomic characterization are encouraging in suggesting that the genomic features of PCa be integrated with their metastatic recurrence in the design of future clinical studies evaluating treatment for prostate cancer [10].

Genomic mutations similarly conducted an analysis of DNA mismatch repair genes for a number of tumors. Mismatch repair is routinely tested in a tumor-agnostic manner through immunohistochemistry (IHC) in different cancer types; however, it is rarely performed in this context, whereas NGS is. A recent study proposed that MMR genes that would have MMR protein loss at higher rates could be detected by using NGS, indicating the clinical utility of post-IHC reflex testing with NGS.

2.1.2 Key Results

- MMR gene mutations were found in 698/15,701, or 4.4%, of patients with mutations observed across tumor types.
- For at least one MMR protein, IHC loss was displayed for 317/4994, or 6.3%, of patients.
- Variation was found in the dMMR rate according to type of mutation. Here, 207/4669, or 4.4%, of patients had no mutations observed, with 110/325, or 33.8%, of patients having mutations.
- Patients with missense mutations represented 69.3% (484/698), followed by frameshift/truncation (171, 24.5%), splice-site (31, 4.4%), and in-frame inser-

tion/deletion (12, 1.7%) mutations. Moreover, 166 patients (24%) had mutations in PMS2, 178 (26%) in MLH1, 216 (31%) in MSH2, and 232 (33%) in MSH6, whereas 76 (10.9%) had mutations in more than one MMR gene.

- Patients with colorectal cancer (CRC) displayed a frequency of 5.5% (119/2,148) of MMR gene mutations, whereas the frequency of endometrial cancer and that of gastric cancer was 6.1% (31/505) and 2.9% (7/244), respectively.

The association of MMRs with NGS was demonstrated through IHC testing as well: "Of the 324 patients with IHC results, 214 patients had intact IHC for MMR proteins and 110 had a loss of MMR proteins."

Although the authors did conclude that IHC screening should routinely be performed, their results provide support for their hypothesis that MMR mutations are found in tumor testing where IHC testing is not performed. They concluded that patients harboring dMMR may be matched with treatment options including known or inferred inactivating mutations through reflex IHC testing [11].

2.2 Biomarkers and Precision Oncology

The detection of biomarkers such as TMB and MSI, overexpressed genes, and germline and somatic variants was the result of the implementation and adoption of NGS and the implementation of gene- and multigene-sequencing panels. Genomic biomarkers include gene amplification, oncogene mutations, and translocation. Oncogene targets include EGFR, ALK, BRAF, MET, KIT, and KRAS. Tumors containing the MSI biomarker have deficient mismatch repair with random insertions or deletions of cancer-related genes in repetitive regions of DNA, resulting in somatic mutations. MSI is considered a predictive biomarker for Lynch syndrome, a hereditary cancer. BRCA1 and BRCA 2 tumors have germline pathogenic alleles and show a loss of HDR proficiency, which plays a role in double-stranded DNA break repair. PARP inhibitors rely on the synthetic lethality of double-stranded break repair. BRCA-deficient tumors can no longer engage in base excision and single-strand break repair mediated through PARPs. Because single-stranded breaks in tumors treated with Poly (ADP-ribose) Polymerse inhibitors (PARPi) cannot be repaired, double-stranded breaks are irreparable, leading to cell death.

Biomarkers are measures of biological phenomena in cells that lead to potential clinical actionability in the diagnosis and treatment of disease. In the form of genetic, epigenetic, metabolomic, proteomic, and transcriptomic biomarkers, the development and validation of biomarkers, although challenging, led to the rise of precision oncology and targeted drug therapy development. Genetic markers include commonly known mutations in tumor suppressor genes and oncogenes (discussed below), such as RAF, EGFR, p53, BRAF, and HER2, that implicate molecular signaling pathways or cell-cycle regulation. Tumor-agnostic drugs rose from the development of the MSI-high/-low biomarkers in NSCLC, among other tumor types. Transcriptomic biomarkers include miRNA molecules that regulate gene expression relevant to tumor cell growth. Epigenetic markers include patterns of DNA methylation on genes that regulate their expression. Biomarkers can be both prognostic and predictive and monitor disease progression. Other noted biomarkers include PD-L1, tumor mutational burden (TMB), and minimal residual disease.

Challenges in the advancement of precision oncology in the context of biomarkers are the result of the tumor heterogeneity and complexity, the availability of biomarkers, and resistance to targeted therapies. The complexity of tumor biology is reflected in the concept of tumor heterogeneity, which is both spatial and temporal, leading to distinct phenotypes and genotypes in cell subpopulations and posing many challenges to the treatment of cancer, especially when based on a single biomarker that in many cases guides targeted treatment. The accuracy, sensitivity, and specificity of biomarkers are also at issue given that biomarker detection could lead to false positives and false negatives. The power of precision medicine has revolutionized cancer treatment as well, improving outcomes and reducing toxicities, and as the field continues to evolve, the impact on oncology will also grow because more-effective targeted therapies will emerge. The medical model allows for the consideration of individual profiles that include genetic biomarkers, environment, and lifestyle. Efficacy in one patient may not be relevant for efficacy in another patient, and very little translation of causation factors in cancer has occurred among patients, involving the collaboration of healthcare workers such as oncologists, pathologists, and geneticists to gather information about the patient's malignancy to use that information to design a personalized treatment plan. Biomarkers derive from the omics analysis of patients and give rise to the development of targeted therapies, being mainly genetic, transcriptomic, epigenomic, metabolomic, and proteomic. As noted earlier, genetic biomarkers include oncogenes such as HER2, BRAF, and KRAS; tumor suppressor genes such as TP53, BRCA1, and BRCA2; DNA repair genes such as BRCA1 and BRCA; and microsatellite instability (MSI high), commonly seen in colorectal cancer and gastric cancer. Transcriptomic biomarkers include the widely characterized microRNAs and noncoding long microRNAs. In highlighting biomarkers in cancer, HER2 overexpression is targeted by trastuzumab and pertuzumab and EGFR in NSCLC is targeted by gefitinib, erlotinib, afatinib, and the third-generation osimertinib as resistance to these agents developed. BRAFV600E is a driver alteration for melanoma, with targeted agents vemurafenib, dabrafenib, and encorafenib developed for the cancer. These biomarkers are relevant for cancer prognosis and the prediction of the clinical outcome of these therapies. Imaging such as positron emission tomography (PET) scans and magnetic resonance images (MRIs) can assess responses to tumors and liquid biopsy (Chap. 3) can play a key role in treatment decisions. Also important is the complexity of tumor biology, in which as a result of the numerous genetic alterations that can arise over tumor progression, multiple subclones with distinct parts of the tumor having distinct molecular characteristics can also emerge, complicating the selection of biomarkers targeting a single cellular pathway that is driving tumor growth. Tumors evolve both spatially and temporally, with distinct genotype and phenotypic characteristics. These new subclones can pose "significant challenges to the diagnosis, prognosis and treatment of cancers." Drug resistance emerges from the numerous interacting cell-signaling pathways, hampering the identification of a single targeted therapy for robust clinical outcomes. There are other challenges in the discovery of clinically actionable alterations, including the high cost of therapies and resistance to them and the risk of misinterpretation. Healthcare disparities may emerge from differential access as a result of socioeconomic factors. As one observer concludes, "[t]argeted therapies are transforming cancer treatment"; however, clinical trials and treatments need to be optimized to improve the accuracy of matching the tailored treatments with a patient's biomarker profile. The authors also claim that artificial intelligence will come to play a large role in analyzing huge amounts of clinical data [3].

Precision oncology for bladder cancer through the discovery and development of diagnostic, prognostic, and predictive biomarkers was described in a review in 2017 by Kojima et al., in which important biomarkers were investigated. These include transcriptomic biomarkers such as microRNAs, "of which 11 were upregulated (miRNA-96, miRNA-138, miRNA-126, miRNA-182, miRNA-143, miRNA-222, miRNA-21, miRNA-133b, miRNA-518c-5p, miRNA-452, and miRNA-129) and four were downregulated (miRNA-200c, miRNA-99a, miRNA-100, and miRNA-29c)" and in which mutations such as the FGFR3 gene associated with a higher risk for intravesical recurrence were detected via NGS. These authors also reported that a combination of mutated FGFR3 and wild-type PIK3CA led to a statistically significant risk of recurrence, demonstrating how genetic analysis of multiple genes could predict disease outcomes. The hemizygous and homozygous deletion of CDKN2A was associated with disease progression as an independent predictor alteration. Everolimus was found in a phase II trial to lead to tumor regression in patients who harbored the TSC1 mutation that negatively regulates the mechanistic target of rapamycin (mTOR). The authors concluded that molecular biomarkers were promising for the early detection of disease and predicting tumor progression and clinical recurrence that would be facilitated by using NGS, WES, and WGS. The authors also note in terms of the future implications for biomarkers that molecular subtypes of malignancies could be categorized according to the identification of genes that are "responsible for tumor development" and "treatment response." They also posited that the predictive accuracy of candidate biomarkers would be enhanced through validation in diverse patients for clinical application, realizing the revolutionary potential of "predictive molecular biomarkers" for bladder cancer and other urologic cancers [12].

One report highlighted the development of the integrated Clinical and Genomic Information System (CGIS), which will aid precision oncology by providing the systematic interpretation of genomic alterations derived from NGS data. The methodology involves a web-based CGIS that processes NGS data, annotates variants, and integrates clinical information to recommend therapies and support patient cohort exploration. Key findings include the ability of the system to identify actionable genomic targets, stratify patient cohorts on the basis of molecular data, and provide interactive tools for variant exploration and survival analysis. The conclusion emphasizes that the CGIS software is designed for both clinicians and medical scientists, integrating diverse genomic resources to facilitate biomarker development and clinical decision-making. Potential implications include improving precision medicine through an enhanced understanding of genomic data, patient stratification, and targeted therapy options. The integration workflow is shown Fig. 2.6. Like similar prior studies, the development of the CGIS was an early example of establishing the importance of NGS for oncology and the processing of clinical information for determining effective therapies through actionable genomic targets [13].

Ohnmacht et al. revealed in a report in *Nature Communications* their development of an oncology biomarker discovery framework, or OncoBird, for analyzing randomized controlled trials (RCTs) to show the molecular biomarker landscape of tumors. In a statistical analysis, they identified single gene-based biomarkers or mutually exclusive genetic alterations in isolation that led to a predictive model. Focusing on the randomized trial for metastatic colorectal cancer (mCRC) , OncoBird in the study evaluated responses to EGFR-targeted agent cetuximab and anti-VEGF agent bevacizumab. Five biomarkers with predictive components were identified, and chr20q-amplified tumors or tumors that lack mutually exclusive ERK signaling alterations were shown to benefit from anti-EGFR therapy when compared to bevacizumab. In the FIRE-3 trial, patients harboring the KRAS exon 2 mCRC were randomized to receive bevacizumab and cetuximab in combination with chemotherapy and with no prior therapy. A "gene-expression-derived consensus molecular subtype," or CMS, is proposed that identifies molecular subtypes that reflect distinct tumor biology and that has prognostic value, through which patients with wild-type RAS show significantly longer OS when treated with cetuximab. This potentially leads to the CMS classification of CRC that yielded insight into the elucidation of complex biomarkers by applying a model based on interactions between tumor subtypes and their somatic alterations, highlighting the urgent need

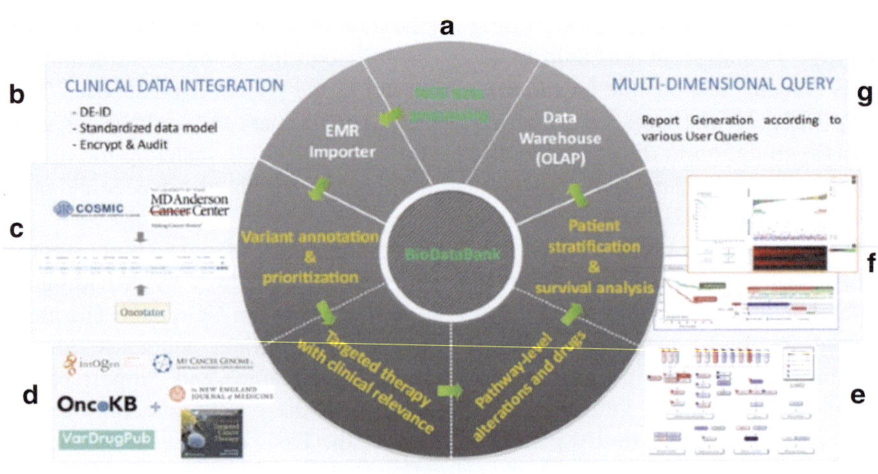

Fig. 2.6 Information flow of BioDataBank. (Adapted from Jang et al. [13]. Permission to reuse by Creative Commons CC BY 4.0)

to present meaningful information from data emerging from computational frameworks by systematically deciphering the molecular landscape of tumor subtypes and biomarkers. OncoBird leads to "systematic identification not actionable biomarkers for clinical trials in oncology." In a five-step process, molecular subtypes and mutations are investigated, and treatment is based on genetic alterations and identified biomarkers and is evaluated for its "predictive component across treatment arms" when applied to RCTs. Furthermore, mCRC with wild-type RAS displayed superior OS: hazard ratio (HR) = 0.53 (0.38–0.073). In the example of the FIRE-3 clinical trial, 31 frequently altered cancer genes were observed, including SRC, TOP1, GNAS, and ARFRP1 and chr20q amplifications. In total, 453 gene expression profiles were also analyzed. Regression modules assessed single genes and mutually exclusive gene modules as biomarkers for cetuximab. BRAF mutations were found to be mutually exclusive with RAS mutations. The gene module that included mutations in SOX9 and MYC amplification tumors displayed worse prognostic according to OS. In terms of genetic biomarkers for bevacizumab, regression models showed that the mutually exclusive module of BRAF and KRAS mutations demonstrated a lower OS. Wild-type adenomatous polyposis coli (APC) served as a superior predictor for OS. The predictive components of biomarkers were shown in a comparison of cetuximab and bevacizumab when their genetic alterations and treatment arms between tumor subtypes were assessed. The predictive value of chr20q amplification was found in CMS2 tumors, whereby the largest predictive component was demonstrated by ARFRP1 amplifications. By analyzing the statistical power of biomarkers, the authors concluded on how the OncoBird is able to characterize the biomarker and molecular landscape of RCTs that is generalizable across tumor types [14].

Solid tumors, including cholangiocarcinoma, biliary tract cancer, renal cell carcinoma, and ovarian carcinoma, were the subjects of studies conducted to elucidate clinically actionable biomarkers. One on cholangiocarcinoma, an aggressive biliary tract cancer, sought to identify serum metabolite biomarkers as a result of metabolic mechanisms, including amino acid and lipid metabolism, to predict recurrence in the malignancy for screening and disease management. Using high-performance mass spectrometry (MS), liquid chromatography, and support vector modeling (SVM) to develop predictive frameworks for the metabolite biomarkers, alterations were revealed across cholangiocarcinoma (CCA) recurrence subtypes and lipidomics and metabolomics enabled predictive accuracy that was compatible with current clinical diagnostic standards for preoperative detection. This study was significant also because cholangiocarcinoma is usually detected at late stages of the disease. In the study, 88 cholangiocarcinoma (CCA) patients were divided into a testing cohort and a training cohort ($n = 28$ and $n = 60$, respectively) after undergoing surgical resection and experiencing disease recurrence. The RFS categories were early recurrence and late recurrence, with 2369 metabolites identified in positive mode and 1872 in negative mode after identification in MS and further filtration into early and late recurrence groups in both modes. These were further categorized into common metabolites involved in energy production and amino acid biosynthesis (positive mode) and lipid metabolism including energy storage (in negative mode) that enabled the further analysis of distinct metabolic pathways. In terms of the results, distinct metabolic profiles between recurrence subtypes, among which were 39 lipids and 26 metabolites, were elevated in late recurrence, and five lipids and 20 metabolites were upregulated in early recurrence, suggesting that they have potential for use as biomarkers for preoperative screening, predicting recurrent patterns, guiding treatment decisions, and improving patient monitoring. Kaplan–Meier analysis showed a diagnosis of shorter RFS and OS in early versus late recurrence (RFS = 200 vs. 786 days; OS = 264 vs. 960 days). Pathway analysis further highlighted that global changes in metabolism lead to recurrence in CCA patients. MetaboAnalysis 6.0 identified metabolic pathways implicated in common amino acid metabolism, including alanine/aspartate/glutamate metabolism, tryptophan synthesis, arginine biosynthesis, and the Krebs cycle. In terms of lipid metabolism, key pathways such as unsaturated fatty acid biosynthesis and alpha-linolenic acid metabolism were also shown to be affected. In short, strong links to metabolic alterations were demonstrated, and both fatty acid metabolism and amino acid metabolism were significantly involved.

The authors concluded that the current diagnostic standards for CA19-9 and Carcinoembryonic Antigen (CEA) have high false-positive rates and low accuracy; show a low ability to predict DFS and OS, with wide variation; and demonstrate a poor classification of recurrence subtypes in CCA. The methods that they have utilized, including SVM algorithm classification, provide predictive models and valuable tools for identifying recurrence risk in patients, allowing for a high level of robust and interpretable generalizability. Because cancer progression is linked to tumor metabolism, the identified amino acids and lipid metabolism pathways were implicated as being significantly changed and linked to recurrence rates [15].

Plasma proteomic biomarkers were found to predict survival in biliary tract cancer (BTC) patients receiving camrelizumab and the gemcitabine and oxaliplatin (GEMOX) treatment in one study by Cui et al. In that study, 37 BTC patients provided plasma and tissue samples; this was followed by an analysis of 92 proteins for partial responses and for stable disease (SD) and progressive disease (PD). The results included eight proteins, namely IL7, ANGPT2, IL15, HO-1, CXCL1, CXCL5, IL33, and VEGFA, that exhibited signficantly greater expression in SD and PD versus CR and PR. ANGPT2, HO-1 and IL15 demonstrated high accuracy in immune checkpoint blockade (ICB) treatment plus chemotherapy. In the study, camrelizumab plus GEMOX was evaluated as a first-line treatment, and the results demonstrated a PFS of 50%, whereas mPFS and mOS were 6.1 months and 11.8 months, respectively. Due to a lack of a durable treatment response, the identification of predictive biomarkers for screening populations who benefit from this treatment becomes more necessary, and further WGS did not distinguish among response groups or find any meaningful correlation between TMB on one hand and circulating biomarkers and immune cells associated with the tumor microenvironment (TME) on the other, thus mandating a study on predicting treatment response through proteomic analysis. Peripheral blood samples showed that patients were divided into groups on the basis of complete response (CR), partial response (PR), ,

SD, and PD. Differentially expressed proteins were shown to have observable differences among PR, SD, and PD groups, where interaction effect, response effect, and time effect were relevant and were analyzed at each time point and among the 92 proteins; 10 showed significant proteins with response effect, and 11% of plasma proteins were shown to have significant changes among SD, PD, and PR groups. The eight differentially expressed proteins were CXCL1, CXCL5, ANGPT2, IL15, HO-1, IL33 and VEGFA, with proteins CXCL1 and HO-1 being at T1. In patients experiencing PR, proteins PDCD1, TNFRSF4, DCN, CRTAM, ADA, and VEGFR-2 were associated with immune cell activity that also exhibited distinctive expression patterns. Among patients experiencing SD and PD, altered expression profiles in PDCD1, CD28, IL10, PTN, and ADA were displayed. A prognostic model that was created by combining genomics with proteomics found associations with PFS and OS. Genomic analysis led to the identification of differentially expressed genes. In view of plasma samples, the NTRK1 gene and the CD27 and CRTAM proteins were protective factors in PFS, whereas BAI3, CTCF, CDKN1A, and Akt1 were high-risk factors for PFS. The BRIP1, GRM3, and TET2 genes were relatively high-risk factors for OS, whereas IL1 and VEGFR2 were protective factors. The authors concluded that their results of analyzing the predictive effect of proteomics for finding differentially expressed proteins on the basis of response effects (as well as time and interaction) would complement the existing repertoire of biomarkers for ICB treatment, including PD-L1, TMB, and dMMR, and MSI, that are related to the curative effects of immunotherapy. The study took into consideration that proteins levels exhibit dynamic behavior involving an intricate regulatory network of proteins with a three-time-point baseline. The proteins that exhibited difference after 6 weeks of treatment were LAP TGF-β-1, MUC-16, IL-15, ANGPT2, and FGF2, being closely related to tumor cell growth. Among them, the differential expression of MUC-16(CA125) was evaluated as having value for having a curative effect, for being prognostic and recognized as a tumor marker, and for serving as the most distinct marker. Through the synthesis of three time points, consistent differentially expressed proteins (DEPs) were obtained (IL-15, ANGPT2), and while patients were undergoing treatment, predictive factors with curative effects may reflect the fluctuations in the patients' internal environment.

Due to a change in signaling pathways, Cui et al. (2025) posited that DEPs change with the development of the disease course and the time effect. The expression profiles of DEPs, specifically ADA, CD28, IL10, PDCD1, and PTN, changed according to SD and PD status, whereas PR changed according to changes in the expression profiles of ADA, CRTAM, DCN, PDCD1, and TNFRSF4. Among them, in distinguishing between SD or PD and PR groups, CD28, DCN, CRTAM, IL10, PTN, and TNFRSF4 may be valuable DEPs. ANGPT2, HO-1, and IL15 were three cytokines that play important roles in immunotherapy response, were found in this study to be the most significant DEPs, and at all three time points were higher in the PR groups compared to the SD or PD groups. The study authors concluded that focusing on proteomic analysis for BTC provides a "novel perspective for targeted therapy of BTC" and improves the sensitivity of immunotherapy with some limitations for inevitable bias due to confounding facts and a small sample size [16].

Clear cell renal cell carcinoma (ccRCC) is a disease treated with an antiangiogenic treatment such as VEGF inhibitors for low-risk disease and immunotherapy such as immune checkpoint inhibitors (ICIs) for high-risk disease; however, no biomarkers exist to guide treatment. In the IMmotion150 study, outcome predictions were conducted through RNA-sequencing-based gene expression signatures. In a phase 2 study, 305 patients were randomized to receive atezolizumab and atezolizumab plus bevacizumab. Gene sets were used to subdivide tumors into biological categories, where CD8A, EOMES, PRF1, CD274, and IFNG were the five genes related to cellular immunity, and their expression defined the T-eff cell 'Gene Expression Signature (GES) and allowed for the subdivision of tumors into T-eff-low and T-eff-high cell groups, with T-eff-high cell tumors demonstrating increased PD-L1 expression, CD8+ T cell infiltration, and improved PFS when treated with sunitinib versus atezolizumab plus (HR 0.55, 95% confidence interval (CI) 0.32–0.95). To enable a clustering of predictions on disease and therapy patterns and to guide precision oncology for this disease to guide responses to treatment, a gene signature for ccRCC was created. Specifically, a refined-66 gene signature for improved subclassification was constructed on the basis of analyzing the gene expression profiles of 469 ccRCC patients and to distinguish stromal from immune cells with a novel comprehensive expression profile, which is further significant as a result of low TMB and a high immune infiltration score with high proportions of indels from a pan cancer analysis. Although other gene expression classification studies have been done to show how the gene-expression-based subclassification of disease played a role in response to treatments, they were not empirical data analyses, and these studies showed that the TME played a role when 1500 genes were analyzed. In this study, ccRCC samples ($n = 469$) from the TCGA dataset and cBioPortal were analyzed for their expression profiles. VHL, BAP1, SED2, PBRM1, and TP53, frequently mutated genes in ccRCC, were analyzed to form different patient clusters, and they improved the understanding of this association. In the analysis, mutations in VHL, BAP1, SETD2, PBRM1, and TP53 were isolated to different patient clusters to assess the association of frequently mutated genes in ccRCC. A statistically significant association was found between the angiogenic and T-eff groups with TP53, BAP1, and PBRM1 mutations. In this study, 415 patients subclassified as the Angio cohort ($n = 150$, 90.4 months) had a longer OS than that of the T-effector gene cohort ($n = 187$, median 62.8 months). As the study authors state, in assessing the prognositc ability of the 66-gene signature, a high HR ratio in the mixed (exp (coef)) = 1.7433, $p = 0.0386$) and T-effector (exp (coef)) = 2.2091, $p = 0.0201$) groups was observed compared to the angiogenic group as part of their Cox regression analysis on DFS time and status in the same patient cohorts. The analysis of invasion genes that were identified showed that half clustered with the angiogenic group and half clustered with the T-effector group, demonstrating the novelty of their study. This separation analysis of the distinct genes implicated in the migration of angiogenic stromal cells from immune cells, leading to tumor cell migration and metastasis, had not been conducted before. Compared to the IMmotion150 32-gene signature, the 66-gene signature showed a change in the K = M plots, with the angiogenic stratified patients having longer OS. As the authors conclude, the 66-gene panel encompasses crucial genes with both clinical and therapeutic value in clear cell renal cell carcinoma [17].

Through a systematic review, Wang et al. identified predictive biomarkers for the efficacy of PARP inhibitors in ovarian cancer. PARP inhibitors have shown benefits in a number of clinical trials, including OlympiAD (olaparib) and EMBRACA (talazoparib) for HER2 metastatic disease, and the role of predictive biomarkers becomes important for epithelial ovarian cancer. The Study 19 phase 2 trial showed olaparib efficacy for recurrent epithelial ovarian cancer (EOC) in patients harboring BRCA1/2 pathogenic variants. The phase 3 SOLO2 trials showed a 19.2-month PFS benefit for BRCA1/2-variant patients in recurrent ovarian cancer (OC), and NOVA and ARIEL 3 also showed the advantages of PARP inhibitors in platinum-sensitive recurrent EOC with the BRCA1/2 variants, as well as in PAOLA-1, PRIMA, and VELIA. BRCA1/2 and HRD are being developed as candidate predictive biomarkers for PARP1 effectiveness due to their role in HRR pathways. HRD cells employ DNA reparative mechanisms through nonhomologous end joining and MMEJ and through the error-prone mechanism for repairing double-stranded DNA breaks through microhomology-mediated end joining, allow for greater PARPi escape while further disrupting single-stranded DNA repair. DNA damage accumulation leads to cell death and synthetic lethality, and this makes selecting EOC patients for PARP1 on the basis of the presence of HRD and BRCA1/2 status and establishing universally accepted biomarkers for patient stratification even to maximize PARPi benefits even more necessary and challenging. Their systematic review, including 62 research articles, revealed that 89%, or 55, of HRR-related genes can be categorized into gBRCA and sBRCA variants, pathogenic variants of HRR-related genes, and HRR-related gene-promoter methylation. BRCA 1and BRCA 2 proteins were also found to have complex interactions with CHEK2 and PALB2, with significant roles played by RAD51, CHEK1 and CHEK2, ATM, and ATR. Furthermore, 77% of the studies utilized the BRCA allele, both germline and somatic, to assess the effectiveness of PARPi, including the use of the Myriad MyChoice CDx kit and FoundationOne CDx kits. Other pathogenic variants included hMOB2, CCDC6, EMSY, RAD51C and RAD51D, and PALB2, where hMOB2 and CCDC6-PP4 required further validation. However, effectively predicting PARPi efficacy for EOC patients is difficult because these "gene panels do not adequately capture the multifaceted nature" of HRR-related genes and BRCA1/2 variants. Mutational signatures, including DNA copy number alterations (CNAs) and loss-of-heterozygosity (LOH) scores, were also probed. Functional assays for detecting HRD were also shown to have predictive power, providing "real-time insights into the capacity" of HRRd by assessing the active repair capacity of tumors. Reversion mutations are also detectable thanks to the restoration of mechanisms of HRR proficiency for a more positive identification of HRD-positive tumors. The RAD51 assay was found to evaluate the role of RAD51 in double-stranded DNA breaks in the HRR pathway and was shown to be a superlative method for assessing HRD. However, there was insufficient evidence of clinical validity, even though improved survival for patients with low RAD51 levels was demonstrated, and RAD51 was not shown to consistently predict treatment in the

TOPACIO phase 2 trial. Additional biomarkers, including KELIM or CA-125 ELIMination Rate Constant K, with an HR of 0.67 (95% 0.50–0.91) for two phase 2 trials, showed a favorable KELIM score with a significant reduction of PD or death in EOC rucaparib-treated patients. SLFN11 is emerging as a predictive biomarker for ovarian cancer because it induces irreversible replication block and shows a positive correlation between the effectiveness of PARP1 and level of objective response. A classification score of HRD greater than or equal to 42 was also revealed to guide treatment. The authors conclude that genomic assay for detecting BRCA 1/2 can be widely used as a predictive biomarker for PARP1 efficacy in ovarian cancer patients; assays such as those described can provide valuable insights into HRD and assessing the real function of HRR; and novel biomarkers such as KELIM scores and SLFN11 expression also offer potential, but they need validation for clinical applicability and reliability [18].

2.2.1 Urothelial Cancer

In the RANGE study, ramucirumab, an anti-VEGFR2 mAB, was evaluated for predictive biomarkers for platinum-refractory urothelial cancer (UC) through the use of transcriptomic analysis and PD-L1 IHC, revealing angiogenic and OS-immune pathway association with molecular subtypes. The OS of ramucirumab treatment was found to be associated with higher immune pathway scores and higher PD-L1, but not angiogenesis scores. They show data indicating the utility of using multiple biomarkers to identify UC patients who might derive greater clinical benefit from ramucirumab therapy. Because KEYNOTE-45 and JAVELIN 100 showed that responders to ICIs were in the low PD-L1 category, further studies are needed to analyze a complex tumor type treatment such as ramucirumab to reveal biomarkers. The 2017 RANGE trial, a phase 3 study, showed significant benefit in PFS in the intention-to-treat (ITT) population from ramucirumab + docetaxel vs. docetaxel only, with an exploratory biomarker analysis showing a significant association between the expression level of PD-L1 and R + D administration.

2.2.2 Key Results

- The retrospective analysis suggested the putative role of the utility of predictive biomarkers with ramucirumab, with higher baseline PD-L1 expression (CPS greater than or equal to 10) in patients with PD-L1 CPS $\geq$ 10 (vs. HR 0.999, $p = 0.9955$), whereas in patients with a PD-L1 CPS < 10, increased OS was seen in the ramucirumab + docetaxel cohort (HR 0.51).
- Longer OS was also associated with higher PD-L1 CPS in the ramucirumab arm (CPS $\geq$ 10 vs. < 10, median OS 9.03 vs. 7.92 months) in the TR1 population. In addition, when compared to CPS < 10 (stratified HR, 0.926, 95% CI 0.604 to

1.42; interaction p-value = 0.063), CPS ≥ 10 was predictive of OS benefit for ramucirumab vs. placebo (stratified HR, 0.451, 95% CI 0.275 to 0.74; $p = 0.002$, Benjamini–Hochberg-adjusted $p = 0.047$).

- High PD-L1 is associated with greater OS outcomes in UC (CPS greater than or equal to 10), which are correlated with immune signatures and angiogenic pathways. The study authors note that the heterogeneity of tumor tissue and the low sample size would have further affected the analysis, but the study represents an important step in the associated OS response with antiangiogenic therapy using and assessing biomarkers in UC [19].

2.2.3 KRASG12C Mutant Cancers

The RAS oncogene is the most frequently mutated oncogene in human cancers, and after its discovery in 1982, in 2013, researchers also discovered that the G12C mutation in the KRAS gene could be targeted. Sotorasib is a targeted agent that received approval when it was found to directly target the KRAS oncoprotein in KRAS-mutant cancers. Kwan et al. conducted a comprehensive review of KRAS G12C inhibitors, describing their path to the clinic from the discovery of the clinical KRAS G12C mutation with the structure and function of RAS oncoproteins. NIH/3 T3 mouse cell lines revealed that transformations had an activated KRAS oncogene, and the molecular basis for RAS gene activation later identified in patient tumors was codon 12. The G domain of the RAS protein is composed of six B-sheets and five alpha helices and binds GTP for activation, where the GTPases cycle in their GTP-bound (active) and GDP-bound (inactive) states, which play roles in cell proliferation and survival and drive transformation and tumor progression. Data from the TCGA, cBioPortal, and the International Cancer Genome Consortium show that ~19% of cancer patients have the RAS mutation, leading to ~18 million new cancer diagnoses a year, and KRAS mutations are found in ATC (8.6%), cholangiocarcinoma (23%), lung adenocarcinoma (32%), colorectal cancer (CRC) (50%), and pancreatic cancer (88%). The KRAS G12 C mutation is found in colorectal cancer (25.8%), lung adenocarcinoma (5.9%), and pancreatic cancer (29.9%). The breakthrough in targeting the KRAS G12C mutation, once considered a completely undruggable mutation, was the discovery of the switch II pocket, and that led to the discovery and development of a series of compounds that are irreversible and that covalently bind the cysteine residue of KRAS G12C, to which the switch II pocket and binds allosterically. These compounds are "preferentially bound to Ras in the GDP conformation" and decrease RAF affinity for GTP relative to GDB by blocking the interaction of RAS in KRAS G12C mutant cells while sparing the wild-type KRAS protein, minimizing toxicities. Subsequent to the discovery of the compound, four preclinical studies were performed that evaluated KRAS inhibition in cells, including ARS-853, ARS-1620, AMG510, and MRTX849. ARS-853 rapidly bound to KRAS G12C and blocked nucleotide exchange, potently inhibiting mutant cell growth with the blocking of downstream signaling pathways through the specific binding of KRASG12C. MS studies demonstrated specific binding to KRASG12C with the blockade of downstream signaling through the PI3K-AKT and RAF-MEK-ERK signaling pathways. However, because ARS-853 was found to have limited potency in vivo and poor plasma stability, ARS-1620 was developed and was found to be well tolerated in mice while being also potent and selective. ARS-1620, having improved pharmacologic properties and potency, showed efficacy in human cancer cell lines and patient-derived mouse xenograft models.

Combinations of AMG510 with various inhibitors of the AKT and MAPK signaling pathways included HER kinases, MEK inhibitors, and AKT, EGFR, SHP2, and PI3K inhibitors. The synergistic activity of these multiple combinations were a result, particularly the MEK inhibitor trametinib, which in combination led to enhanced antitumor activity in spheroid, monolayer cell culture, and mouse tumor models compared to administering each agent alone. Because a prevalence of KRASG12C mutations exist in lung adenocarcinoma, the treatment of carboplatin, a standard-of-care (SOC) chemotherapeutic for NSCLC and other lung cancers, with AMG510 investigated, was found to significantly inhibit tumor growth, and resulted in increased antitumor activity. Both drugs had the same activity when administered alone in KRASG12C-mutant NCI-H358 (NSCLC) xenograft mice models, though therapy in combination was more effective, demonstrating that the clinical combination of MAPK inhibitors or chemotherapy with AMG510 can bypass compensatory resistance mechanisms and lead to increased potency in its therapeutic effects, creating a durable treatment response.

In vivo, MRTX849 led to a 30% reduction in volume from baseline in 17 of 26 preclinical models. Sotorasib was one of the first KRASG12C inhibitors to be investigated in human clinical studies and to show clinical efficacy and safety. In total, 129 patients were enrolled in a dose escalation and dose expansion study on NSCLC ($n = 59$), CRC ($n = 42$), and 28 other tumor types. Safety served as the primary end point, and no dose-limiting toxic effects were observed. Specifically, 73 patients, or 56.6% of them, had TRAEs with grade 3 gastrointestinal (GI) and hepatic events occurring. Moreover, 19, or 32.2%, of the NSCLC patients had confirmed objective response rate (ORR), and disease control occurred in 52 patients, or 88.1% of them; mPFS was 6.3 months. Three CRC patients, or 7.1% patients, had disease control, and 31 patients, or 73.8% of them, had a confirmed response; mPFS was 4 months. Overall, the authors concluded on the favorable safety profile exhibited with few dose-limiting and toxic effects, most of which were low grade. In a heavily pretreated KRASG12C mutant population, sotorasib demonstrated promising antitumor activity—especially in NSCLC, and to a lesser extent in CRC. In the CodeBreak 100 phase 2 trial, ORR was observed in 46 patients, PR in 42 (33.9%), and CR in four (3.2%). Median duration of response (DOR) was 11.1 months, (95% CI 6.9 could not be evaluated), and 124 patients had a value of 6.8 months (95% CI 5.1 to 8.2) and 12.5 months (95% CI 10.0 could not be evaluated) for mPFS and mOS, respectively. Biomarker analyses revealed comutations in TP53, STK11, and KEAP1, with KRAS mutations in NSCLC. Sotorasib gained FDA approval, and ongoing clinical trials are evaluating adagrasib in the KRYSTAL-1 trial and combination approaches in other clinical trials and preclinical investigational compounds. The authors conclude on the fast-moving research and development into direct KRAS G12C inhibitors [5].

Adagrasib was evaluated in a report by Yaeger et al. in the NEJM in KRASG12C-mutated CRC, where 2.5–3.5% harbor the mutation and are associated with worse prognosis. An ORR of 19% and an mPFS of 5.6 months was reported among 46 evaluable chemorefractory patients in the phase II KRYSTAL-1 study. In contrast, 9.7% of 62 patients were heavily pretreated with sotorasib in the CodeBreaK100 basket trial. The BRAFV600E mutation, which formed the basis of an effective target for melanoma, had slight effectivity in CRC due to primary adaptive resistance as a result of the reactivation of the RAS-MAPK signaling pathway through the feedback stimulation of EGFR and that of the RTK. This is also responsible for the relatively low efficacy in KRAS G12C-mutant CRC tumors and led investigators to combine adagrasib with cetuximab in the KRYSTAL-1 trial, which led to OR in 13/28, or 46%, of evaluable patients in this cohort with an mDOR of 7.6 months. In 15 patients, a disease control rate (DCR) of 100% was observed. Grade 3 or 4 TRAEs were seen in 34% of patients (15 of 44) with mCRC in KRYSTAL-1 because monotherapy and the safety profile were not substantially altered by the addition of cetuximab. Predictive biomarkers were not found, and the authors proclaimed that the features of tumors—including sidedness, transcriptomic and methylomic signatures, metabolomic profiles, and the influence of the microbiome and immunoscore—would be considered in correlative analytic studies in the future. Nicolantonio and Bardelli conclude that in a heavily pretreated KRAS12GC-mutant mCRC patient population, the clinical data from KRYSTAL-1 underscore the PRs achieved in approximately 20% of patients through adagrasib monotherapy. They also add that cetuximab provides concomitant EGFR blockade that more than doubles ORR. They conclude, however, that although "this therapeutic strategy is clearly a relevant step to advance precision oncology for mCRC, the success of targeted therapies—including EGFR, HER2, BRAF and KRAS inhibitors—remains incremental and is not yet transformative for patients with mCRC" [20].

2.3 Targeted Therapies Become the Standard of Care

Targeted therapies (Table 2.2) are small molecular inhibitors or biologics that take the form of monoclonal antibodies that target signaling pathways in the cell, resulting in apoptosis and the inhibition of tumor cell proliferation. Some of the most notable FDA-approved targeted therapies for several tumor types and associated targeted mutation and companion diagnostic tests are shown in Table 2.2.

Table 2.2 Targeted therapies by tumor type and biomarker (Biomarker)

Tumor type	Therapy type	Target	Agent
Bladder cancer	Kinase inhibitor	FGFR enzymes	Erdafitinib
Breast cancer	Cell-cycle inhibitor	CDK4 and CDK6	Abemaciclib, Ribociclib, Palbociclib
	Kinase inhibitor	PI3K	Alpelisib
	Kinase inhibitor	HER2 and EGFR	Lapatinib
	PARP inhibitor	BRCA1/HRD	Olaparib, Veliparib, Rucaparib
	Monoclonal Ab	HER2	Pertuzumab, Herceptin
	Kinase inhibitor	HER2 and HER3	Tucatinib
Colorectal cancer	EGFR antagonist	EGFR	Cetuximab Panitumumab
	Kinase inhibitor	BRAF V600E	Encorafenib
	VEGFR2 antagonist	VEGFR2	Ramucirumab
Endometrial cancer	Kinase inhibitor	VEGF receptors	Lenvatinib
Kidney cancer	Kinase inhibitor	VEGFR-1, −2,-3	Axitinib
	mTOR inhibitor	mTOR	Everolimus
			Sunitinib
			Sorafenib
Hepatocellular carcinoma	Kinase inhibitor	EGFR	Afatinib
	Kinase inhibitor	ALK and RET	Alectinib
Hepatocellular carcinoma	Kinase inhibitor	FLT-3, IGFR-1R, ROS1, and ALK	Brigatinib
Hepatocellular carcinoma	Kinase inhibitor	MET	Capmatinib
Hepatocellular carcinoma	Kinase inhibitor	EGFR	Dacomitinib Erlotinib, gefitinib
Hepatocellular carcinoma	Kinase inhibitor	MET	Tepotinib
Hepatocellular carcinoma	Kinase inhibitor	MEK1, MEK2	Trametinib
Melanoma	Kinase inhibitor	BRAF V600E	Vemurafenib
Non–small cell lung cancer	RAS GTPase inhibitor	KRAS	Sotorasib
Prostate cancer	PARP inhibitor	HRR/BRCA1/2	Olaparib, veliparib, rucaparib
Ovarian cancer	PARP inhibitor	HRR/BRCA 1/2	Niraparib

Adapted from Joshi [21]

2.4 The Limitations of Targeted Therapies

The limitations of targeted agents have been elucidated in certain adaptive trials, such as NCI-MATCH and basket trials, that enroll multiple cohorts of patients with refractory cancers and administer targeted therapies according to their DNA mutation testing. The results from the "National Cancer Institute–Molecular Analysis for Therapy Choice ECOG-ACRIN Trial (EAY131) Subprotocol EAY131-B" showed that the afatinib, an orally available small molecule inhibitor with a high degree of potency in the HER2 family of irreversible inhibitors that were approved for metastatic NSCLC, did not meet in ERBB2-mutated advanced solid tumors the prespecified threshold for antitumor activity. The results reported confirmed ORR in only 2.7% of patients (n = 1/37; 90% CI 0.14 to 12.2), and they confirmed PR and a 6-month PFS in 12.7% of patients (90% CI 5.6 to 25.8) with extra-mammary Paget disease of the skin (n = 1). The investigators concluded that only its activity against the rare tumor Paget disease in patients with tumors with HER2-activating mutations was particularly notable in this phase II trial. Other studies have shown that CDK4/6 inhibitors are less effective against tumors of high heterogeneity, like soft-tissue sarcomas, leading to high resistance [22].

Sadee et al. describe how counterstrategies due to parallel pathway genes and acquired resistance develop, and they describe reversion mutations and activation ESR1 mutations in treatment-naive ER+ breast cancer treated with aromatase inhibitors. In addition, tumor heterogeneity is due to selective pressure induced by the therapy that results in correcting the initial defect and restoring protein functionality derived from a reversion mutation in germline BRCA1 and BRCA 2 pathogenic variants. Tumor heterogeneity arises from mutations, epigenetic factors, and stromal cell-type diversity and immune cells, and as revealed by NGS, worse outcomes and frequent tumor resistance are associated with immune and stromal cell-type diversity. NGS also shows that secondary mutations arise from subclones in untreated tumors. Single-cell sequencing shows rapid tumor evolution with high tumor heterogeneity and neoantigen diversity that is less responsive to immune checkpoint inhibitors and that can be mitigated by combination therapies targeting both genes in subclones and driver events. This increases the possibility of producing tumor responses to therapy. This possibility has been further revealed by single-cell sequencing, which showed rapid tumor evolution and showed that high neoantigen diversity and heterogeneity confer less of a response to immune checkpoint inhibitors [23].

2.5 Precision Oncology Clinical Trials

With the advent and implementation of NGS, matched targeted therapies (Chap. 4), liquid biopsy (Chap. 3), and omics, the design of clinical trials evolved from tumor type–centered trials to "gene-directed and histology-agnostic trials," namely basket, umbrella, platform, and N-of-1 trials (Table 2.3). Precision oncology trials rely on data from genomic markers and are based on mutation status such as NTRK fusions, yielding tumor-agnostic approaches. Improved response rates for OS and PFS have been associated with biomarker-based trials. Basket trials are tumor-agnostic trials including NTRK fusions for larotrectinib and entrectinib and dMMR/MSI-H for pembrolizumab and were the first agents to receive tumor-agnostic approval from the FDA

Table 2.3 Characteristics of precision oncology clinical trials

Table 2 Challenges and opportunities by trial design				
Trial design	Features	Advantages	Disadvantages	Challenges
Basket	One molecular alteration, multiple histologies	Rare molecular alterations Test treatment in diverse tumor types in parallel	Alterations are not drivers in every tumor type Different mechanisms of resistance are based on tumor type A lack of comparative arm	Recruiting rare subsets across multiple disease types
Umbrella	One histology, multiple molecular alterations	Biomarker assessment Improved enrollment rates when biomarker prevalence is low Parallel evaluation of multiple treatment agents Flexibility of dropping failing drugs	Inadequate sample size Multiple treatments matching molecular alterations Suboptimal selection of treatment targets	Intrapatient heterogeneity of molecular findings, hampering the categorization of patients
Platform	Combines umbrella and basket features to create a broad-based trial	Allows the addition or exclusion of new investigational arms during the trial Enables evaluation of multiple hypotheses in a single protocol Shortens time Lowers costs	Complicated design Administrative and logistical complexity Long-term nature High execution costs	Complexity of statistical analysis and of the monitoring of extremely heterogeneous patient groups

(continued)

Table 2.3 (continued)

Table 2 Challenges and opportunities by trial design				
Trial design	Features	Advantages	Disadvantages	Challenges
Adaptive	During the course of the study, the trial is changed as data are collected and analyzed	Drops ineffective arms early Modifies patient randomization to more-effective treatments Improves biomarker selection Requires fewer participants Requires shorter follow-up time	Complicated design Administrative and logistical complexity Misses important secondary outcome data due to early elimination of treatment arms	Dependent on intense statistical monitoring; the constant need to adapt the design may make the interpretation of the results difficult
Telescope (seamless)	Seamless transition from phase I to II and sometimes to III	Combines learning and confirmatory stages Shortens duration of drug development and approval Reduces administrative costs Reduces effort Focuses on promising treatments to be used in later trial stages Drops failing treatments early Focuses on responding subpopulations in later trial stages	Design complexity	Designing all phases of the trial (I, II, and III) without taking into consideration preliminary data from phase I trial The long time period required to complete the study, which may be associated with change in practice and experimental drugs that gain regulatory approval in the interim, therefore making the interpretation of the results challenging

(continued)

Table 2.3 (continued)

Table 2 Challenges and opportunities by trial design				
Trial design	Features	Advantages	Disadvantages	Challenges
N-of-1	Personalized combination therapy; patient-centric trial where each patient gets a customized therapy The efficacy of the matching strategy rather than the individual therapies is evaluated	Based on unique patient characteristics and tumor profile Addresses molecular complexity and heterogeneity Customized treatment	The lack of a comparator Heterogeneity of treatments Complexity of analysis/ statistical algorithms	Difficult fit between individualized therapy and the way clinical oncology is practiced, wherein physicians often specialize in specific types of cancer Rarity of patient characteristics Need to analyze the robustness of the strategy (algorithm) for matching, rather than drug combinations, because the latter differs from patient to patient

Adapted from Fountzillas [24]

(KEYNOTE-016, -163, -012, -028, and -158). Larotrectinib also received FDA approval on the basis of the SCOUT and NAVIGATE trials. Umbrella trials evaluate multiple treatments for a single histology on the basis of biomarker subsets, with the significant advantage of being able to address interpatient heterogeneity, differentiating between outcomes that reflect underlying disease and predictive effects that reflect biomarker impact on therapies, in addition to the concurrent evaluation of multiple distinct treatments for their efficacy. Examples are the Lung-MAP, whereby patients were matched to a 200-gene molecular profiling assay in multiple trial sub-studies. The Lung-MAP trial exemplified the performance of genomically driven treatments performed in large-scale platform studies that led to the evaluation of talazoparib for HRR deficient in lung cancer and durvalumab and tremelimumab for advanced NSCLC. In 2016, the Targeted Agent and Profiling Utilization Registry (TAPUR) began and served as the one of the first clinical trials in precision medicine and was conducted across multiple institutions, evaluating both the side effects and efficacy of FDA-approved therapies. Another phase II nonrandomized trial launched by the NCI trial in the precision medicine category is NCI-MATCH, which, as alluded to earlier, targets specific molecular alterations by evaluating treatments in a heavily pretreated patient population with advanced malignances regardless of the tumor type they have. Available targeted treatments are evaluated in patient tissue samples that underwent testing for molecular alterations. According to the study, NCI-MATCH and TAPUR trial enrollment and the accrual of new arms opening for enrolling patients whose molecular abnormalities are matched with targeted therapies across large national networks are rapidly expanding, offering drugs to patients at no cost while demonstrating and promoting the feasibility of large-scale sequencing efforts and collaboration between large academic and medical centers, and community settings are encouraging all this. One of the most recent innovations from these trials is the N-of-1 cancer trial that includes multiple patients with a deep understanding of each patient's tumor biology, treated according to their targetable alterations. As the authors state, "[t]he strategy of drug assignment, rather than the drug regimens themselves, is assessed. N-of-1 oncology trials therefore differ fundamentally from other trial designs in that they are patient-centered—the drugs are fitted to the patient—rather than drug centered—the patient is fitted to the drug trial. N-of-1 oncology trials are also fundamentally different from trials denoted as 'N-of-1' in non-oncology patients, despite the similar name, because the non-oncologic trials involve multiple crossovers in the same patient." As the authors conclude, "[r]emarkable advances in molecular technology, almost unimaginable a few years ago, now permit deep interrogation of tumor biology and customization of patient therapy, which has enabled a revolution in clinical trial design" [24].

Regarding the NCI-MATCH trial, the BRAF study demonstrated an impactful and revealing result in which patients harboring the BRAF V600E mutation received the targeted therapy combination of dabrafenib, a BRAF inhibitor and trametinib, and a MEK inhibitor that inhibited the MAP kinase signaling pathway through dual treatment. Targeting the RAF oncogene is also effective in melanoma but is ineffective in colon cancers harboring the BRAF V600E mutation. Precision oncology was a result of efforts to characterize molecular alterations that led to significant benefit for specific patients. One example is the treatment of NSCLC and melanoma patients with precision medicines, which has led to dramatically decreasing death rates when administered with EGFR- and ALK-directed therapies and tumors treated with BRAF inhibitors. These effective molecular drugs have changed standards of care in oncology and revealed the limitations of traditional chemotherapy and existing standard-of-care treatments that have been observed for many years. As an example, an ORR of 10.3% was seen in NCI-MATCH, which was seen as a meaningful result. Both trial design specificities and the therapeutic strategies specific to trial design are implicated from these results, leading to the implementation of cancer tissue sequencing to target the potential vulnerabilities of a tumor as well as their treatment. The trial proves the need for the early treatment of tumors according to the patient time course with the recognition of the limitations of single-agent treatments that require combination treatments to overcome resistance in settings that are aiming for potential cures. Intrinsic resistance to cancers, such as epigenetic, metabolic, and transcriptional and DNA damage response aberrations, and extrinsic resistance evolving from the tumor microenvironment, such as CAFs and immune cells that contribute to tumor growth and progression, are plausible targets. Targeted therapies and cancer immunotherapies form treatments that when combined lead to markedly enhanced activity. Cabozantinib is an example of what is being investigated in trials when it is combined with anti-PD-1 Abs such as nivolumab and the anti-CD20 antibody rituximab in hairy-cell leukemia. These immunological treatments, which are targeted according to the patient's molecular characteristics after collecting appropriate specimens, form one basis of precision cancer studies and trials, where these combinations are directed to "genomically defined subsets," which is a critical goal with considerable potential for developing precision medicine drugs [25].

2.6 Clinical Studies

Other studies attempting to identify biomarkers for solid tumors have shown limitations in HRD biomarker detection for other types of breast cancer. One such study, the phase II PETREMAC study, involved the analysis of 360 genes derived from the pretreatment biopsies of 201 patients with primary breast cancer. Through BRCA1 methylation analysis and a targeted gene panel, homologous recombination deficiency, typically seen in triple negatives, was identified in 5% of cases not featuring triple-negative breast cancer (TNBC), possibly implying that HRD testing should be expanded to include a wider set of the breast cancer population other than triple negatives. TNBC tumors also had higher PD-L1 expression and tumor-infiltrating lymphocyte (TIL) content when compared with non-TNBC, in which these markers are significantly lower. Given other evaluated measures discussed in the study, RAD51 foci staining and determining HRD are also recommended as the most suitable and accurate predictive biomarkers to evaluate PARP1 inhibitor therapy in non-TNBC cases. Alternative criteria such as determining basal-like subtypes via PAM50 or BRCAness via Multiplex Ligation-dependent Probe Amplification (MLPA) are less useful for screening and have less accuracy [26].

Targeted gene panels revealed the mutational landscape of an anaplastic thyroid carcinoma tumor that present with aggressive disease, showing the commonly occurring mutations TP53 (59%), BRAF (41%) and TERT promoter (37%) and the RAS gene family (22%).

The BRAFV600E mutation was associated with better OS (median OS: 24 months), whereas RAS mutations were associated with lymph node involvement and worse OS (median OS: 6 months). Patients receiving BRAF-directed therapy (BRAF and MEK inhibitors) had lower PFS, of which 48%, or 29 out of 60, developed disease progression, which determined the best prognosis of mOS for 31 patients. The study authors concluded that these driver mutations were associated with survival outcomes and were characterized by clinicopathologic features that reflected tumor heterogeneity.

CDK4/6 inhibitors are established therapies for metastatic breast cancer (mBC) patients, as shown in the phase III MONARCH-2; in MONALEESA-2, MONALEESA-3, MONALEESA-7; and in PALOMA-3, in chemotherapy-naive patients, and many studies have revealed predictive biomarkers determining PFS for this malignancy. Intrinsic resistance and acquired resistance to CDK4/6 inhibitors are frequent and significant clinical problems in patients with partially understood mechanisms. One review was conducted by Bui et al., titled "Biomarkers for Cyclin-Dependent Kinase 4/6 Inhibitors in the Treatment of Hormone Receptor-Positive/Human Epidermal Growth Factor Receptor 2-Negative Advanced/Metastatic Breast Cancer: Translation to Clinical Practice."

In an analysis of phase II and III clinical studies evaluating CDK4/6 inhibitors in HR+/HER2- mBC, the performance of biomarkers with predictability for PFS was determined. Biomarker results collected from 22 articles with 12 clinical studies yielded the following:

- Cyclin E1 mRNA expression and retinoblastoma protein (RB) status were shown to be promising baseline biomarkers.
- PIK3CA ctDNA ratio, plasma thymidine kinase activity, and CTC were potential dynamic response biomarkers.
- Despite a strong mechanistic rationale, other biomarkers were considered unsuccessful.

As the authors state, efforts are ongoing to validate biomarkers and conduct exploratory studies to reveal novel mechanisms of action.

In this population, the categories of low levels versus high levels of baseline protein tyrosine kinase A (PtkA) did not distinguish between values of mPFS, regardless of cutoff. Liquid biopsy analysis of the relative change in PIK3CA mutation abundance (mutant copies/mL) was predictive of PFS in the treatment of palbociclib and fulvestrant, as shown by levels on cycle 1 day 15 of treatment relative to baseline. Specific results included worse PFS in patients with PIK3CA CDR15 above the median value of 0.034 (n = 26) compared with those below median (n = 26; HR = 3.94, 95% CI 1.61 to 9.64). However, biomarkers such as CCND1 amplification and p16 loss do not predict PFS for treatment with CDK4/6 inhibitors and have not demonstrated it, despite what would be indicated by mechanistic rationale, and tumor heterogeneity determines biomarker performance. HR+/HER2+ breast cancer patients shown distinct signaling pathways that are responsible for tumor growth that prevent the discovery of universal biomarkers for this tumor subtype. Tumor evolution also can lead to high intratumoral heterogeneity in response to therapy and lead to resistance [27].

2.6.1 MSH/MSI-H as a Biomarker for CRC

MSH/MSI high serves as a prognostic biomarker for metastatic colorectal adenocarcinomas. This study performed an epidemiological analysis of the data to show outcomes for the United States.

Key Results
- In 2018–2019, 101,259 colorectal adenocarcinomas were shown to be MMS/MMR proficient.
- 3.8% were characterized as MSI low and 14.2% MSI high/MMR deficient.
- 16.6%, 19.9%, 12.4%, and 7.3% of stage I, II, III, and IV cancers were MSI high/MMR deficient, respectively.

The evaluation of MSI high/MMR deficiency in locoregional cancers revealed an interesting result. An association was found with female sex, bimodal age distribution, wild-type KRAS, prior cancer diagnosis, and right-sided colonic origin, illustrating that these findings associate national-level epidemiology and genomic features with the prognostic implications of MSI high and MMR deficiency in colorectal adenocarcinoma. The study arrived at a further confirmation of MSI high/

MMR deficient as a predictive biomarker for immunotherapy in these solid tumors [28].

Another study found that high PD-L2 predicts the early recurrence of ER+ BC and has higher affinity for PD-1 than for PD-L1. The marker was isolated through quantitative immunofluorescence histocytometry, correlated with PFS ($n = 684$) and validated in another cohort ($n = 273$). That study found that when high PD-L2 protein expression levels are detected in cancer cells in treatment-naive ER+ breast tumors, they are validated for being an independent predictor for early recurrence in this tumor type after adjusting for associated clinicopathological variables. High PD-L2 expression was associated with poor outcomes and a shorter PFS hazard ratio (HR), 1.8 (95% CI 1.3 to 2.6; $p = 0.001$), with further evidence of an increased risk of recurrence in ER+ BC, providing a rationale for the use of ICIs in this tumor with this molecular classification and warranting future studies on the role of PD-L2 in ER+ breast cancer tumor progression [29].

One study "hypothesized that the principal categories of tumor somatic mutations might also portend survival," using the Pan-Cancer Atlas with the evaluation of the burden of major mutation categories; also, cancer type, stage, and grade had prognostic capabilities for disease-specific and overall survival. These mutation categories included indels (small insertions, or SMs), short substitutions, gene fusions, and copy number alterations that drive tumor progression. CNA fraction and SM count were shown to be predictors of survival, being key indicators of clinical utility independent of histologic grade and anatomic stage, and were shown to be distinct from the neoantigen load for immunotherapeutic treatment. The study also quantified the effects; its statistical analysis is beyond the scope of the book [30].

2.6.2 *TP53 as Prognostic Stratifier*

TP53 has been shown to be a prognostic stratifier for colorectal cancer. A study by Pan et al. determined whether TP53 could also define the prognosis for pancreatic ductal adenocarcinoma (PDAC). As the study points out, "TP53 gain-of-function (GOF; R175H, R248Q, R248W, R249S, R273H, R273L, R282W) and non-GOF (the rest of mutations) mutations on the basis of previous definition by literature review stratified the prognosis of metastatic colorectal cancer." The study investigators probed whether advanced PDAC and its prognosis in clinical studies can be stratified, and the impact on patients with KRAS, SMAD4, and CDKN2A along with co-mutations between TP53 GOF and non-GOF could be assessed. NGS can be performed with utility on these locally advanced, recurrent, and de novo metastatic pancreatic ductal adenocarcinoma (mPDAC) tumors.

Key Results

- GOF mutp53 (R175H, R248W, R248Q, R249S, R273H, R273L, and R282W) was associated with worse OS than non-GOF mutp53 (HR, 1.27; 95% CI 1.02 to 1.59).

- Non-GOF was not associated with worse OS than wtp53 (HR, 0.95; 95% CI 0.80 to 1.13).

The study authors concluded that, according to their findings, advanced PDAC could be stratified into molecular categories on the basis of GOF and non-GOF mutp53 and that tumors were associated with differential prognoses, potentially proving useful in the design of clinical trials and clinical practice and providing "new insight for further mechanistic studies" [31].

2.6.3 *Exome Sequencing as Prognostic and Predictive*

Likewise, exome sequencing was revealed to be prognostic and predictive of paired CRC synchronous with liver metastasis. Tumor sample pairs underwent WES and were derived from 20 patients diagnosed and treated at the center. The study authors also note that the COAD-READ dataset from TCGA (n = 380) were involved with in silico validation, where possible.

Key Results

- APC was shown to be the most frequently altered oncogene driver mutation in 55% of primary cancers and 60% of metastatic lesions. TP53, TRIP11, FAT4, and KRAS were identified alterations in 50/45, 30/5, 20/125, and 15/25 cancers/metastatic lesions.
- KRAS variants were shown to be in primary tumors "with a high or moderate predicted functional effect," and in both single and validation datasets, they were shown to be significantly associated with poor RFS, underlining the fact that primary tumors differ from their synchronous metastasis, influencing the effectiveness of treatments and providing future therapeutic opportunities [32].

2.6.4 *Oncogenic Drivers in Melanoma*

Several pathway alterations, such as NRAS, NF1, and BRAF, have been sufficiently established as clinically actionable genomic alterations in melanoma. Other oncogenic drivers were explored in one study that entailed a retrospective cohort of cases that provided specimens collected from an international consortium using primary samples from the InterMEL study. TP53, cell cycle, and Pi3K were frequently signaling pathways (31%, 30% and 18%), whereas (other than the three common genes) no positive significant trend in the analysis of co-occurring different pathways was exhibited.

Key Results

- Finding the opportune time for additional pathways to be targeted is limited due to excess mutual exclusivity, implying that a single-pathway mutation enhances tumor growth.

- Out of 453 cases with at least one pathway alteration, 33.1% are "singletons having exactly one pathway altered (the majority of which are RTK-RAS singletons), 28.3% have two pathways altered (most frequently RTK-RAS and cell cycle), and 18.3% harbor three concurrent pathways" [33].

2.6.5 BRCA-HRRm Testing in Advanced Ovarian Cancer

One study suggested that non–BRCA HRRm testing should not necessarily be done in advanced ovarian cancer patients. The PAOLA-1 trial established the use of olaparib plus bevacizumab in BRCA HRRm–mutated ovarian cancer patients; however, this line of treatment has not been evaluated in non–BRCA HRRm–mutated patients.

Key Results

- 152/806 patients, or 18.9%, had non-BRCA1 or non-BRCA2 mutation HRD-positive tumors. Depending on the gene panel used, the non–BRCA HRRm prevalence "ranged from 30 of 806 (3.7%) to 79 of 806 (9.8%)."
- "The majority of tumors harboring non–BRCA HRRm had a low median GIS (Genomic Instability Score) ; however, a GIS of > 42 was observed for tumors with mutations in five HRR genes (BLM, BRIP1, RAD51C, PALB2, and RAD51D)."

The study authors concluded that in PAOLA-1, only a small proportion of HRD-positive tumors were captured by non–BRCA HRRm, and gene panels that were non–BRCA HRRm were not predictive of PFS on the maintenance treatment of olaparib plus bevacizumab, regardless of gene panel testing, implying that existing gene panels "exploring non–BRCA HRRm" are not substitutes for "HRD as determined by BRCA mutation status and genomic instability in newly diagnosed advanced OC" [34].

One study identified somatic mutations among patients with early-onset and late-onset endometrial cancer (EC) through the identification of TMB values and genomic patterns. According to the study authors, early-onset EC has a significantly lower TMB when compared with late-onset EC among patients with nonhypermutated tumors, and FGFR2 and PIK3Ri mutations showed inverse associations with early-onset EC compared with late-onset disease. BRCA2 and CTNNB1 displayed a significant positive association with early-onset EC. The study authors concluded that their study "supports future clinical investigations to develop and test personalized therapeutic modalities tailored to young women diagnosed with this malignancy" [35].

2.6.6 HER2 Aberration in a Pan Tumor Analysis

A real-world study was performed to investigate the nature of HER2 aberration in metastatic cancer through IHC, which revealed a putative correlation between HER2 overexpression and amplification in a pan-tumor analysis. The most prevalent tumor types included were CRC ($n = 702$; 33.1%), gastrointestinal cancer (GC) ($n = 481$; 22.7%), and sarcoma ($n = 180$; 8.5%). "In all, 189 patients (8.9%) had HER2 aberration in their tumor specimen." Mutations in the form of single nucleotide variations (SNVs), amplifications in the form of copy number variations (CNVs), and fusions were determined through NGS.

Key Results

- Of 2119 patients, 189, or 8.9% of patients, harbored the HER2 aberration, 113 patients harbored the HE2 amplification, 82 patients harbored the HER2 mutation, and 11 had the HER2 fusion.
- NGS demonstrated a strong relationship between HER2 protein overexpression and HER2 amplification.
- NGS revealed 74 patients with HER2 amplification, and IHC showed 64 patients with HER2 overexpression. The study authors concluded that when NGS is applied to metastatic cancer, it reveals HER2 aberration in the tumor, with most patients harboring the HER2 amplification and an even smaller percentage having the HER2 fusion, and a great majority of these patients with HER2 amplification or fusion were HER2+ through IHC for "future guidance in designing HER2 inhibitor trials."
- The case study described a "39-year-old woman with metastatic CRC, who has failed to three lines of chemotherapy including irinotecan, oxaliplatin-based chemotherapy, had HER2 amplification in her tumor specimen. The NGS result of her CRC specimen showed a very high copy number (111.7) of HER2 amplification and concurrent HER2 fusion (RBBP8-HER2). The HER2 IHC showed 100% positivity in tumor cells tested. The patient was enrolled onto trastuzumab deruxtecan trial and achieved dramatic partial response to HER2 inhibitor for > 4 months. Her computed tomography result of lung/chest showed tumor volume in the lung was dramatically reduced. Taken together, it is clinically very important to identify HER2 aberrations and treat the patients with targeted therapy during the course of treatment," the study authors concluded [36].

The above study shows how mutations detected through NGS are able to complement the amplifications and overexpression of HER2 identified through an IHC test and validate its results in tumor specimens.

2.6.7 *Validated Gene Expression Testing in Melanoma*

The risk of recurrence, metastasis, and death for the cases of melanoma (1A, low, 1B/2A, intermediate, or high (class 2B)) can be established through a validated gene expression test, called the DecisionDx-Melanoma gene expression profile, or 31-GEP. This decision tool is able to determine clinical survival outcomes and prognosis at the population level. In one study involving the clinical testing of a melanoma cohort and using the 31-GEP risk category and Kaplan–Meier curves (among other statistical indicators), the investigators could analyze the OS and melanoma-specific survival differences of 31-GEP stratified patients and determine their risk of dying from melanoma.

Key Results

- "Patients with a 31-GEP class 1A result had higher 3-year MSS (genetic stability indicating a normal mismatch repair system (MSS)) and OS than patients with a class 1B/2A or class 2B result (MSS: 99.7% vs. 97.1% vs. 89.6%, $p < 0.001$; OS: 96.6% vs. 90.2% vs. 79.4%, $p < 0.001$)."
- "A class 2B result was an independent predictor of MSS (HR, 7.00; 95% CI 2.70 to 18.00) and OS (HR, 2.39; 95% CI 1.54 to 3.70). 31-GEP testing was associated with a 29% lower MSS mortality (HR, 0.71; 95% CI 0.53 to 0.94) and 17% lower overall mortality (HR, 0.83; 95% CI 0.70 to 0.99) relative to untested patients."

The study authors concluded that clinical utility of 31-GEP served as a prognostic factor for survival outcomes and leads to a "more personalized clinical management decisions for patients with [melanoma]." [37].

2.6.8 *Measuring Relative Gene Expression Levels for Prognosis*

A retrospective study identified a tool that measures relative gene expression, called digital display precision predictor (DDPP). Lazar et al. determined the association of DFS with measured relative gene expression levels in primary tumor samples and compared them with normal bronchial tissues derived from a 120 NSCLC patient cohort who underwent curative surgical resection, noting that identifying the prognostic state of NSCLC patients who underwent surgery was an urgent unmet need.

Key Results

- Associated with decreased DFS were a high coexpression of PD-L1 with CTLA-4, two immune checkpoints, and an inducible T cell costimulator (ICOS) in a normal lung (28 of 120 patients), which was considered statistically significant ($p = 0.0013$) and suggested an immune tolerance to tumor neoantigens in certain patients.
- For 29 patients with stage 1 or 2 cancer and a low DDPP score, improved DFS ($p = 0.0041$) was associated with adjuvant chemotherapy.
- For patients with a low DDPP score, the shortest DFS was shown in immunotolerant tissue.

The study authors concluded that 'Tumor Node Metastasis (TNM) stage, DDPP score, and immune competent status in normal lung tissue serve as independent prognostic factors when they identified key tumor-specific transcribed genes associating with adjuvant DFS on the basis of differential mRNA expression between tumor tissues from patients with resected NSCLC and normal tissue [38].

2.7 Diagnostics and Molecular Testing

One study revealed fascinating results on using targeted sequencing to diagnose HRD in tumor types. The original report focused on HRD in ovarian tumors through the sequencing of genome-wide single nucleotide polymorphisms (SNPs) that inferred LOH events, leading to the diagnosis of HRD. The methods, according to the study authors, were adaptable for HRD diagnosis in other tumors and readily generalizable to other targeted gene assays, and these authors concluded that their approach requires minimal sequence reads and "can be readily integrated into targeted gene capture workflows already in use for molecular oncology."

Details of the methods include the development and validation of a cost-effective strategy that is also efficient for HRD determination. HRD would be determined on the basis of a genome-side LOH score through NGS and targeted hybridization capture with 3000 common polymorphic SNPs with genome-wide distribution. Furthermore, 99 ovarian neoplasms with their normal pairs were interrogated with this method and compared to mutated genotypes to orthogonally predict HRD as derived from whole-genome mutational signatures.

Diagnosing HRD in OCs involved the empirical selection of a threshold for LOH scores that ranged from 11% to 28.6% (average, 20.47%), with the selection of greater than 11% for determining LOH-high samples. This was performed through the random selection of 10 HRD-positive samples to establish them as a training set. This led to a sensitivity of 86.9% as a strong correlation between HRDetect probability scores and LOH scores.

An independent validation set of 24 HRD-positive samples consisting of the remainder identified "20 as LOH-high ($r(51) = 0.5881$; $p < .00001$; Pearson's correlation coefficient), evidencing concordance between the two approaches." Inferred "negative specimens by HRDetect had significantly lower HRD scores (average, 10.87%) than inferred HRD-positive samples (average, 22.62%; $p = .552 \times 10–6$; two-tailed T test)." As the study authors state, if "we are to accept HRDetect results as accurate, gold standard diagnoses, an LOH score of $\geq$ 11% provided 96.7% sensitivity for correctly identifying HRD-positive tumors, whereas specificity was 50%."

These data were compared and confirmed with the targeted gene-sequencing panels that are most widely used for HRD detection. However, correlation between treatment scores and LOH scores was not achieved, because although the LOH score is clinically useful for determining HRD status, it cannot serve as a predictor for platinum therapy in the first line. The authors concluded that an "LOH score of $\geq$ 11% can identify OCs with molecular alterations implicated in producing defective HRD with a high sensitivity (aggregate sensitivity > 90%)" [39].

A prognostic model reported by Safdar et al. in *JCOPO* was identified and validated for determining TME bladder-associated genes. In one analysis, scRNA-sequencing datasets were shown to identify potential biomarkers. The differentially expressed genes identified through gene expression profiles in normal versus bladder cancer cells could be "subsequently assessed for prognostic significance by patient follow-up data."

2.7.1 Key Results

- "A hazard ratio of 2.97 (95% CI 2.28 to 3.9, $p < 0.001$) [was found]. In the validation cohort, the [area under the curve (AUC)] at 1, 2, and 3 years is 0.74, 0.74, and 0.72, respectively."

Their analysis showed also immune cell infiltration associated with high-risk tumors, including B cells, both CD4+ and CD*+ T cells, M2 macrophages, and Th2 and Treg cells, that characterize immune-rich areas with the TME.

According to the study authors, precision oncology can enhance the treatment of bladder cancer with their findings that the immune landscape in high-risk patient may foster a TME conducive to tumor progression, with the development of a prognostic model capable of reliably predicting patient outcomes. Precision medicine, allowing for a deeper understanding of genes associated with BLCA (bladder cancer) , validates the efficacy of the model through immune cell infiltration assessment and gene set enrichment analysis [40].

2.8 Pharmacogenomics

Pharmacogenomics has had an impact on the determining treatment outcomes of certain cancers. As early as 2016, a report published in the ASCO Educational Book by Calvo et al. discussed pharmacogenomics and the role of interindividual variation in the dosing of TKIs for CRC, OC, prostate cancer, and NSCLC. When a malignancy sample undergoes molecular, IHC, and FISH analysis in narrowing specific treatment options through its prognostic and predictive value and determines expected outcomes, the selection of a targeted agent begins. For CRC, the sequencing of the KRAS mutations (downstream of EGFR) distinguishes whether panitumumab or cetiximab is to be administered. Unlike the case for trastuzmab, EGFR overexpression did not serve as the predictive biomarker for the EGFR inhibitor but rather for mutations in KRAS in CRC. Wild-type KRAS patients receiving panitumuab had an mPFS of 12.3 weeks compared to 7.3 weeks when they had the best supportive care. KRAS-mutated patients receive greater benefit from cetuximab. PARP inhibitors such as olaparib take advantage of synthetic lethality in BRCA1- and BRCA2-deficient tumors, and because PARP compensates for this loss of homologous repair, the PARP inhibition would result in apoptosis and would be approved for use in ovarian cancer in 2014 and mCRPC in prostate cancer. EGFR TKIs also targeted NSCLC and "activating mutations in exons 18 to 21 predict a response" to afatinib, erlotinib, and gefitinib with novel ones such as the third-generation TKI osimertinib, which has affinity for the T790M mutation. ALK C1156Y confers resistance to crizotinib; however, treatment options remain with aceritinib and other non-ALK-directed therapy or with another ALK inhibitor, namely lorlatinib. As the authors conclude, basket trials for tumor-agnostic, biomarker-driven trials should be accompanied by molecular analysis; liquid biopsy will also play relevant roles in standard-of-care clinical management; and "[p]harmacogenomic analysis of tumor tissue has evolved from focused interrogation of select genes to guide targeted therapies to multigene panels being used in conjunction with molecular tumor boards to help direct optimal therapy for patients" [41].

One study analyzing genetic subtypes between both pediatric and adult B cell acute lymphoblastic leukemia and leukemia genomics showed differential drug sensitivity between molecular subtypes, with acute lymphocytic leukemia (ALL) "drug sensitivity profiling [providing] new insights into pharmacological heterogeneity." Furthermore, 21 therapeutic agents in 767 children and 309 adults were evaluated, and drug sensitivity was quantified as LC(50). Of the 21 drugs, seven showed different activity for asparaginase, prednisone, mercaptopurine, daunorubicin, and inotuzumab, to which children were more sensitive, and dasatinib and nelarabine, to which adults were more sensitive. The investigators also found "age–drug sensitivity, using leukemia gene expression profiling." Adult cases "displayed mainly BCR::ABL1 (90%) like transcriptomic signature and IGH::CRLF2 (78%) rearrangements." DUX4 ALL adults displayed high CEBPA expression. In pediatric populations, "adult-like leukemia exhibited marked resistance to mercaptopurine and prednisolone." These results indicate how although both adult and pediatric ALL is curable, the adult patients have significantly worse prognoses, with this prognostic effect seen in age [42].

Another pharmacogenomic study reported on outcomes of childhood ALL. Genomic determinants of relapse in children with standard risk or standard risk (SR) ALL were identified with the genomic and transcriptomic sequencing of diagnostic and remission samples of children with SR ALL or high-risk ALL ($n = 1381$). A case-control study was also done on 439 patients who relapsed and 1057 patients who remained in complete remission. The PAX5-altered ALL genomic subtype (odds ratio (OR) 3.31 (95% CI 2.17 to 5.03)) was associated with relapse with a 50% prevalence.

2.8.1 Key Results

- "Gain of chromosome 10 with disomy of chromosome 7 was associated with favorable outcome (OR, 0.27 (95% CI 0.17 to 0.42)). Disomy of chromosomes 10 and 17 with gain of chromosome 6 was associated with relapse (OR, 7.16 (95% CI 2.36 to 21.51)).
- "Other genomic determinants include INO80 in ETV6::RUNX1 ALL, IKZF1, and CREBBP in hyperdiploid ALL and FHIT in BCR::ABL1-like ALL."

In short, new genomic predictors of relapse in SR ALL pediatric patients result in this case-control study design. One result reported that 50% of children with PAX5alt rearrangements and IKZF1 plus relapsed, with the latter having higher rates of relapse. One implication is the minimization of toxicity through deintensification strategies given that the study identified current risk predictors. MRD was not found to be associated with any clinical features; however, genomic alterations occurring at translocation breakpoints had an association with clinical outcomes, where the highest risks of relapse were observed in TCF3/4::HLF translocations, compared with ETV6::RUNX1 ALL. The study authors concluded that "genetic subtype, patterns of aneuploidy, and secondary genomic alterations determine the risk of relapse in childhood ALL, and comprehensive genomic analysis is required for optimal risk stratification" [43].

A recent study showed that APOBEC mutational status (Table 2.4) accounted for tumor heterogeneity in several cancers, including breast, by analyzing 29,833 BC samples for TMB through comprehensive genomic profiling. "APOBEC or apolipoprotein B mRNA-editing enzyme catalytic polypeptides [belong] to a family of cytidine deaminases which protect against viral infection by degrading viral genomes via cytosine deamination. Dysregulation of APOBEC has been shown to serve as a major driver of tumor mutations in human cancer leading to intratumoral heterogeneity, clonal evolution, and tumor adaptation in response to therapy in multiple tumor types."

A study on the prognostic signature of miRNA biomarkers analyzed from the TCGA database and validated in a HNSCC cohort, as conducted by Worakitchanon et al., developed a miRNA signature (hsa-miR-10b, hsa-miR-148b, hsa-miR-99a, hsa-miR-127, hsa-miR-370, and hsa-miR-500a) from TCGA database, which

Table 2.4 The clinical benefit of immune checkpoint inhibition in a series of APOBEC+ patients [44]

APOBEC status	Cohort	Clinical end point	Key data	ICI efficacy
+		Shorter TTD on ET + CDK4/6i compared to APOBEC -	7.8 (95% CI 4.3 to 14.6) versus 12.4 months (95% CI 11.2 to 14.1; HR, 1.6; 95% CI 1.03 to 2.39; $p = 0.0036$)	
HR+/ HER2- APOBEC+	4/9 CGDB patients	TMB high TTD 0.3–11.3 months		Clinical benefit
	4/6 Duke/ Mayo cohort	(TTD 0.9–40.5 months) with a TTD of ≥ 3 months		
16.7% lobular, 10% metastatic HR+/HER2 tumors APOBEC+		Shorter time to treatment discontinuation, shorter OS on first-line ER and CDK4/6i relative to APOBEC- patients		

places low-risk and high-risk categories in locally advanced head and neck squamous cell carcinoma (HNSCC) patients.

The overexpression of miR-99a in HNSCC was found to inhibit the PI3K/AKT signaling pathway from the overexpression of miR-99a in HNSCC, resulting in a reduction in cellular proliferation, apoptotic induction, and migration through the post-transcriptional suppression of IGF1R and mTOR genes. Moreover, miR-99a expression was downregulated in HNSCC when compared to normal tumor tissue, as well as miR-127 in HPV-positive pharyngeal cancer. Additionally, two miRNAs in the prognostic miRNA signature, namely miR-148b and miR-500a, were upregulated. Validating this candidate miRNA signature took place through an independent Ramathibodi (RA) cohort by using droplet digital polymerase chain reaction (ddPCR), finding that "hsa-miR-10b, hsa-miR-148b, hsa-miR-99a, hsa-miR-127, hsa-miR-370, and hsa-miR-500a expression were independently associated with overall survival (OS)." The miRNA signature risk score led to the characterization of the TCGA cohort into low- and high-risk groups according to "median OS, in which the median OS of patients in the high-risk group was significantly shorter than that in the low-risk group (36 vs. 68 months; HR, 1.7 [95% CI 1.3 to 2.3]." This further validation of this miRNA signature panel was in the RA cohort ($n = 87$) and served as an "independent prognostic factor" for OS in this cohort (HR, 1.958; 95% CI 1.006 to 3.812; $p = 0.048$) in multivariate analysis. The sensitivity and specificity values were 70.08% and 57.86%, respectively.

According to the authors, in HNSCC, the dysregulation of miRNAs has been identified, and their upregulation in tumor tissues, after analysis, demonstrates their potential targets for six enriched miRNAs in signaling pathways associated with the progression of HNSCC [45].

2.9 Transition from One Size Fits All to a Personalized Treatment: The Case Study of Triple-Negative Breast Cancer

Triple-negative breast cancer (TNBC) has the HR-/PR-/HER2- molecular subtype and is recalcitrant to most therapies. The KEYNOTE-522 established a standard of care in stage II/III TNBC patients that consists of neoadjuvant pembrolizumab with neoadjuvant anthracycline/taxanes/carboplatin followed by adjuvant pembrolizumab. The pathologic complete response (pCR) rate is 7% (absolute improvement), and the EFS showed a 9% improvement compared with chemotherapy alone. Data from the phase III KEYNOTE-522 trial demonstrated a pCR rate of 63% vs. 56% for chemotherapy alone. A few questions surrounded this personalized approach, namely treatment duration optimization and a lack of predictive biomarkers, while questions on the efficacy of pembrolizumab were left unanswered. In the pembrolizumab cohort, 18.7% had an event, suggesting a lack of clinical benefit from the immunotherapy regimen while still being exposed to potential toxicities. As Kok et al. write in the *Journal of Clinical Oncology*, the "ideal predictive marker would define a marker -positive population whose outcomes improved with pembrolizumab while there is now improvement in the marker-negative subset." Biomarkers such as TMB and tumor-infiltrating lymphocytes (TILs) were not prospectively validated for this tumor type. The value of the adjuvant therapy is still not completely evident either given its consequent potential adverse events and financial toxicity [46].

At the 2024 European Breast Cancer Conference, ImPRINTTN, a single-sample classifier, was revealed, and it could predict a response to immunotherapy that was developed by researchers who had enrolled patients in the ISPY2.2 trial. Validated and tested for TNBC patients in the I-SPY2 trials that evaluated 23 therapies in 2118 patients, the tool showed an association between polymerase chain reaction (PCR) and immunotherapy arms with twofold–threefold increased efficacy and a 5-year 95% recurrence-free rate in HR-/PR-/HER2-negative tumors that characterize the TNBC molecular subtype. ImPRINTTN-positive patients show response to immunotherapies, whereas a negative test predicts a less favorable response in comparison to PD-L1 and TILs [47].

2.10 Conclusion

Precision oncology is increasingly making progress through the discovery and clinical validation of genetic alterations and advances in the field of cancer genomics. NGS, WES, and WGS are complementing diagnostic techniques, including IHC. Pharmacogenomic tests that led to novel understandings of gene–drug interactions are playing ongoing roles in oncology as well, and new clinical trial designs in basket and umbrella adaptive strategies are beginning to play important roles in increasing options for treating cancer patients with personalized cancer medicines.

References

1. Riedl JM, Moik F, Esterl T, Kostmann SM, Gerger A, et al. Molecular diagnostics tailoring personalized cancer therapy—an oncologist's view. Virchows Arch. 2024;484:169–79.
2. Moore DC, Guingundo AS. Revolutionizing cancer treatment: harnessing the power of biomarkers to improve patient outcomes. J Adv Pract Oncol. 2023;4:4–8.
3. Gadade DD, Jha H, Kumar C, Khan F. Unlocking the power of precision medicine: exploring the role of biomarkers in cancer management. Future J Pharm Sci. 2024;10:5.
4. Yildirim A, Akalin H, Dundar M. Oncogenic genomic changes in cancer. In: Tuli HS, Aycan MBY, editors. Oncology: genomics, precision medicine and therapeutic targets. Singapore: Springer Nature; 2023. p. 25–38.
5. Kwan AK, Piazza GA, Keetori AB, Leite CA. The path to the clinic: a comprehensive review on KRAS(G12C) inhibitors. J Exp Clin Cancer Res. 2022;41:27.
6. Gibbs SN, Peneva D, Carter GC, Palomares MR, Thakkar S, et al. Comprehensive review on the clinical impact of next-generation sequencing tests for the Management of Advanced Cancer. JCO Precis Oncol. 2023;7

7. Feng X, Li H, Fourquet J, Brahmi M, Dufresne A, Meurgey A, et al. Refining prognosis in localized gastrointestinal stromal tumor: clinical significance of phosphatase and Tensin homolog low expression and gene loss. JCO Precis Oncol. 2022;6
8. Boye K, Gorumova L, Gunawan B, Hompland I, Sander B, et al. Genomic complexity as a biomarker to De-escalate adjuvant Imatinib treatment in high-risk gastrointestinal stromal tumor. JCO Precis Oncol. 2023;
9. Almassi N, Whiting K, Toubaji A, Lenis AT, Jordan E, et al. Clinical and genomic characterization of bladder carcinomas with glandular phenotype. JCO Precis Oncol. 2022;6
10. Fonseca NM, Van der Eaken K, Herberts C, Verbeke S, Ng SWS, et al. Genomic features of lung-recurrent hormone-sensitive prostate cancer. JCO Precis Oncol. 2022;6
11. Holla VR, Kahle MP, Kim S-H, Ronaghy A, Yang RK, et al. Genomic alterations in DNA mismatch repair genes across different cancer types. JCO Precis Oncol. 2024;8
12. Kojima T, Kawai K, Miyazaki J, Nishiyama H. Biomarkers for precision medicine in bladder cancer. Int J Clin Oncol. 2017;22:207–13.
13. Jang Y, Choi T, Kim J, Park J, Jihae S, et al. An integrated clinical and genomic information system for cancer precision medicine. BMC Med Genet. 2018;
14. Ohnmacht AJ, Stahler A, Stintzing S, Modest DP, Holch JW, et al. The oncology biomarker discovery framework reveals cetuximab and bevacizumab response patterns in metastatic colorectal cancer. Nat Commun. 2023;14:5391.
15. Prajumwongs P, Titapun A, Thanasukarn V, Jareanrat A, Khuntikeo N, et al. Identification of serum metabolite biomarkers and metabolic reprogramming mechanisms to predict recurrence in cholangiocarcinoma. Sci Rep. 2025;15:12782.
16. Cui S, Zheng H, Xu Y, Wu Q, Liu W, et al. Plasma proteomic biomarkers predict therapeutic responses in advanced biliary tract cancer patients receiving Camrelizumab plus the GEMOX treatment. NPJ Precis Oncol. 2025;9:102.
17. D'Costa NM, Cina D, Shrestha R, Bell RH, Lin Y-Y, et al. Identification of gene signature for treatment response to guide precision oncology in clear-cell renal cell carcinoma. Sci Rep. 2020;10:2026.
18. Wang Y-W, Allen I, Funingana G, Tischowtitz M, Joko-Fru YW. Predictive biomarkers for the efficacy of PARP inhibitors in ovarian cancer: an updated systematic review. BJC reports. 2025;
19. Van der Heijden MS, Powles T, Petrylak D, Wit R, Necchi A, et al. Predictive biomarkers for survival benefit with ramucirumab in urothelial cancer in the RANGE trial. Nat Commun. 2022;13:1878.
20. Nicolantonio FD, Bardelli A. Precision oncology for KRAS(G12C)-mutant colorectal cancer. Nat Rev Clin Oncol. 2023:355–6.
21. Joshi H. Precision medicine: translation of individualistic treatment in oncology. In: Tuli HS, Aycan MBY, editors. Oncology: genomics, precision medicine and therapeutic targets. Singapore: Springer Nature; 2023. p. 77–149.
22. Hsu JY, Seligson ND, Hays JL, Miles WO, Chen JL. Clinical utility of CDK4/6 inhibitors in sarcoma: successes and future challenges. JCO Precis Oncol. 2022;6
23. Sadee W, Wang D, Hartmann K, Toland AE. Pharmacogenomics: driving personalized medicine. Pharmacol Rev. 2023;75:789–814.
24. Fountzilas E, Tsimberidou AM, Vo HH, Kurzrock R. Clinical trial design in the era of precision medicine. Genome Med. 2022;14:101.
25. O'Dwyer PJ, Gray RJ, Flaherty KT, Chen AP, Li S, et al. The NCI-MATCH trial: lessons for precision oncology. Nat Med. 2023;29:1349–57.
26. Yndestad S, Engebrethsen C, Herencia-Ropero A, Nikolaienko O, Vintermyr OK, et al. Homologous recombination deficiency across subtypes of primary breast cancer. JCO Precis Oncol. 2023;7
27. Bui TBV, Burgering BMT, Goga A, Rugo HS, van't Veer LJ. Biomarkers for cyclin-dependent kinase 4/6 inhibitors in the treatment of hormone receptor-positice/human epidermal growth factor receptor 2-negative advanced/metastatic breast cancer: translation to clinical practice. JCO Precis Oncol. 2022;6

28. Gutierrez C, Ogino S, Meyerhardt JA, Iorgulescu JB. The prevalence and prognosis of microsatellite instability-high/mismatch repair-deficient colorectal adenocarcinomas in the United States. JCO Precis Oncol. 2023;7
29. Chervoneva I, Peck AR, Sun Y, Yi M, Udhane SS, et al. High PD-L2 predicts early recurrence of ER-positive breast cancer. JCO Precis Oncol. 2023;7
30. Smith JR, Park FE, Dupont WD. Mutation burden independently predicts survival in the Pan-cancer atlas. JCO Precis Oncol. 2023;7
31. Pan MP, Jiang C, Zhang Z, Achacoso N, Alexeeff S, et al. TP53 gain-of-function and non–gain-of-function mutations are associated with differential prognosis in advanced pancreatic ductal adenocarcinoma. JCO Precis Oncol. 2023;7
32. Hlavac V, Cervenkova L, Susova S, Holy P, Liska V, et al. Exome sequencing of paired colorectal carcinomas and synchronous liver metastases for prognosis and therapy prediction. JCO Precis Oncol. 2023;7
33. Kostrzewa CE, Luo L, Arora A, Seshan VE, Ernstoff MS, et al. Pathway alterations in stage II/III primary melanoma. JCO Precis Oncol. 2023;7
34. Pujade-Lauraine E, Brown J, Barnicle A, Wessen J, Lao-Sirieix P, et al. Homologous recombination repair gene mutations to predict Olaparib plus bevacizumab efficacy in the first-line ovarian cancer PAOLA-1/ENGOT-ov25 trial. JCO Precis Oncol. 2023;7
35. Choi J, Holowatyj AN, Du M, Chen Z, Wen W, et al. Distinct genomic landscapes in early-onset and late-onset endometrial cancer. JCO Precis Oncol. 2022;6
36. Jung J, Kim ST, Ko J, Hong JY, Park JO, et al. Clinical implication of HER2 aberration in patients with metastatic cancer using next-generation sequencing: a pan-tumor analysis. JCO Precis Oncol. 2023;7
37. Bailey CN, Martin BJ, Petkov VI, Schussler NC, Stevens JL, et al. 31-gene expression profile testing in cutaneous melanoma and survival outcomes in a population-based analysis: a SEER collaboration. JCO Precis Oncol. 2023;7
38. Lazar V, Girard N, Raymond E, Martini J-F, Galbraith S, et al. Transcriptomics in tumor and Normal lung tissues identify patients with early-stage non-small-cell lung cancer with high risk of postsurgery recurrence who may benefit from adjuvant therapies. JCO Precis Oncol. 2022;6
39. Krumm N, Khasnavis NS, Radke M, Banda K, Davies HR, et al. Diagnosis of ovarian carcinoma homologous recombination DNA repair deficiency from targeted gene capture oncology assays. JCO Precis Oncol. 2023;7
40. Safder I, Valentine H, Uzzo N, Sfakianos J, Uzzo R, et al. Identification and validation of prognostic model for tumor microenvironment-associated genes in bladder cancer based on single-cell RNA sequencing datasets. JCO Precis Oncol. 2024;8
41. Calvo E, Walko C, Dees C, Valenzuela B. Pharmacogenomics, Pharmacokinetics and pharmacodynamics in the era of targeted therapies. Am Soc Clin Oncol Educ Book. 2016;35:e175–84. ASCO Educational Book.
42. Yoshimura S, Li Z, Gocho Y, Yang W, Crews K, et al. Impact of age on pharmacogenomics and treatment outcomes of B-cell acute lymphoblastic leukemia. J Clin Oncol. 2024;42(29)
43. Chang T-C, Chen W, Ou C, Cheng Z, Hedges D, et al. Genomic determinants of outcome in acute lymphoblastic leukemia. J Clin Oncol. 2024;42(29)
44. Sammons S, Raskina K, Danziger N, Alder L, Schrock A, et al. APOBEC mutational signatures in hormone receptor–positive human epidermal growth factor receptor 2–negative breast cancers are associated with poor outcomes on CDK4/6 inhibitors and endocrine therapy. JCO Precis Oncol. 2022;6
45. Worakitchanon W, Panvongsa W, Siripoon T, Kitdumrongthum S, Wongpan A, et al. Six-MicroRNA prognostic signature in patients with locally advanced head and neck squamous cell carcinoma. JCO Precis Oncol. 2023;7
46. Kok M, Gielen R-J, Lennerz JK, Sharma P, Loibl S, et al. Academic uphill Battle to personalize treatment for patients with stage II/III triple-negative breast cancer. J Clin Oncol. 2024;42(30)
47. Helwick C. New genetic test may predict response to immunotherapy in triple-negative breast cancer. The ASCO Post. 7.25.2024. https://ascopost.com/issues/july-25-2024/new-genetic-test-may-predict-response-to-immunotherapy-in-triple-negative-breast-cancer. Accessed 28 Apr 2025.

Chapter 3
Liquid Biopsy: A New Clinical Tool for Cancer Prognosis and Biomarker Detection

Liquid biopsy (LB), wherein molecular detection could be facilitated with a blood draw, became a crucial component of personalized cancer care. LB could be in the form of exosomes, circulating tumor DNA, or other types of circulating biomarkers, such as mRNA, and is called a multimodal diagnostic technique, a groundbreaking method yielding quantifiable results. Due its high specificity, liquid biopsy can acquire reliable data in an easy, noninvasive fashion through a simple blood draw. Although not implemented in clinical practice and not a standard procedure, its applications are quickly being implemented in the monitoring of surgical outcomes, the quantification of minimal residual disease (MRD), diagnosis through genomic profiling, and evaluating reaction and feedback to systemically administered treatments [1] (Fig. 3.1).

The main categories of liquid biopsy are circulating tumor cells (CTCs), circulating tumor DNA (ctDNA), and exosomal vesicles (EVs), all encompassed by cell-free DNA (cfDNA). Lone et al. performed an analysis of LB and its clinical applications in their review on status and future challenges. The review reported that the EGFR gene was shown to be a "secondary point mutation" in the detection of T790M that confers resistance to gefitinib and erlotinib in patients with lung adenocarcinoma. When CTCs are isolated from patients and undergo genetic and molecular profiling, more-effective and newer therapeutic responses can result because the evolving changes in tumor genotype can be detected in real time and are not detectable through conventional tumor biopsy. Also having applications in the screening of mutations, LB has in effect added extraordinary value to clinical oncology in the overall monitoring and detection of alterations and the personalized prognosis of clinical efficacy and has boosted the validity of clinical results.

Peripheral blood is the main source for obtaining liquid biopsy samples, and different methods and techniques are available for isolating CTC, ctDNA, and exosomes from blood. Other liquid biopsy analytes, such as platelets and sampling sources, including urine, cerebrospinal fluid, saliva, and sputum, are less well characterized but are also potential sources of obtaining and isolating CTCs, ctDNA,

P. Hays, *Personalized Medicine in Oncology*,
https://doi.org/10.1007/978-3-032-14437-9_3

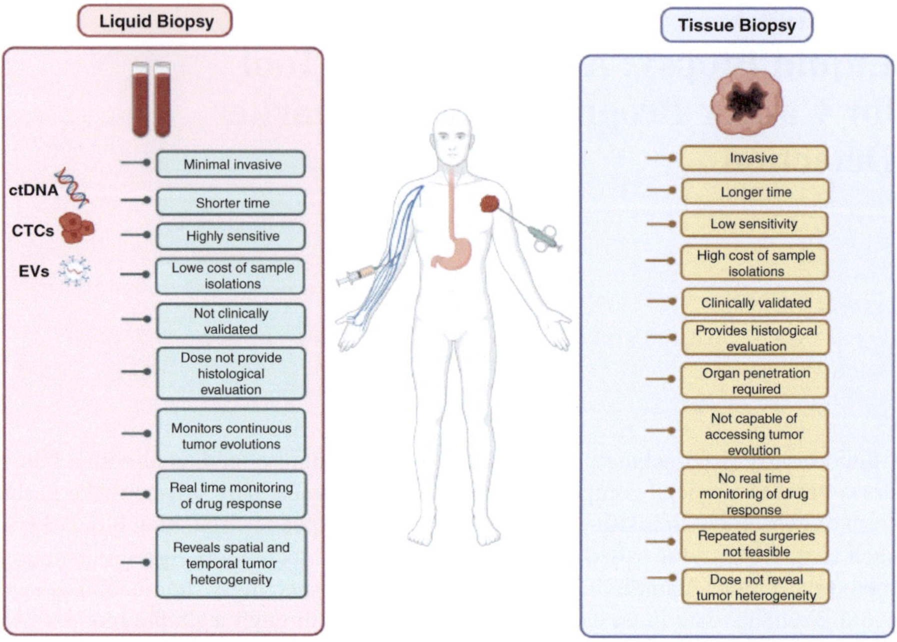

Fig. 3.1 Comparing CTCs, ctDNA, and tumor EVs that were isolated, undergoing surveillance, and derived from liquid biopsy with traditional tissue biopsy. (Adapted from Lone [2]. Permission to reuse by Creative Commons CC BY 4.0)

and exosomes. Liquid biopsy, especially its noninvasive nature, becomes more relevant because tissue biopsy depends on the accessibility of the tumor and the condition of the patient and may be more difficult in locally advanced and metastatic cases. For example, in non–small cell lung cancer (NSCLC), 31% of cases may not have accessible tissue, and most cases of pancreatic cancer are locally advanced and metastatic and are diagnosed at asymptomatic and late stages. Problems also arise as a result of tumor heterogeneity and the sampling of biopsied tissue that involves limitations in technical ability, and the ability to sample genetically distinct, newly evolving tumors that require the standard protocol for the periodic monitoring of progression and recurrence becomes paramount. Tissue biopsy may also incur expense and patient discomfort, whereby patients avoid a repeat biopsy. Liquid biopsy emerged when challenges such as obtaining adequate tumor tissue arose, and a minimally invasive and sensitive technology to capture the tumor and its genome was required. The nature of circulating cancer cells as they detach from a solid tumor circulating in peripheral blood led to the possibility of the "capture and molecular analysis of diverse tumor-derived materials," the clearance debris resulting from necrosis and apoptosis that results in DNA accumulation that is released into the blood as a result, which is an effective process in cells that come from the tumor. An early report by Abraham et al. describes how investigators aimed to develop liquid biopsy to predict drug efficacy and monitor tumor progression.

Liquid biopsy operates on the principle that as cancer stage advances, the probability of finding DNA in blood increases because the shedding of tumor cells and fragments of cancer-causing DNA into the circulation gives an adequate window into the existing tumor mutations at the time of sampling [3].

3.1 Circulating Tumor Cells (CTCs)

CTCs are intact viable tumor cells and became of interest when CTC counts with high values in peripheral blood came from metastatic breast cancer (mBC) patients whose prognosis was poor. Occurring at a frequency of 1 in 100 million cells and extremely rare in healthy subjects, CTCs are released as clusters or single cells into blood circulating during metastasis, and thus, the spreading cancer cells, which present as single cells or clusters, are released into the bloodstream during the metastatic spread of the cancer. Next-generation sequencing (NGS) revealed CTCs to carry druggable and driver mutations such as APC, KRAS, TP53, and ERBB [3].

3.2 Cell-Free DNA (cfDNA)

In plasma circulation, cfDNA appears as small DNA fragments, and its molecular profile has been shown to be similar to that of tumor tissue DNA. NGS became the advancement central to the identification of cfDNA. In NSCLC and pancreatic cancer, the DNA sequencing and RNA sequencing of liquid biopsy samples were implemented in a clinical trial to investigate correlations of mutations in cfDNA and disease progression. Patients with metastatic disease with circulating DNA were at significantly high levels when compared to patients without metastatic disease. Originating from apoptotic cells and considered relatively stable, they are usually 170–500 bp and outnumber CTCs by 50 to 1 with a higher abundance of mutations [3].

3.3 Obtaining Molecular Information from Liquid Biopsy Samples (Figs 3.2 and 3.3)

Due to the small size of CTCs and cfDNA and their relatively low abundance in the blood, they must be enriched and purified to augment specificity and sensitivity from other components of blood. As an example, CTC can be positively and negatively enriched on the basis of cell surface markers such as epithelial cell adhesion molecule (EpCAM). Analysis through real-time polymerase chain reaction (RT-PCR) and droplet digital polymerase chain reaction (ddPCR), and microfluidic

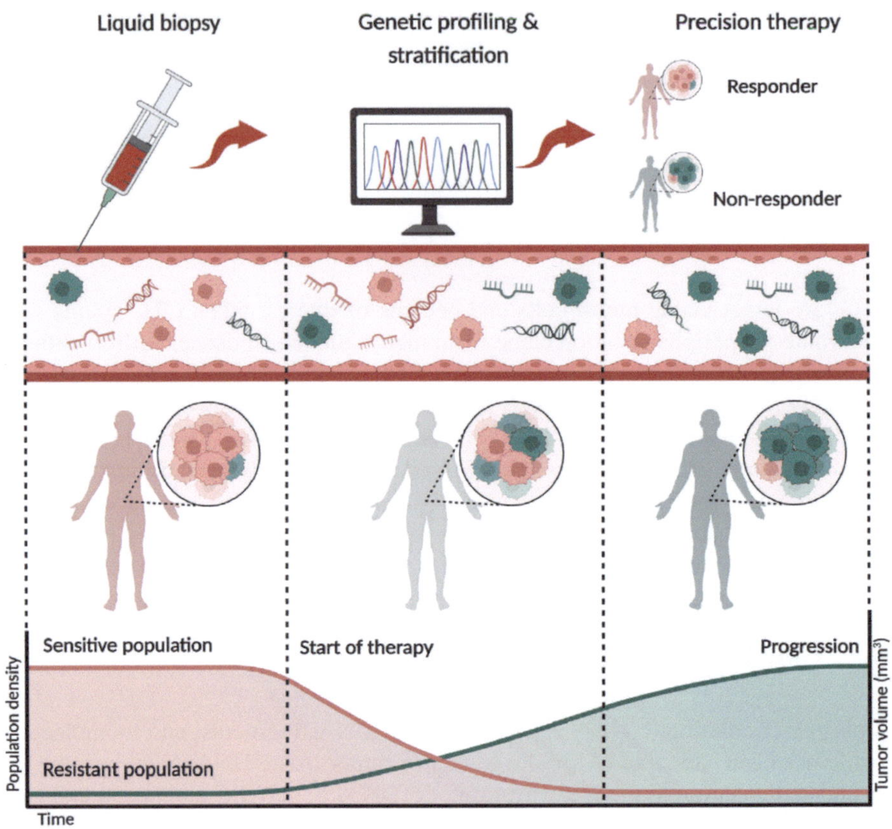

Fig. 3.2 Liquid biopsies capturing tumor heterogeneity before tumor clinical progression. (Adapted from Gruen [4]. Permission to reuse by Creative Commons CC BY 4.0)

platforms leads to the detection of these rare ctDNA sequences without requiring reference standards [3] (Fig. 3.4).

Many studies have outlined methods that target druggable mutations and alterations in cfDNA and that have been validated though concordance with tissue biopsy samples. Detecting EGFR mutations in lung cancer becomes feasible when testing purified cfDNA. Exon19del and L858R missense mutations on EGFR were shown to be strong predictors of efficacy in mAB cetuximab; TKIs gefitinib, afatinib, and erlotinib; or TKI-resistant mutations in T790M, and they required the use of third-generation TKIs. Purified cfDNA detected 29 somatic mutations in EGFR by using real-time PCR, with a mutation rate of 60.5% in plasma. Furthermore, patients with cfDNA+ status for EGFR mutations became cfDNA- patients. Serum EGFR L858R, a mutation that is associated with improved outcomes with afatinib, was correlated with overall survival (OS), progression-free survival (PFS), and the objective response rate (ORR) in erlotinib therapy in NSCLC in the EURTAC trial. Using quantitative ddPCR, EGFR mutations were detected in the cfDNA of NSCLC patients, and

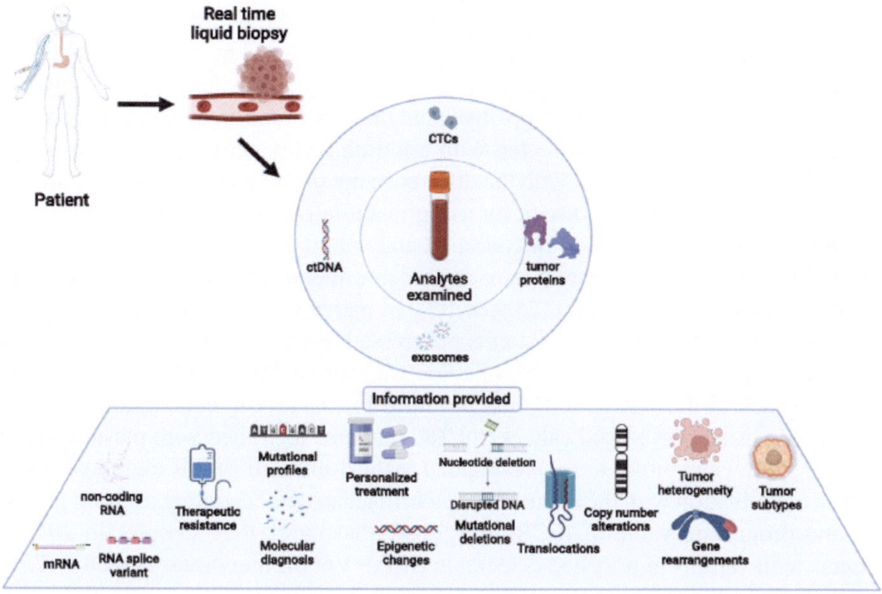

Fig. 3.3 LB analytes involved in the diagnosis, monitoring, and treatment of tumors. (Adapted from Lone [2]. Permission to reuse by Creative Commons CC BY 4.0)

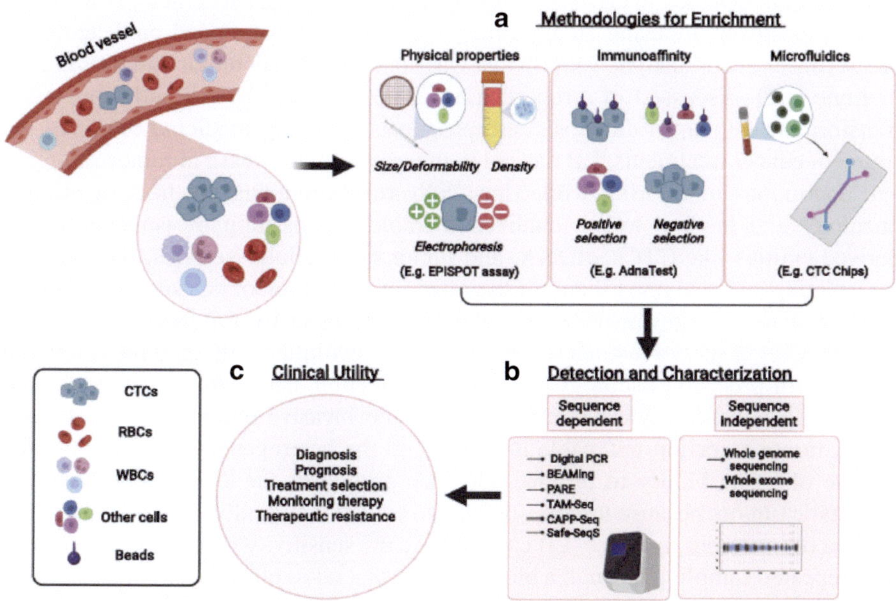

Fig. 3.4 The clinical utility in detecting and isolating CTCs derived in this process. (Adapted from Lone [2]. Permission to reuse by Creative Commons CC BY 4.0)

fluctuations in EGFR mutations in cfDNA in plasma collected serially over 2 months correlated with the size of the tumor changes, as determined by imaging. Using polymerase chain reaction (PCR), EGFR mutations were detected in study cohorts taking erlotinib versus placebo, which showed that at least one activating EFGR mutation (Del9, L858R, L861Q) as cfDNA positive, and these erlotinib-treated patients harboring an EGFR mutation when treated with erlotinib had better outcomes versus placebo (13.1 versus 6.0 months), with the difference not observed with cfDNA- patients. Comparable results were also seen by using quantitative polymerase chain reaction (qPCR) with a KRAS mutation in codon 12 and one in codon13 in newly diagnosed NSCLC treated with a chemotherapy as the sole therapy or when combined with bevacizumab. Prior to treatment, 7/69 or 10% of patients were shown to have plasma KRAS mutations; however, two patients progressed that harbored no mutations at the start of treatment. Furthermore, 60% of colorectal cancer (CRC) patients who showed the emergence of the KRAS mutation developed resistance to cetuximab or panitumumab. Metastatic colorectal cancer (mCRC) patients identified with plasma KRAS status (in contrast to tumor tissue) responded to third-line anti-EGFR treatment cetuximab in combination with the chemotherapy irinotecan demonstrating a strong predictive and prognostic value of mCRC response. Plasma cfDNA samples in 29% of patients with various tumors had detectable BRAF V600E mutations, and 88%, 73%, and 98% rates of success were seen in terms of tissue concordance, sensitivity, and specificity, respectively. Percentage rates of BRAFV600E that were higher were aligned with shorter times to treatment failure and shorter OS (10.7 months versus 4.4 months) when receiving BRAF/MEK inhibitors. Alterations in ER1 and ERBB2 of mBC were detected in cfDNA with rates of sensitivity and specificity at 86% and 82%, respectively, by using an algorithm, which when incorporated predicted early breast cancer at this analytic validity that was not detectable in tumor tissue (Fig. 3.5).

Lone et al. discussed in a report in *Molecular Cancer* how liquid biopsy is a transformative force in diagnosis and prognosis, bringing medicine closer to the future of cancer treatments. LB has led to the capabilities of ease in tumor sampling and continuous monitoring while drastically revolutionizing the field of clinical oncology and leading to personalized therapies. Consisting of isolated tumor-derived entities like CTCs, ctDNA, and tumor extracellular vesicles, the methods for isolating and analyzing them for their genomic and proteomic uses have evolved over the years, and they provide data on tumor heterogeneity, progression, and staging; the level of mutations in a tumor; and clonal evolution, and they provide more leverage for precision oncology's role when detecting, determining prognosis, and monitoring outcomes when treating cancer. The invasive nature of tissue biopsy makes tumor resection untenable at times, and the heterogeneity of tumors limits the use of tissue biopsy to provide adequate prognoses for locally advanced and metastatic tumors because tumors spread and evolve temporally and spatially in the context of treatment response. LB can enhance the sensitivity in diagnosis and facilitate repeated sampling through a blood sample that takes place in a noninvasive and convenient way and can lead to the early detection of tumors through both the assessment of genomic and proteomic analyses of tumor analytes, including CTCs, ctDNA, and exosomal subcellular vesicles composed of miRNAs and nucleic acids and proteins, providing crucial longitudinal information and data for accurate

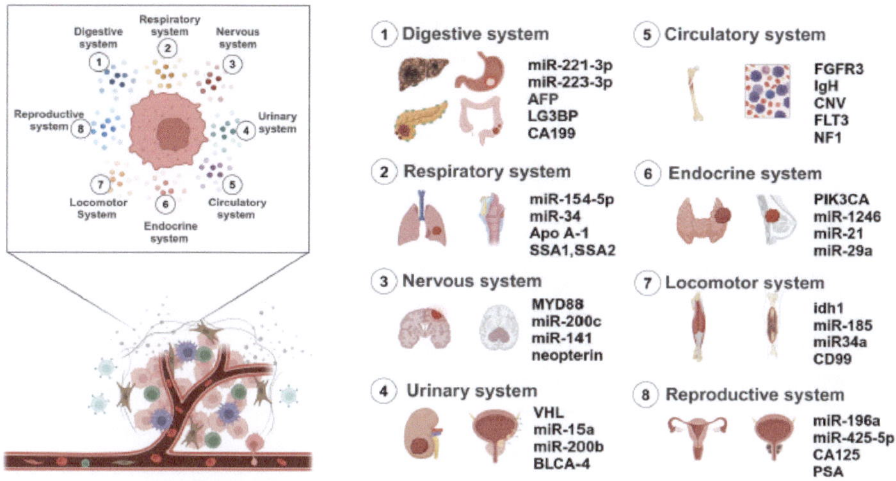

Fig. 3.5 The liquid biopsy biomarkers of systemic tumors. (Adapted from Ma [5]. Permission to reuse by Creative Commons CC BY 4.0)

diagnosis. Copy number alterations (CNAs) and transcriptomic and proteomic profiling can be performed. As an example, CTC levels change in a dynamic way that runs more parallel to tumor condition than usual blood biomarkers because they offer a better indication of response to treatment, with reduced levels correlating with superior OS. CTCs have a number of technologies available to isolate them. EPISPOT assay detects CTCs in a single cell, has shown clinical validity in BC, colorectal cancer, melanoma, and prostate cancer (PCa), and targets the EpCAM, having prognostic relevance in charactering the CTCs from BC. The CellSearch system that pulls down CTCs also targets EpCAM and demonstrates a correlation between predicting patient survival in PCa and CTC cell counts. AdnaTest uses PCR to detect the AR-V7 transcript that is overexpressed in prostate cancer and tumor-specific mRNA transcripts against PSA and determines its upregulation of androgen receptor (AR) modulation genes. CellSearch also targets the ER, BCL-2, and EGFR; Ki67 can predict response to endocrine treatment and is relevant in the development of the relatively new CTC-endocrine therapy. The metastasis-initiating cell (MIC) assay analyzes a tumor's invasive properties by obtaining CTCs and thus providing detail on the staging and subtypes of tumors when designing novel precision oncology drugs targeting tumors. The mutational profiling capability of CTCs is used to reveal the characteristics and outcomes of response from, for example, the EGFR gene, where the T790M mutation is associated with the relapse of the tumor and confers resistance to normally used therapies such as gefitinib and erlotinib in NSCLC. The mutational profiling of KRAS and PIK3CA indicates a therapeutic outcome for CRC and reveals the heterogeneity of genomic mutations in genes identifying the individual mutation responsible for treatment response variability, demonstrating that the genetic and molecular profiling of CTCs isolated from patients can, unlike tissue biopsy, in real time detect genotypic changes in tumor evolution [2] (Figs 3.6 and 3.7).

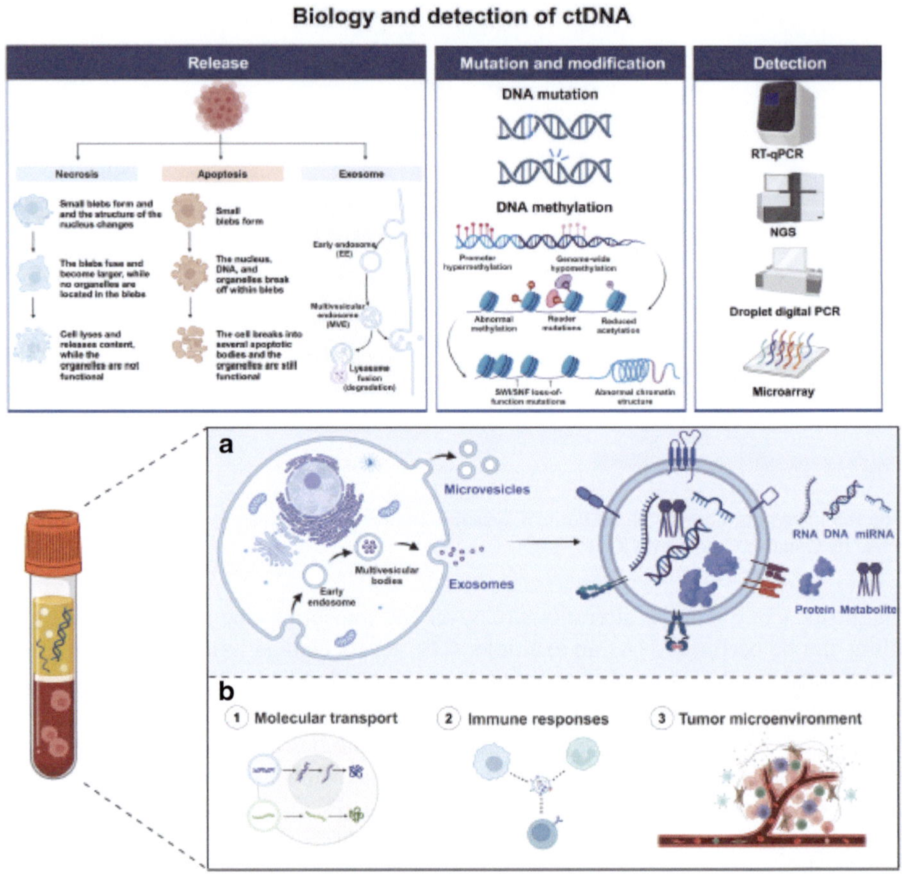

Fig. 3.6 Liquid biopsy ctDNA and exosome markers depicting formation process and detection contents. (Adapted from Ma [5]. Permission to reuse by Creative Commons CC BY 4.0)

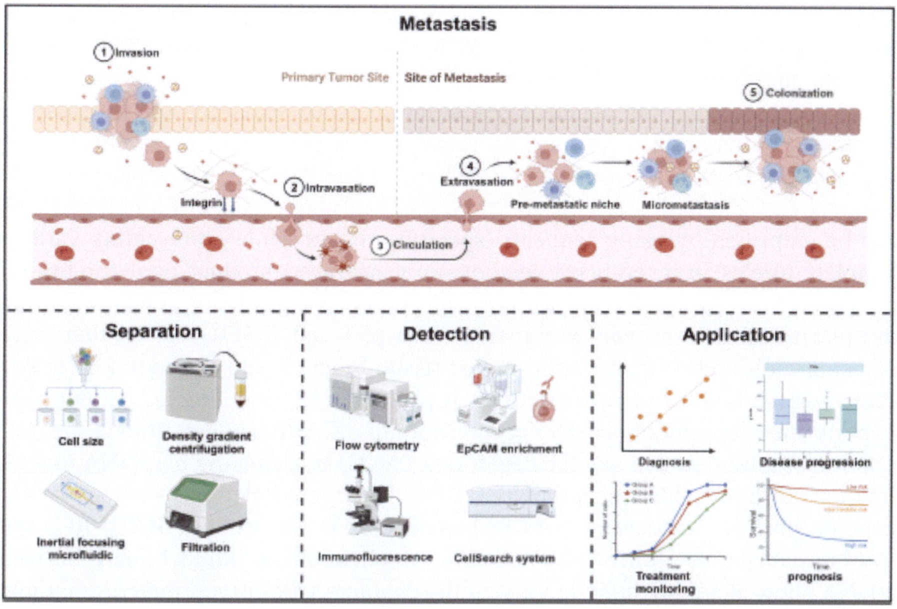

Fig. 3.7 Liquid biopsy CTC markers indicating metastasis, separation detection, and application. (Adapted from Ma [5]. Permission to reuse by Creative Commons CC BY 4.0)

3.4 Circulating Tumor DNA (ctDNA)

Early studies revealed how ctDNA was detected in the serum of pancreatic cancer patients, which decreased after therapy. The sequences were altered too and contained oncogenes such as KRAS. Also, ctDNA was shown to lead to host cell genetic changes and promote cellular metastasis and transformation through a horizontal transfer of apoptotic moieties released by tumorigenic cells; ctDNA varies with tumor stage and therapeutic response. ctDNA in precision oncology allows for the detection of ctDNA of 20–50 bp and their analysis in plasma, with other reports stating that ctDNA differed in length from circulating cfDNA. There was a difference of in length when comparing ctDNA and circulating cfDNA by 20–50 bp, as shown through the analysis of plasma ctDNA variants in from a recent study. In addition, ctDNA analysis is complicated by major hurdles involving the methods in sample handling and isolation. However, a deficit in full standardization and a lack of analytical consensus remain. The observed variation in quality and quantity must reflect the biological changes attendant to the tumor and not artifact generation as a result of sample-handling variation. Gene mutations that lie within genomic regions and rearrangements of genes as well are templates for variation hotspots in selected tumor types. Targeted approaches rely on this variation, whereas untargeted approaches, such as CNAs and nucleotide variation, offer a broader analysis of tumor genome monitoring. These include ddPCR (targeted approaches) and BEAMing (targeted approach). In patients with advanced CRC, BC, or PCa, digital PCR detects ctDNA in more than 75% of patients, and a personalized analysis of rearranged ends (PARE), has sufficient sensitivity to successfully detect levels as low as 0.001% in CRC and BC samples of plasma by using primers flacking breakpoint regions. Tagged amplicon deep sequencing (TAm-seq) can detect ctDNA mutations derived from a plasma allele frequency of 2% with a sensitivity of >97%. Multiple regions of a targeted area can be amplified by using sequence-specific primers while representing various template alleles in a template, leading to a narrowed product pool for further enrichment amplification, adaptor tagging, and deep sequencing. Also detected in the plasma of ovarian cancer patients were p53 and EGFR regions that were detectable through invasive solid tumor tissue biopsies and through a TAm-seq screening method for tumor mutations of plasma in BC and NSCLC patients that is performed longitudinally over several months. CAPP-seq determined the correlation of tumor burden and the detection of MRD by detecting of ctDNA mutant fractions of a low value, specifically 0.02%. Untargeted methods such as whole-genome profiling detected CNAs in hepatocellular carcinoma (HCC), BC, and ovarian cancer. In clinical oncology, the application of liquid biopsy–derived ctDNA showed a more holistic view of the characteristics of a primary tumor and its progression to form primary and metastasize tumor foci. The genome sequencing of ctDNA assisted in detecting tumor-specific CNAs in PCa genes, revealing the dynamic "changing nature of cancer cell genomics," whereby gene amplification led to cancer progression. Also, ctDNA genotyping assists in detecting in B cell lymphoma patients tumor subtypes that can predict clinical outcomes while personalizing treatments, negating the use of CTCs that are required in high number from multiple solid tumor biopsies. In contrast to CTCs, ctDNAs are can serve as biomarkers indicative of tumor burden in lung cancer studies. Studies also revealed the therapeutic response and signification of ctDNA in the prognosis of cancer progression and response to treatment, where its detection was found to correlate with relapse and relatively poor clinical outcomes. When CRC and BC patients have their ctDNA profiles, MRD can also be detected following treatment and a risk of relapse, thus allowing for subsequently modified therapy. Furthermore, ctDNA analysis via the plasma-seq analysis of ctDNAs identified a large set of varied mutations and alterations that can predict treatment in cancer with KRAS and BRAF mutations when detected in samples derived from plasma. Isolating ctDNA from mCRC patients led to the identification of five to six mutations that drive primary resistance and determine post-EGFR treatment such as cetuximab and panitumumab. Mutations in PIK3CA RB1 proteins and EFGR that confer resistance to chemotherapy in advanced cancer through mechanisms of intrinsic and acquired resistance develop over time; they have different genetic origins, but they converge at crucial signaling foci leading to the conclusion that "numerous applications of ctDNA in the diagnosis, prognosis, therapy and drug resistance associated with precision oncology" are available [2].

3.5 The Potential of Liquid Biopsy for Guiding Therapy

Liquid biopsy has gained traction for its role in earlier prognostication, the monitoring of recurrence, and its impact on clinical efficacy, leading to personalized treatments (Fig. 3.8). Circulating tumor cells (CTCs) are uncommon cancer cells in the bloodstream when compared to ctDNA, and are detected in peripheral blood while circulating, as well as being derived from fragments shed into the vasculature from tumors either at earlier stages or when metastasized. The known methods for detecting CTCs are whole-genome sequencing (WGS) and whole-exome sequencing (WES), which are crucial for the detecting tumor heterogeneity. Originating from healthy leukocytes, in cancer patients, the source of cell-free DNA is the tumor, which becomes ctDNA. Early studies showed that in AML, NRAS, and KRAS mutations were found in blood cfDNA, and ctDNA in 18 patients had a number of alterations, such as PIK3CA, APC, TP53, and KRAS, which by monitoring the process of tumor burden dynamics led to the identification of acquired resistance to cancer treatments, as shown through the ctDNA mutation rate. CTC testing potential is a marker of temporal heterogeneity, reflecting the personalization of individual therapy, the monitoring of the cancer patients' prognosis, and primarily the detection of tumors. High specificity is the goal because it confers the benefits of reproducibility and high efficiency. As an adjunct to the detection of MRD postsurgical resection, pivotal clinical trials have been performed to evaluate the analytic validation and clinical utility of liquid biopsy.

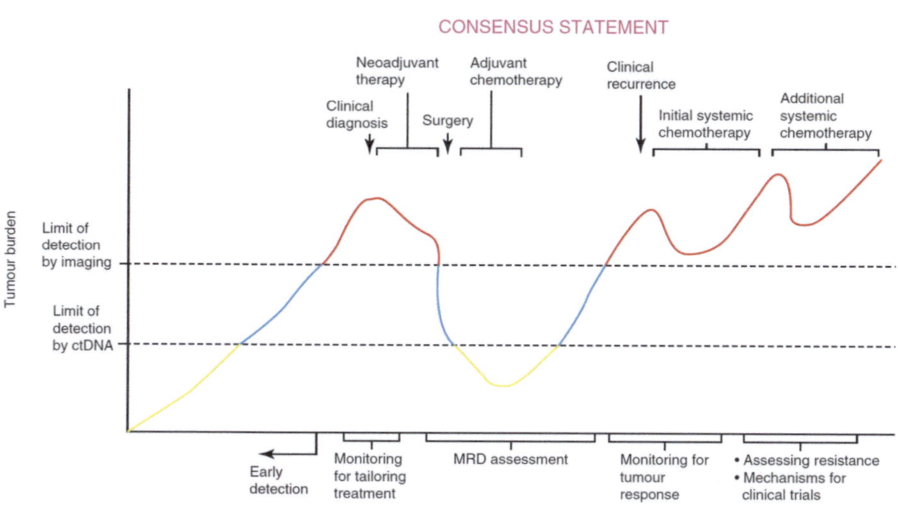

Fig. 3.8 LB timeline according to clinical stage. (Adapted from Snyder et al. [6]. Permission to reuse by Creative Commons CC BY 4.0)

When the Cellmax platform was applied to detect CTCs, it showed rates of 86.9%, 97.3%, and 0.88 for sensitivity, specificity, and area under the curve (AUC), respectively, in CRC patients alongside identifying additional CTC subgroups, including M-CTCs, which were associated with Tumor Node Metastasis (TNM) stage, T stage, vascular invasion, and Carcinoembryonic Antigen (CEA). M-CTC values were greater than 1, and CTCs were associated with worse disease free survival (DFS) and had a strong correlation with poor OS and with aggressive progressive disease (PD) (OS: HR = 2.36, 95% CI 1.87–2.97; PFS: HR = 1.83, 95% CI 1.42–2.36). T-cell activation is inhibited when anti-PD-1 inhibitors are combined with anti-PD-L1, leading to tumor cell immune escape. However, when PD-L1 assessment takes place, it incurs a risk of sampling bias and immunotherapy evasion and prevents representing the entire tumor.

One of the reviews on liquid biopsy reported on commonly altered genes in CRC, such as APC, BRAF, KRAS, PIK3CA, and TP53, that are implicated in NGS and become feasible for clinical implementation and the rapid integration of NGS in the development of using somatic mutations for CRC. The phase III ASPECCT study showed that CRC responded to EGFR-targeted therapy along with KRAS mutation status with the detection of RAS ctDNA that was not prognostic for poor prognosis [7].

NGS remains one of the main detection methods for the analysis of liquid biopsy in terms of detecting mutations. However, recently, disease monitoring and MRD sensitivity identification have been advanced by omics platforms and epigenomics, such as through the utilization of experimental techniques for determining histone modifications and methylation patterns [8].

3.6 NGS and Liquid Biopsy Analysis

Notably, ctDNA detection through next-generation sequencing has been shown in tumors such as colorectal cancer to detect MRD with evidence for its clinical utility and eventual integration into routine clinical settings. Most ctDNA platforms, such as Liquid CDx, AVENIO, and TAm-seq, have focused on prevalent genomic variation such as single nucleotide polymorphisms (SNPs) and CNVs. MRD detection requires a high level of sensitivity to detect low levels of ctDNA, necessitating benchmarking that can assess limit of detection (LOD), precision, and accuracy and can reference standards in plasma-in-plasma such as the BLOODPAC consortium to validate assay LOD. The use of contrived samples to assess tumor-naive and tumor-informed MRD assays is highly commutable to clinical trial samples [9].

Another report analyzed ctDNA to predict gastric and esophageal cancer in patients and the risk of recurrence through tumor-informed assays, revealing real-world data showing that they could be used in enhancing patient-risk stratification and demonstrating prognostic ability to predict recurrence in early gastric cancer (EGC) that has a high patient morbidity with a usual median DFS of 11 months. Here, ctDNA rates were determined preoperatively and postoperatively. The key results were that the recurrence rate was 88.2%, or 30/34 patients, in ctDNA+ patients and 5.5%, or 5/91, of ctDNA- patients, exhibiting, according to the study authors, a median relapse-free survival (RFS) of 9.6 months for ctDNA+ patients, constituting a marked reduction versus the median not reached in ctDNA- patients, with values of 85.7%, or 30/35, and 95.5%, or 85/89, for sensitivity and specificity, respectively (HR = 23.6; 95% CI 100.2 to 66.0). However, selection bias and patient heterogeneity posed as limitations in the real-world study [10].

Another study also showed additional evidence of ctDNA as a prognostic tool for mCRC patients for estimating the risk of relapse with the establishment of ctDNA as a post-adjuvant surrogate for MRD. In this cohort, ctDNA-positive patients had a decreased RFS compared to that of ctDNA- patients (median RFS 12.7 vs. 27.4 months, HR = 2.09). The study authors concluded that detecting postsurgical ctDNA served as an independent prognostic marker and can be utilized to identify high-risk relapse in CRC patients after liver resection metastasis [11].

The prognosis of cancers is typically carried out via radiologic imaging within 6–10 weeks after treatment has been initiated. Given the short half-life of ctDNA (and other types of molecular analysis), it may allow for the assessment of therapeutic response and lead to the evaluation of tumor prognosis, as evidenced by numerous studies reported in precision oncology journals and other literature. Dynamic changes in the quantity of ctDNA are demonstrated by early indicators of outcomes, as shown by numerous reports, as described below.

The MD Anderson Cancer Center conducted a study in advanced solid tumor cancer patients who had comprehensive analysis conducted on their blood samples and ctDNA detection through a liquid biopsy protocol in which peripheral blood sample collection took place serially before, during, and after systemic therapy. They found that among 260 patients receiving systemic therapy, ctDNA was higher in progressor patients compared with nonprogressor patients, who had either stable disease (SD), partial response (PR), or complete response (CR). Key results in the detection of ctDNA and therapeutic responses are as follows:

- Patients who experienced progression had higher rates of ctDNA detection than nonprogressor patients when compared to the baseline (77.4%, or 72/93, vs. 60.2%, or 77/128; $p = 0.007$).
- Nonresponders presented with higher ctDNA detection rates than responders did (patients with PR or CR at first restaging) at "mid-treatment (107/148 [70.9%] vs. 7/21 [33.3%]; $p = 0.001$) and first restaging (91/137 [66.4%] vs. 2/17 [11.8%]; $p < 0.001$) but not baseline (133/194 [68.6%] vs. 16/27 [59.3%]; $p = 0.334$)."

The study authors concluded that median time to treatment failure rates should be separated by qualitative groups and quantitative groups. The qualitative groups were as follows: (G1) the cohort of patients with ctDNA that was detectable and remained detectable while on treatment; (G2) the cohort of patients that had ctDNA that was undetectable but upon therapy became undetectable; (G3) the cohort of patients who upon receiving treatment had undetectable ctDNA but who upon treatment had detectable ctDNA; and (G4) the cohort of patients that had undetectable ctDNA throughout the course of treatment. The quantitative groups were as follows:

ctDNA CR that was marked after initial detectability with ctDNA clearance; ctDNA PR that was characterized by a decrease of more than 10% in variant allele frequency (VAF); ctDNA PD that was characterized by an increase of more than 10% in VAF or the de novo detection of ctDNA; ctDNA SD that was characterized by less than a 10% increase or decrease in VAF or no increase; and ctDNA nonmeasurable disease, which was characterized by no detectable ctDNA throughout the course of treatment. The G2 group had the longest TTF and ctDNA CRs during the middle of the treatment course and at the first restaging, having worse clinical outcomes. The limitations of this study stemmed from its retrospective nature [12].

KRAS is now considered a targeted mutation whose detection has entered the standard of care in the treatment of solid tumors. One report showed that this mutation was able to be identified by ctDNA across solid tumors. Pancreatic cancers were evaluated in another liquid biopsy study, in which CTCs, cfDNA, and ctKRAS variant allele fraction were assessed. Metastasis was found to be associated with high ctKRAS VAF and worse OS, whereas cfDNA was not. CTC detection was made with the CellSearch antibody-mediated platform. Median OS was 11.9 months (95% CI 9.2 to 15.5) in the overall cohort and 8.5 months (95% CI 7.0 to 12.9) otherwise. Also, cfDNA, ctKRAS, and CTCs were shown to be higher in patients with PDAC as compared to locally advanced cancer patients. The detection rate of KRASG12C was 7.5% in adenocarcinoma. The compound AMG510 has been found to be clinically active in these mutated cancers and received FDA approval. The study was found to have limitations in that the ability to separate treatment-naive and previously treated patients to compare detected rates from previously studies with similarly reported detected rates was not conducted [13].

The evidence for the prognostic ability and predictability of liquid biopsy as a minimally invasive biomarker has further augmented debates within the field of oncology and the management, especially temporal, of tumors, with a risk of recurrence and diagnostic accuracy being the main parameters. One study on the monitoring and prognostic implications of ctDNA in Merkel cell carcinoma (MCC) showed high accuracy in prognosis when detecting recurrence in MCC, showing a 95% sensitivity and 90% specificity, and the prognostic and predictive value was deemed high in the analysis of tumor-informed ctDNA. This led to the authors to describe ctDNA analysis as a stratification method, identifying high-risk MCC patients with a risk of recurrence, validating its clinical utility. Furthermore, ctDNA analysis at enrollment discriminated between no evidence of clinical disease and disease that was clinically evident in the discovery cohort. The results indicate the following:

A gradual increase in positive predictive value (PPV) was observed. Positive ctDNA detection was associated with a PPV for 1 year of recurrence at 69% discovery (95% CI 32 to 91) and 94% validation (95% CI 71 to 100). Negative ctDNA detection was associated with negative predictive value (NPV) at 95% discovery (95% CI 90 to 97) and 93% validation (95% CI 89 to 97) at 135 days after the test. The time between NPV and PPV was also evaluated. The authors suggested that these positive results in MCC might reduce the need for imaging surveillance [14].

Tissue-based assays were compared with liquid biopsy for assessing prognosis and predictive aspects of tumors. For one druggable mutation, KRASG12C, a comprehensive analysis through ctDNA was done in the form of KRASG12C testing. Previously treated and treatment-naive cancer patients with metastatic solid tumors were enrolled in a 5-year retrospective study harboring KRASG12C mutations and undergoing Guardant360 testing, and this testing revealed the mutation in 3.7% of patients, or 2985 of 80,911, across >40 tumor types [14].

The rates of KRASG12C mutation detection in these tumors appear in parentheses in the following: NSCLC (7.5%), NSCLC of all subtypes (6.9%), cancer of unknown primary (4.1%), colorectal cancer (3.5%), squamous NSCLC (2.0%), pulmonary neuroendocrine tumors (1.9%), pancreatic ductal adenocarcinoma (1.2%), and cholangiocarcinoma (1.2%). The highest rate of detection in NSCLC showed the feasibility of the ctDNA approach in detecting KRASG12C alterations across the various tumor types. Additionally, KRASG12C wild-type lung cancer exhibited the enrichment of the EGFR and TP53 mutations, and the STK11 mutation was the most commonly occurring mutation in KRASG12C-mutated NSCLC that had concordance with 84 NSCLC and 39 CRC patients, with tissue and ctDNA results available.

The cohort was grouped into two categories on the basis of the time elapsed between the analysis of ctDNA and the tissue biopsy. Time asynchronous was defined as greater than 6 months, whereas time synchronous was defined as less than 6 months between the analysis of ctDNA and the tissue biopsy within 81 patients and 48 patients, respectively. Between the two groups, greater discordance, including 11% in NSCLC, 38% in CRC, and 33% overall, was shown in the time asynchronous group, whereas high concordance (98%, or 47 of 48) was shown in the time synchronous group. The concordance rates between the analysis of ctDNA and the tissue biopsy was 100% for CRC and 98% for lung cancer in the time synchronous group. Within tests conducted more than 6 months apart, the overall concordance rate was lower, at 77%. CRC patients had the highest discordance rate, 38%, and for lung cancer patients, the discordance rate was 11%. However, as the authors point out, a key limitation of the study is that the Guardant360 database includes both previously treated and treatment-naive patients, so it lacks the ability to compare detection rates with previously published prevalence rates due to its lack of the necessary details for analyzing them separately. However, this study remains remarkable, being the first of its kind to compare tissue biopsy and ctDNA analysis across 80,000 unique patients with metastatic solid tumors [15].

Another study, the SCRUM-Japan GOZILA substudy, conducted a similar tumor biopsy–liquid biopsy analysis comparison; using Guardant360, the investigators did a similar tumor assay–liquid biopsy analysis and determined the clinical validity of assessing microsatellite instability (MSI) between plasma-based genotyping and tissue-based genotyping. They performed plasma-based MSI assessment and provided comparisons with tissue-based MSI assessment by using a PCR-based method in patients enrolled in the GOZILA study with advanced GI cancers while performing a nationwide ctDNA profiling study.

Positive percent agreement (PPA), negative percent agreement (NPA), and overall percent agreement (OPA) served as primary end points, and immune checkpoint inhibitor therapy efficacy was also evaluated. Precisely 658 patients who had MSI, PPA, and NPA assessment through plasma and tissue biopsy resulted in values of 98.2% (95% CI 96.8 to 99.1), 71.4% (95% CI 47.8 to 88.7), and 99.1% (95% CI 98.0 to 99.7), respectively. In patients with a ctDNA fraction of ≥1.0 the PPA was 100.0% or 15/15; 95% CI 78.2 to 100.0). PFS ranged from 4.3 to 16.7 months in three patients who underwent ctDNA genotyping and with detectable MSI-high (MSI-H) tumors, after which anti-PD-1 therapy conferred clinical benefits. The quick detection of MSI-H through ctDNA genotyping in another patient harboring aggressive malignancy of unknown primary site also benefited from pembrolizumab. OPA, PPA, and NPA were 98.2%, 71.4%, and 99.1%, respectively, and high concordance rates between ctDNA genotyping and validated tissue-based MSI testing were observed, especially in patients with tumors that had ctDNA shedding. ICI therapy benefit was conferred in these patients who underwent ctDNA genotyping, which led to the identification of MSI-H tumors in patients [16].

A series of studies on solid tumors demonstrated that ctDNA was able to genotype metastatic sites in colorectal cancer, wherein ctDNA genotyping also revealed a relationship between the site of metastasis and the detection of ctDNA. NGS ctDNA assays were performed on mCRC patients with single-organ metastasis by using the Guardant360, as was applied in the SCRUM-Japan GOZILA study. The tumor type status of 138 patients who were eligible divides into 49 with liver-only, 47 with lung-only, 27 with peritoneum-only, and 15 with lymph node–only metastases. Additionally, ctDNA fraction was 23%, or five in liver-only metastasis; 6.0%, or five, in lymph node–only metastasis; 0.4%, or three, in peritoneum-only metastasis; and 0.4%, or three, in lung-only metastasis. The study also reported that lymph node–only metastasis (13.3% with a max VAF of less than 0.2%) was present with liver-only metastasis at a rate of 2.0%, and only a few patients were required for the detection limit of 95%. However, a max VAF was more frequently in lung-only metastasis at a rate of 27.7% and peritoneum-only metastasis at a rate of 29.6%. The study showed that when the NGS ctDNA assay was applied to lung-only/peritoneum-only cases, it should undergo evaluation, and concurrent plasma-based and tissue-based tests should be considered only in low (<0.2%) cases of max VAF [17].

In another study, circulating cfDNA was used in multinodular HCC to capture intratumor heterogeneity. For HCC, liver biopsy is the gold standard for diagnosis; however, serial collections of multiple liver biopsies are considered untenable with multinodular disease. In multinodular HCC, ctDNA analysis and its utility in capturing intratumoral heterogeneity were investigated. The experiment consisted of the synchronous collection of tissue and cfDNA biopsy from HCC patients who were prospectively recruited during systemic therapy. High-depth targeted sequencing with molecular barcoding was used in the analysis of plasma-derived cfDNA and matched germline samples. In the experimental method, seven HCC patients who underwent systemic therapy were prospectively recruited for collecting plasma and tumor biopsies synchronously before and during treatment. WES from matched tumor biopsies was compared with the cfDNA mutational profile. When compared to mutations detected from tumor biopsies, cfDNA detected a majority of mutations at a level significantly greater than that of tumor biopsies. Standard-of-care biomarkers indicating targeted therapy response in addition to the driver mutations CTNNB1 S33C, NRAS Q61R, ARID1A R727fs, and NF1 E2368fs were identified only through cfDNA analysis, and the study authors concluded that cfDNA could serve as a surrogate for the genetic profiling of multinodular HCC [18].

A similar study on advanced clear cell renal cell carcinoma (ccRCC) was also conducted, where tumor tissue was compared to cfDNA with matched molecular profiling. The assessment of whether ctDNA could serve as a biomarker and have clinical utility was also performed. The NGS of primary tumor tissue was performed, which assisted in determining cfDNA-based genomic profiling's validity through the analysis of a large cohort of ccRCC patients. On the basis of tumor volume determined through radiographic analysis, clinical data were collected to find correlations between treatment response and tumor burden. According to the investigators, the MSK-IMPACT platform was utilized to provide a paired NGS analysis of plasma cfDNA and tumor DNA in a cohort of 110 metastatic clear cell renal cell carcinoma (mccRCC) patients. Tissue profiling revealing variants and CNAs was conducted and compared with germline testing, and thus, a comparison between cfDNA tumor tissue was conducted through manual cross-genotyping. However, negative conclusions were reached, and little support was available for the routine cfDNA panel testing provided, limited by its applications in biomarker efforts because of the low rates of detection through cfDNA-based NGS profiling in mccRCC patients. A low concordance rate with tumor profiling was reached, even for von Hippel–Lindau (VHL) mutations, and there was also the risk of detecting clonal hematopoiesis rather than mutations in peripheral blood. According to the authors' analysis, "the overall low concordance and detection rate using this panel-based cfDNA assay do not support the broad use of this assay testing as a clinical tool for patients with metastatic RCC" [19].

One study by Gerratana et al. showed that the interrogation of the mutational landscape of tumors through ctDNA analysis in solid tumors can lead to new insights and novel hypotheses, generating data and integrating histology-agnostic workflows and biomarkers such as tumor mutational burden. In that study, 1763 patients retrospectively identified with advanced cancers underwent NGS for ctDNA and tumor tissue with a commercial assay at Northwestern University. The authors found high utility in the ctDNA analysis while identifying FDA-approved targeted therapies for clinical use and while demonstrating high concordance between variants found by ctDNA analysis and tissue biopsy. High clinical utility was shown for ctDNA analysis, which had the potential to identify targeted therapies, with robust clinical value in finding emerging and established clinically actionable and targetable alterations across several tumor types, including the most frequent TP53 in all tumor types; the PIK3CA, ERBB2, BRCA1, and FGFR1 alterations that were associated in breast cancer; the KRAS and APC mutations in CRC; and common mutations in NSCLC, such as the KRAS, EGFR, PIK3CA, and BRAF mutations [20].

Additional reports have shown that ctDNA analysis could lead to cost- and time-reduction benefits. As one study declared, MRD could be detected in ctDNA analysis, as shown in trials that stratified patients into low- and high-risk categories for ongoing treatment assignment. These reports concluded that these studies could have a high impact on the conduct and design of clinical trials and the treatment and management of cancer and concluded that these tests have sensitivity and specificity. Clinical trial design can be based on the reliability of MRD detection, substantial reductions in trial sample size, and increasing statistical power by enriching trials with patients likely to recur through the reliable detection of MRD through ctDNA analysis, and such a design remains a substantial implication of these data. When conventional biomarkers for determining treatment response are unavailable, the potential role for ctDNA increases because it can serve as a surrogate end point for treatment response in the adjuvant setting [21].

A Bayesian model was developed by Napolitano et al. to distinguish false negatives from true negatives in ctDNA analysis and the detection of KRAS mutations in CRC targetable by monoclonal antibodies cetuximab or panitumumab. For this model, 172 subjects had tissue and ctDNA tumor samples collected to find information on the probability of finding KRAS false negatives. True negatives and false negatives were able to discriminated by their tool, as shown through their validation studies, with further utility confirmed by simulation studies. A reference mutation such as TP53 should be observed. Although the statistical methods are beyond the scope of this book, Napolitano et al.'s model for calculating the probability of KRAS false negatives is valid and has clinical utility in ctDNA samples of CRC [22].

3.7 Key Results: Detectable Alterations through cfDNA

- The most commonly detected alterations in genes were the TERT promoter (57%), TP53 (47%), CTNNB1 (37%), ARID1A (18%), and TSC2 (14%), where the rate of genomic alteration detection was at 92.2% for all HCC patients.
- When compared with the mutation rate in patient-matched plasma samples in which 37% or 73% of patients had paired tumor NGS performed on them, the mutation rates were as follows, in parentheses: TERT (83%), TP53 (94%), CTNNB1 (92%), ARID1A (100%), and TSC2 (71%), showing high concordance. However, alterations as detected through ctDNA analysis in 10 of 37 tumor-plasma samples, or 27% of the samples, were not detected in the patient-matched tumors.
- Oncogenic and likely oncogenic alterations in TSC1/2 (18%), BRCA1/2 (8%), and PIK3CA (8%) were detected and identified as potentially actionable, confirming tumor heterogeneity.

  Clinically actionable mutations were also identified:

- TSC1/2 in 18%, cfDNA in 37%, BRCA1/2 in 8%, and PIK3CA in 8% of cases were identified through cfDNA analysis, whereas as tissue biopsy genomic alterations were not identified in 10 patient samples. Of those 10 patients, 40%, or four of 10, had an OncoKB actionability level of 3b.

- In third- and fourth-line settings, two patients received everolimus on the basis of alterations detected in the MTOR-AKT pathway, which were first shown in tissue-based NGS and then confirmed through cfDNA analysis.
- One patient with a stable disease of 5.4 months had a TSC2 splice site mutation, and a second patient with PD after 2.5 months had a frameshift deletion. According to the analysis, VAF showed an association between outcome and tumor burden.

As the study authors concluded, for advanced HCC patients who could not undergo regional therapies, surgical resection, or liver transplant, a feasible genomic landscape could be characterized through the targeted NGS of cfDNA, with a rate of 92.2% for the detection of tumor-associated clinically actionable alterations [23].

Other issues, such as assessing the significance of minimal or measurable residual disease, are undergoing evaluation and analysis, an example being understanding the significance of BCR::ABL1 MRD in Philadelphia chromosome-positive (Ph+) acute lymphocytic leukemia (ALL), which was initially found in chronic myeloid leukemia. MRD is considered to be the most powerful prognostic factor in ALL and informs treatment strategies such as allo-HSCT, the "driver BCR::ABL1 lesion [being] the gold standard marker." One study has challenged this with strong evidence that immunoglobulin/T-cell receptor MRD better reflects response to treatment and is a predictor of clinical outcomes. In the GRAAPH-2014 study, 264 patients with Ph + ALL were enrolled, and central molecular analysis was performed.

While BCR::ABL1 <0.01% was not associated with adverse DFS regardless of allo-HSCT status, IG/TR MRD >0.01% after cycle 2 was associated with a "significantly lower DFS" (HR, 2.49 (95% CI 1.40 to 4.40)). Suboptimal lymphoblast clearance represented a slow-responding patient population, and those not "in IG/TR molecular remission before transplant had a dramatically higher risk of a DFS event (HR, 8.96)," with no significant impact on BCR::ABL1 status before transplant. This study is significant in its assessment of lymphoid-specific markers as determining DFS and MRD status and "challenges the use of BCR::ABL1 as a marker," with implications for clinical practice determining allo-HSCT status and obviating the need for therapeutic escalation based on BCR::ABL1 MRD as toxic and unnecessary in Ph + ALL (Table 3.1) [24].

The International Society for Extracellular Vesicles defined *extracellular vesicles* (EVs) as "particles naturally released from cells that are delimited by a lipid bilayer and cannot replicate." They are released into the extracellular space (EXS) from normal and malignant cells and lead to communication between nearby cells and cells at distant sites. Results from mBC tumor analysis whereby the prospective clinical trial SWOG0500 used open-source ACCEPT software applied to archived CellSearch images led to the enumeration of CTCs and tumor-derived extracellular vesicles (tdEVs) prior to and subsequent to one cycle of chemotherapy. Clinical data included worse OS in patients with increased tdEVs, who had values of 17.1 vs.

Table 3.1 BCR::ABL1 minimal residual disease and corresponding immunoglobulin/T-cell receptor MRD

Treatment cycle	BCR::ABL1 MRD	IG/TR MRD
1	16%	51%
2	43%	77%
3	48%	87%
4	61%	93%

Adapted from Kim [24]

29.0 vs. 43.3 months for median overall survival (mOS) in high, medium, and low groups, respectively, and this was independently associated with poorer OS in CTC counts of <5 CTC/7.5 mL blood. Longer OS was experienced in patients with detectable low tdEVs after one cycle of CT with an mOS of 10.8 vs. 17.8 vs. 26.7 in high, medium, and low groups, respectively. The evaluation of CTCs could complement tdEV analysis, and the combination of these two factors could result in more-accurate measurements of tumor load and disease aggressiveness and could provide clinicians with the ability to predict patient responses to therapy [25].

In mCRC samples, ctDNA analysis was conducted and evaluated for its role in routine clinical practice for monitoring MRD during the course of treatment and predicting prognosis. One retrospective exploratory study showed a role in mCRC patients for ctDNA monitoring when receiving first-line chemotherapy and bevacizumab. The Oncomine Colon cfDNA Assay on the Ion S5 XL instrument was utilized for ctDNA analysis.

3.8 Key Results: ctDNA for Monitoring MRD in mCRC

- In 44 patients whose plasma levels were ascertained at baseline, RAS, BRAF, or PIK3CA mutations were detected in 44 patients, with high concordance between tumor tissue and ctDNA mutations, at rates of KRAS 100%, NRAS 97.9%, BRAF 97.9%, and PIK3CA 90%. At baseline, low VAF was associated with longer median progression-free survival (mPFS) when compared to high VAF (15.9 vs 12.2 months).
- At first evaluation, patients with a large decline in VAF had both higher PFS rates and higher OS rates, which were 12.29 months (95% CI 9.03 to 17.9) vs. 8.15 months (95% CI 2.76 to not available (NA)) and 34.1 months (95% CI 21.68 to NA) vs. 11.1 months (95% CI 3.71 to NA; $p = 0.003$), respectively.

The study authors concluded that because the mPFS and mOS of all patients were 12.9 months and 25.3 months, respectively, druggable gene alterations with low baseline VAF were associated with longer PFS, and a decrease in VAF at first evaluation was found to be associated with both PFS and OS at baseline [26].

Even with the development of innovations in cancer genomics, diagnostics, and liquid biopsy, precision oncology has "more work ahead," according to one review. Although targeted therapies are transforming cancer treatment, precision medicine

(PM) "needs better clinical guidelines, trials and biomarkers to enhance patient outcomes, demanding new practices and tools. Biomarkers improve treatment by matching patients' right therapy, saving costs. PM fights drug resistance through new targets and tailored treatments based on tumor characteristics, boosting outcomes" [27].

One study identified incidental pathogenic germline variants (PGVs) in liquid biopsy samples. The study authors maintain that the genetic testing of germline DNA has not been replaced by cfDNA sequencing, because percentages of the prevalence of incidental PGVs through liquid biopsy are between 1.4% and 1.9%. In ovarian cancer patients, gBRCA1/2 was observed in 7% of the patients. In terms of molecular profiling, 47% of PGV carriers had tumors with at least one somatic driver mutation, ALK, ROS1, NTRK1/3, RET fusions, or ERBB2/MET amplifications, in addition to EGFR, BRAF, KRAS, MET, and ERBB2 mutations. Furthermore, cfDNA genotyping expands the scope of precision oncology by leading to avenues for genetic counseling in previously excluded patients who have inherited cancer [28].

Bragadin et al. conducted an interesting study on how longitudinal liquid biopsy samples could have predictive value for NSCLC. In their study, ctDNA modeling led to the predictive modeling of the clinical efficacy of immunotherapies, and these authors posited that longitudinal liquid biopsy would be improvement over the detection of the PD-L1 expression. Also, 113 NSCLC patients were analyzed for longitudinal liquid biopsies.

3.9 Key Results: Longitudinal LB as Predictive Value for NSCLC

- At baseline, 67/110 patients, or 60.9% of patients, had detectable mutations, with 39.1% having no detectable patients; nine were positive at T2 and four at T3. Baseline ctDNA quantification yielded 10.03 ng/mL (Q1–Q3: 6.68–15.18).

Tumor genetic testing had the following concordance rates with NGS of plasma cfDNA:

- Of the patients, 20/36, or 55.5%, underwent tissue and liquid biopsy analysis, revealing at least one mutation.
- At baseline, max VAF was associated with relative risk (RR), especially in patients experiencing PD. Patients experiencing the best RR had both a higher maxVAF and a higher cfDNA when compared to patients who experienced PR or SD.

The study authors concluded that although a practical model needs to be developed and tested for clinical applications, the predictive value of ctDNA dynamic analysis can be confirmed [29].

Lin et al. [30] conducted a study on identifying novel gene rearrangements and clinically relevant alterations in lung adenocarcinoma for obtaining accuracy when comparing the results of liquid biopsy with those of solid tissue sequencing. With the sequencing of 100 lung adenocarcinoma patients, sensitivity, specificity, and accuracy values were obtained with the concurrent testing of plasma-based assay and tissue-based NGS assay, with 83% having stage IV disease. Key results include plasma NGS identifying 41 clinically relevant mutations with a sensitivity of 52.6% and tissue NGS identifying 74 clinically relevant mutations with 52 targets for therapeutic agents. Higher sensitivity and higher accuracy were achieved for tissue NGS in newly diagnosed and previously diagnosed patients and for metastatic and nonmetastatic lesions in such patients, including those with actionable fusions such as EGFR, ALK, and NTRK1. The authors concluded that when compared to plasma-based NGS, tissue-based NGS detects significantly more clinically relevant mutations and targeted therapies due to the low sensitivity of liquid biopsy. According to the National Comprehensive Cancer Network and the College of American Pathologists, a substantial NGS panel is recommend by both for "broad molecular profiling such as NGS for the goal of identifying both common and rare mutations that are associated with targeted treatment as determined by clinical trials." The authors posit some of the traditional challenges of solid tumor biopsy, including its invasive nature, its insufficient nucleic acids, and its inability to reveal spatial molecular heterogeneity in tumors without also being able to monitor molecular changes over time to detect molecular targets. However, a serial assay could be used to monitor the temporal development of alterations leading to resistance while tracking tumor burden over the duration and course of treatment. Commercial and hospital laboratories are already implementing plasma-based ctDNA testing and analysis to detect clinically actionable mutations in tumors. In their study, median time between sample collections was 12 days, whereas concurrent testing took a greater period of time, specifically 16 weeks. Within 8 weeks, 96% of total sample collection took place.

3.10 Key Results: Tissue-based NGS versus Plasma-based NGS

- Both tissue-based NGS and plasma-based NGS detected a clinically relevant mutation in 78, or 78%, of cases in lung adenocarcinoma, with therapeutically targetable alterations detected in 55 cases. Additionally, 22, or 22%, of cases did not result in any detectable mutations when analyzed.
- An overall concordance of rate of 59% resulted when both tissue assay and plasma assay detected 37, or 47.4%, of the 78 clinically relevant mutations, whereas 47.4% (37) and 5.1% (4) were the concordance rates of tissue-based NGS only and plasma-based NGS only, respectively.
- Both assays had high accuracy rates, with tissue-based NGS being 96% and plasma-based NGS being 63%. Although the sensitivity of tissue-based NGS

was 94.9% across the entire cohort, the sensitivity of plasma-based NGS was only 52.6%.

- The NPV of plasma-based NGS and tissue-based NGS was 37.3% and 84.6%, respectively. When the analysis focused on therapeutically targetable mutations, similar findings were observed for sensitivity values, with 94.5% and 52.7% for tissue-based NGS and plasma-based NGS, respectively. Both tissue-based NGS and plasma-based NGS assays detected clinically relevant alterations in 53/71 patients, or 74.6% of patients; 27 patients, or 38% of patients, had detectable alterations in both assays. However, 26 patients, or 37% of patients, had discrepant results, with 23 detected through tissue-based NGS only and three detected through plasma-based NGS only. In both untreated and untreated cohorts, the accuracy and sensitivity values of tissue-based NGS were significantly higher than those of plasma-based NGS.
- Plasma-based NGS displayed a trend of decreased accuracy in the treated cohort when compared to the untreated cohort, with the accuracy of tissue-based NGS remaining unchanged across both cohorts: 51.7% vs 67.6%, $p = 0.08$, and 95.8% vs. 96.6%, $p = 0.43$.

Plasma-based NGS led to a reduction in accuracy among patients with nonmetastatic disease. EGFR, KRAS, and BRAF were identified in tissue biopsy but not in plasma biopsy. Plasma biopsy also detected one G12C mutation within EGFR exon 19 deletion and two EGFR L858R mutations. Tumor cellularity was thought to account for the false-negative rate in three cases. Several mutations were detected via plasma-based NGS but not tissue-based NGS, which led to concerns over the specificity of the assay given that molecular testing was regarded as useful for identifying resistance mechanisms and actionable mutations missed by prior tests. This was attributed to ctDNA levels in patients who did not have stage IV disease and were identified for accurate clinical assessment. The authors concluded that the data led to the implementation of tissue-based NGS, demonstrating high clinical sensitivity over plasma-based NGS when detecting clinically relevant mutations in lung adenocarcinoma and supporting "the use of the tissue-based multigene NGS panel preferred for the molecular profiling of lung adenocarcinoma carcinoma when tissue is available and a small increase in accuracy" [30]. The analysis was repeated with treated patients and untreated patients to account for tumor burden and who had prior treatment. Here, 25 patients, or 86.2% or them, had clinically relevant mutations, of which two, or 40%, were detected through tissue-based NGS and plasma-based NGS.

Breast cancer liquid biopsy profiling was performed to reveal tumor evolution, leading to the acquired mutations through which they evade targeted agents. Patients were profiled with both tumor biopsy and liquid biopsy, which showed that acquired mutations are polyclonal and associated with lower allelic fractions (AFs). The study authors note that in "addition to well-characterized resistance mutations (e.g., ESR1, NF1, RB1, ERBB2), we observe a diversity of rarer but potentially targetable mutations (e.g., PIK3CA, HRAS/NRAS/KRAS, FGFR1/2/3, BRAF) and fusions (e.g., FGFR1/2, ERBB2, RET), as well as BRCA1/2 reversions through a variety of mechanisms, including splice alterations and structural deletions." BRCA1/2 mutations were also detected across the two platforms (7.1% TBx, 7.4% LBx), with "higher prevalence in LBx for ESR1 (10.6% TBx, 25.9% LBx), NF1 (4.5%, 8.1%), KRAS (2.0%, 4.1%), RB1 (4.6%, 8.0%), and ERBB2 mutations (3.4%, 4.3%)," which have been shown to be associated with drug resistance. Longitudinal TBx and LBx profiling was also done with a comprehensive genomic profiling (CGP) test in a clinical and genomic database that distinguished tumor resistance mechanism for acquired mutations, with "TP53 (246 alterations; 26.8% of acquired alterations), ESR1 (181; 19.7%), NF1 (69; 7.5%), PIK3CA (65; 7.1%), BRCA2 (48; 5.2%), PTEN (39; 4.2%), RB1 (32; 3.5%), and ERBB2 (21; 2.3%)" being commonly observed alterations. A case study was presented where a patient received liquid CGP and received a combination of treatment with fulvestrant and abemaciclib treatment along with the detection of a resistance mutation to a CDK4/6 inhibitor in RB1 (variant allele fraction, VAF 3.8%) and a resistance alteration to endocrine therapy in ESR1 Y537S (0.4%). ATM (VAF 12%), CDK12 (1.4%), TP53 (0.2%), and EGFR A1118T (0.2%) were other variants that were detected. The investigators concluded that tumor biopsy CGP and liquid biopsy CGP reveal a high prevalence of clinically actionable alterations, such as the well-characterized drivers BRCA1/2 and PIK3CA and alterations associated with therapeutic resistance [31].

A study conducted in 2021 may have led to further refinements in liquid biopsy for greater accuracy and sensitivity. A comparison of NGS solid tissue and plasma samples was performed on lung adenocarcinoma patient samples that identified "relevant gene mutations and rearrangements" that resulted in quantitative measurements of sensitivity, specificity, and accuracy. Concurrent assays were conducted, and new diagnoses occurred in 79% of patients with disease progression on treatment in 21% of patients. However, the study concluded that tissue-based NGS has more sensitivity (74 clinically relevant mutations detected with a sensitivity of 94.8%), whereas liquid biopsy had a sensitivity of 52.6% (41 mutations clinically detected). The EGFR, BRAF, and KRAS mutations and MET exon 14 skipping mutations ALK and ROS1 fusions were detected via tissue sequencing but not via liquid biopsy.

Minimal residual disease (MRD), used for guiding clinical decisions in hematologic malignancies, is a target for liquid biopsy in solid tumors. A review article reported details on the biology of MRD, clinical studies revealing ctDNA association with MRD and outcomes, and therapeutic implications for MRD. A number of solid tumors were discussed, including lung cancer, CRC, breast cancer, urogenital cancers, GI cancers, human papillomavirus (HPV)–related cancer, and ovarian cancer. The authors cite that MRD is used to identify the patients that need adjuvant therapy after surgery to eliminate "residual disseminated tumor cells" in secondary organs.

3.11 Lung Cancer

TRACERx study: NSCLC, 1069 plasma samples, 197 patients, 25% ctDNA detection, and 49% clinical relapse.

AEGEAN: NSCLC, double blind, placebo controlled, and ctDNA clearance associated with higher PCR and major pathological response (MPR).

3.12 Breast Cancer

A ChemoNEAR 598 longitudinal analysis of plasma samples featured 76 patients with early-stage BC (23 TNBC, 33 HER2+, HR+ 4). Conducting ctDNA for 76 months showed a high risk of relapse associated with follow-up ctDNA detection (12.5 months (range 1–60 months)), which suggested the use of the assay for the potential risk of de-escalation because MRD was identified in ten relapsed patients and none in 58 ctDNA-negative patients.

Patients with mBC with prolonged FPS harboring the ESR1 mutation (HR 0.70) were enrolled in the phase III EMERALD trial, where the comparative evaluation of elacestrant was conducted versus the standard-of-care endocrine monotherapy (investigators' choice of fulvestrant or an aromatase inhibitor). The study findings indicate that MRD-detected ESR1 alterations in patients might benefit from post-adjuvant treatment with elacestrant.

The AGITG DYNAMIC-Pancreas study group showed a "remarkable prognostic value" through ctDNA analysis detecting MRD in early-stage PCa, with RFS values being significantly longer in ctDNA+ patients versus ctDNA- patients (22 months versus 13 months; HR 0.52). The authors conclude that "[u]ltra-sensitive ctDNA assays of peripheral blood can detect MRD many months before radiological imaging shows metastatic progression in several types of solid tumor[s]" and that "[d]espite some encouraging data on ctDNA-guided MRD detection, widespread clinical implementation will require current technologies and procedures to be standardized" [32].

A brief review of ctDNA applications in breast cancer reported certain alterations associated with ctDNA plasma levels. When liquid biopsy is applied in the clinic, it can identify mutations associated with advanced breast cancer, so a number of clinical strategies were posed, including predicting the early progression, recurrence, and relapse of disease. One study showed "significant correlation" between ctDNA-positive patients (79.3%) and ctDNA-negative patients (20.7%). Advanced HR+/HER2- patients showed that those receiving ribociclib and endocrine treatment (87 patients) exhibited statistically significant differences in PFS when measuring median ctDNA levels (>24 months and <6 months, $p = 0.034$) and PFS 12–24 months ($p = 0.016$). Median time to progression was 83 days prior to radiological analysis. The authors reiterated the guidelines recommended by ASCO and ESMO for HR+/HER2- negative advanced breast cancer. Also, ctDNA testing for PIK3CA, BRCA, and ESR1 mutations was recommended by ASCO and ESMO guidelines, which state that testing for PALB2 progression after CDK4/6 was administered was optimal. The LB detection of ESR1 and HER2 mutations was also shown to be clinically relevant in a phase 2a trial on this molecular subtype [33].

An insightful study was conducted to determine whether quantitative circulating HPV DNA was determinate of the prognosis of cervical cancer. Patient characteristics included 99 patients, or 71.7% of them, had HPV16-positive tumors, whereas 39 patients, or 28.3% of them, were positive for HPV18.

3.13 Cervical Cancer

- HPV DNA was positive in 69/118 patients, or 58.5% of the entire study group, with a 55.8% rate, or 77/138, in the entire study population. Also, 61.0% of HPV16+ and 51.6% of HPV18+ patients were found to have HPV DNA.
- HPV was detectable in 85/138 patients, or 61.6% of them, when combining ddPCR test results for E7 and L1, with no identifiable HPV E7 in eight patients in the first set of ddPCR results, which in the second round of ddPCR results were later found to be positive for the HPV L1 gene in cervical cancer patients. The study found that HPV DNA could serve as a prognostic marker for cervical cancer [4].

3.14 Prostate Cancer (Fig. 3.9)

The most frequent alterations in PCa are TP53 and alterations in the AR gene. There are also amplifications and point mutations, and homologous recombination deficiency (HRD) was identified in up to 30% of PCa patients, where BRCA2 was one of the most commonly mutated genes, followed by ATM, CDK12, and BRCA1. In an analysis of 3334 patients with metastatic castration-resistant prostate cancer (mCRPC) with high rates of BRCA1/2 genes, ctDNA was used for their detection along with HRD. In mCRPC patients, alterations in the PTEN-PI3K-AKT pathway are also frequent, with PTEN loss being prognostic and predictive for AKT inhibitors; 231 mCRPC patients in one study had their mutations profiled through cfDNA assay, which found that 37% and 17% of patients harbored PTEN loss and PIK3CA gain, respectively, in plasma samples. In the phase III PROfound trial, mCRPC patients were found to harbor HRD mutations by using molecular analysis through the FoundationOneCdX tissue test and ctDNA analysis on the plasma samples of 619 patients, which showed tissue/plasma concordance in terms of the detection of BRCA and ATM gene mutations (81% and 92% of positive agreement and negative agreement, respectively). The single arm phase II TRITON2 trial also evaluated rucaparib, and the concordance was 74% for BRCA status among both tissue-based NGS and plasma-based NGS testing platforms. Six patients had the wild-type BRCA mutation according toplasma analysis and tissue testing. However, all of them had a low allele fraction, suggesting low clinical significance despite having PPA between plasma and tissue for BRCA, which was 93.1% for all mutations detected in plasma samples and were also detected in tissue samples.

The predictiveness of a plasma analysis of HRD mutation through ctDNA analysis detection was also shown in TRITON2, with no statistically significant difference with tissue- and plasma-selected HRD mutant patients versus no patients in terms of rates of response tested solely by using the plasma assay. In addition, there was no difference in rates of response in patients identified as BRCA+ according to tissue testing. In the PROfound trial, the efficacy of olaparib was shown through the liquid biopsy of BRCA

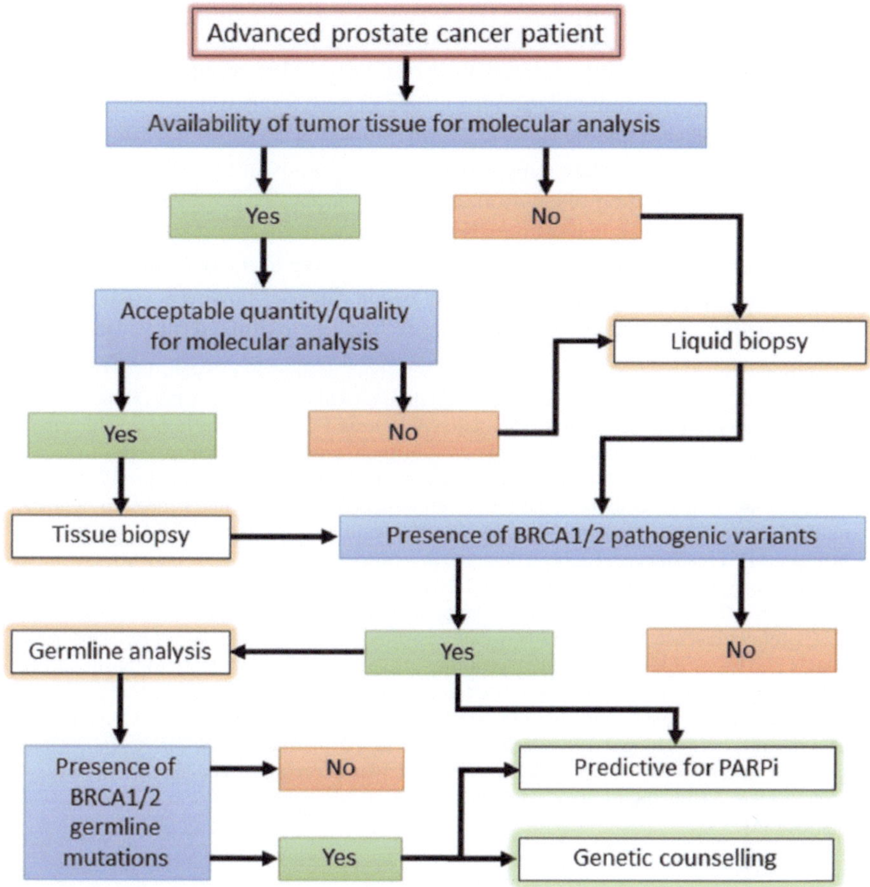

Fig. 3.9 Proposed algorithm for the molecular characterization of prostate cancer patients. (Adapted from Giunta [34]. Permission to reuse by Creative Commons CC BY 4.0)

mutations according to molecular status as shown through radiographic OS and PFS. Similar results were obtained in the PROpel trial, in which patients received abiraterone with or without olaparib and were also molecularly unselected. Tissue and plasma analyses detected an HRD-positive subgroup determined at screening, and the "ctDNA results alone predicted the survival benefit of adding olaparib to the same extent as the overall tissue and plasma results;" moreover, the authors concluded "that given the high failure rate of tissue analysis, a small but significant proportion (around 2%) of false negatives by ctDNA analysis was expected."

The study authors concluded that the liquid biopsy tool has had usefulness in prostate cancer through recent advances and innovations and that diagnosis and response assessment have been enhanced. Recent trends and data analysis from clinical trials and real-world studies have led to its widespread use and rapid adoption despite limitations; however, further efforts should be directed at technique standardization and cost reduction for its precise capillary diffusion methods to implement its use in clinical practice, particularly in low-volume centers, with an "increased level of recommendation for its use in both local and international guidelines. In the precision medicine era, liquid biopsy is an essential tool that could significantly improve prostate cancer patients' outcomes in the near future" [34].

Gruen et al. note in their discussion on "liquid biopsy for prostate cancer the progress and pitfalls, in that LB has contributed to reducing overtreatment and improved detection of PCa and CTCs aim to stratify risk according to the detection of resistance and recurrence markers in patient with metastatic disease; however, costs and a lack of standardization of specialized workflow are barriers to clinical implementation."

> Unfortunately, 20% of patients with lethal metastatic castration-resistant PCa (mCRPC) present with first-line androgen receptor signaling (ARSI) resistance. Clinical biomarkers to stratify this cohort are lacking. The majority of mCRPC patients have detectable circulating tumor DNA fractions (ctDNA%; 2%) in their serum, a known marker of disease burden. Owing to its short half-life, ctDNA reflects the temporal somatic profile of solid tumors, making it an ideal biomarker. Furthermore, ctDNA% is an independent prognostic marker for survival. By identifying specific genomic alterations in ctDNA, markers for primary ARSI resistance have been detected in treatment-naïve mCRPC patients. Owing to the relatively low abundance of tumor DNA in cfDNA, the sequencing depth required represents a financial barrier to clinical implementation of ctDNA profiling. Like ctDNA, CTCs reflect disease burden and facilitate resistance screening via serum biopsies. CTC counts and transcriptomic/genomic "profiling" have shown independent prognostic utility. Targeted genotyping of CTCs captures tumor heterogeneity, allowing early detection of therapy resistance. Neuroendocrine PCa (NEPC)-associated alterations in CTCs are detectable months before biopsy confirmed NEPC status. Furthermore, CTC RNA profiles suggest that sustained AR signaling is the primary driver of progression and mortality next to pretreatment NEPC, highlighting the importance of capturing multiple resistance mechanisms. [35]

3.15 Pancreatic Cancer

Yan et al. conducted a review on advances in liquid biopsy in the detection of pancreatic cancer. The authors found increasing roles for the use of exosomes, cfDNA, CTCs, and miRNA for determining pancreatic cancer stage and differential diagnosis from pancreatitis. They emphasize that having an early diagnosis is crucial for PCa patients, and liquid biopsy may offer the advantage of detecting tumors early. Exosomes, as growing evidence has shown, may contain genetic information in exosomal proteins, lipids, and nucleic acids for indicating early changes in PCa and "molecular species differentially expressed between PC[a] patients and healthy individuals," with certain exosomal markers playing relevant roles in the early diagnosis of PCa. When serum samples of glypican −1 (GPC1) were analyzed (a membrane-anchored protein), they were found to be higher in PCa patients versus healthy controls. In 190 patients, GPC1 was detected with a sensitivity of 100% and a specificity of 100%. Chips used in the detection of tumor-derived exosomes from blood samples have also been developed by researchers in the diagnosis of pancreatic cancer.

The method of using molecular beacons with high luminescence detecting GPC1 with higher sensitivity and specificity in distinguished serum samples from PCa patients and healthy individuals. KRAS and TP53 were also analyzed, showing that of 48 PCa patients, 39.6% had KRASG12D mutations versus 2.6% in healthy controls. TP53 was also distinguishable, with 4.2% detected in PDAC patients and none detected in the KRAS DNA in exosomes. However, no clear consensus exists, because when detecting GPC1 for diagnosing PCa, some studies have found levels with no difference in their expression in exosomes between PCa and healthy controls.

Also, ctDNA has been shown to be a prognostic and predictive biomarker for the early diagnosis of PCa. Digital PCR and deep sequencing have been used to perform mutational analysis to detect KRAS mutation. KRAS was retrospectively analyzed in the plasma of cfDNA in 259 patients. A 60-gene original panel was utilized to perform cfDNA deep sequencing on 48 patients who had a plasma KRAS AF of greater than or equal to 1%, with mutations being identified in the healthy tissue of 14 of 48 patients. Other studies determined minor KRAS AF in ctDNA that could reveal information for the staging of PCa when assaying both KRAS ctDNA and CA 19–9, with improvement in the sensitivity of the early diagnosis of pancreatic cancer. Additionally, 50 oncogene mutation hotspots, 14 chronic pancreatitis patients, and 12 healthy controls were identified by using samples isolated from 26 PDAC patients. When compared to the latter two groups, the median total cfDNA samples were higher in PDAC. Another study showed that, when comparing KRAS mutation between tissue DNA and the ctDNA of 75 patients with PCa, (74.7% versus 62.6%), the survival rate was lower in the latter. Genes associated with PDAC and "related to pancreatic development or function (GATA4, GATA6) and cancer pathogenesis (Yap1, Tead1)" were also detected in ctDNA. In assessing the clinical value of exoDNA and ctDNA in PCa, liquid biopsy samples from patients with localized or metastatic disease after neoadjuvant treatment demonstrated an increase in exoDNA, which correlated with disease progression; however, the levels of ctDNA did not. A greater than 95% concordance existed between liquid biopsy analysis and surgically resected tissues. As the authors state, ctDNA can reveal genetic changes that help in the diagnosis and prognosis of PCa, with the need for further clinical trials, wherein the early diagnosis and screening of PCa have been facilitated through CTCs. Specifically, 72 patients with PDAC were evaluated, the findings showing that the "CTCs in peripheral blood were round/ovoid, ≥6 mm in size, and positive for DAPI, CK, and CEA, but negative for CD45. Based on CTCs, those investigators were able to distinguish between patients with local/regional tumors (I-III, $n = 45$) and those with metastatic tumors (IV, $n = 27$)." The authors conclude that given the complexity in the early diagnosis of PCa involving family history, PCa risk factors, and expensive and invasive imaging, screening using liquid biopsy can be advantageous for "expanding the scope of screening efforts" through liquid biopsy–based assays of CTCs, ctDNAs, and circulating exosomes. Although methods for isolating and analyzing need to be improved, liquid biopsy can be useful in its clinical application to detect biomarkers and assess their prognostic and predictive value [36].

3.16 Hepatocellular Carcinoma (Fig. 3.10)

In an article titled "Targeted Molecular Profiling of Circulating Cell-Free DNA in Patients With Advanced Hepatocellular Carcinoma," a retrospective study analyzing cfDNA from HCC tissue samples showed that cfDNA could identify genomic alterations through NGS and aid in prognosis and treatment.

While conventional tissue biopsy is considered the gold standard for diagnosis and clinical decision-making for HCC, due to tissue biopsy's invasiveness, liquid biopsy is becoming an alternative as a result of its noninvasive, its ability to monitor recurrence, treatment response, and metastasis, and its allowing for repeated analysis, with CTCs and ctDNA drawing increasing attention. CTCs have been shown to have prognostic value, and ctDNA has been shown to have diagnostic value. OS and DFS were shorter in CTC- HCC cohorts, with EpCAM CTCs serving as a "real-time parameter for monitoring HCC recurrence in HCC patients after surgery," where subgroups had AFP levels of less than 400 ng/mL and a low risk of tumor recurrence. Mesenchymal CTC+ serves an independent risk factor for early recurrence when 62 HCC patients in the recurrence group had higher mesenchymal CTCs that those in the nonrecurrence group. Mesenchymal CTC percentages greater than 2% before surgical resection and CTC counts greater than 16 were associated with lung metastasis, early recurrence, and multi-intrahepatic recurrence. Additionally, ctDNA has better clinical correlation and higher sensitivity than other

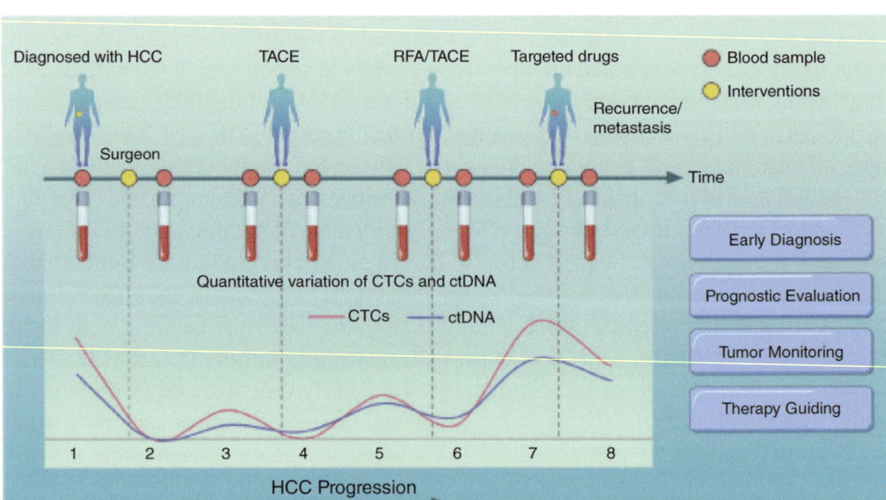

Fig. 3.10 Quantitative CTC and cfDNA analysis and HCC progression. (Adapted from Ye et al. [37]. Permission to reuse by Creative Commons CC BY 4.0)

plasma biomarkers for diagnosing HCC because “cfDNA levels could discriminate between HCC and HCV carriers with a sensitivity of 69.2% and a specificity of 93.3% at a cutoff value of 73.0 ng/mL.” Data revealed that when “using a combined detection of cfDNA and AFP, the sensitivity of cfDNA with two markers (AFP and AFU) was 71.8, 87.2 and 89.7% vs. 56.4, 53.8 and 66.7% for cfDNA, AFP and AFU when used alone, respectively.” The authors concluded that the quantitative analysis of cfDNA is both feasible and sensitive with higher diagnostic value than AFP and concluded that the screening of malignancy with the quantitation of ctDNA somatic mutation analysis is realistic to imagine and may serve as an “independent prognostic factor for HCC recurrence and extrahepatic metastasis.” As the study authors note, intratumoral heterogeneity can be reflected in targeted ctDNA detection and can lead to poor prognosis. TP53, CTNNB1, and TERT served as the “preferred targets for ctDNA detection aberration.” Through ddPCR, 27 of 48 HCC patients, or 56.3% of them, were shown to have intratumoral heterogeneity in HCC in that one kind of circulating mutant detected hotspot mutations TP53, CTNNB1, and TERT. The preferred targets for the identification of ctDNA aberrations detected through targeted ctDNA detection also reflect intratumoral heterogeneity and predict poor prognosis. When ddPCR was applied to 27 out of 48 HCC patients, one type of circulating mutant was detected with an mAF ranging from 0.33% to 23.7%, strongly suggesting a high degree of intratumoral heterogeneity in HCC. The MiSeq system was employed in another study to detect the exact mutations, finding that ctDNA with mutations was more easily detectable in patients with vascular invasion with a predicted shorter DFS time. The authors also state, "li]n addition, pERK+/pAkt- CTCs were more sensitive to sorafenib and remained an independent factor associated with a good prognosis (hazard ratio = 9.389)...Importantly, somatic mutation frequency of ctDNA reflected clinical dynamics corresponding to sequential therapy and might provide a possible solution for monitoring tumor burden and prognosis."

According to one analysis, “ctDNA could track the change in different mutants and therapeutic responses in real-time longitudinal monitoring.” Longer-term multi-institutional trials are needed for the clinical implementation of liquid biopsy because “Currently, most of the data gathered have been within proof-of-concept studies and lack of credibility. Altogether, the liquid biopsy is a critical part of precise medicine, and is believed will become a clinical reality in near future” [37].

3.17 Limitations of Liquid Biopsy [2]

While gaining widespread attention, LBs are considered complementary tests to tissue biopsy and not a standard tool for the confirmation and diagnosis of disease, with limitations such as a lack of sensitivity in identifying tumor type and a lack of clarity in its ability to provide a representative sample of a mutation within a specific region of a tumor. Many of the functions of LB have been successfully addressed via the single-cell analysis of tumor cells, including the diverse features of clonal evolution, the development of drug resistance and genomic changes, and changes in gene expression. Cost-effectiveness is also an issue because a preprofiling strategy is required for preselecting patents due to the lower frequency of target mutation. The occurrence of false negatives and false positives leads to a lack of standardization in methods and protocols for isolation and interpretation. In addition, going from bench to bedside is challenging for EVs due to a lack of precise analysis methods and enrichment technologies. EVs also lead to false negatives as a result of their ability to identify specific tumor-associated biomarkers at various levels, including markers for identification that can be difficult to identify due to downregulation during epithelial-mesenchymal transition (EMT). Wheat germ agglutinin (WGA) is used in generating sufficient quantities of DNA needed for sequencing to be degraded during the template process, leading to new WGA-free techniques, which are needed to augment the required stability [2].

References

1. Srivastava S, Pandey A. Oncology: way forward from clinical and molecular diagnosis to treatment in oncology: genomics, precision medicine and therapeutic targets. In: Tuli HS, Aycan MBY, editors.. Cham: Springer Nature Publishing; 2023. p. 1–24.
2. Lone SN, Nisar S, Masoodi T, Singh M, Rizwan A. Liquid biopsy: a step closer to transform diagnosis, prognosis and future of cancer treatments. Mol Cancer. 2022;21:29.
3. Abraham J, Singh S, Joshi S. Liquid biopsy – emergence of a new era in personalized cancer care. Appl Cancer Res. 2018;38
4. Cheung TH, Yim SF, Yu MY, Worley MJ, Fiascone SJ, et al. Liquid biopsy of HPV DNA in cervical cancer. J Clin Virol. 2019;114:32–6.
5. Ma L, Guo H, Zhou Y, Liu Z, Wang C, et al. Liquid biopsy in cancer: current status, challenges and future prospects. Signal Transduct Target Ther. 2024;9
6. Snyder RA, Dasari A, You YN. Liquid biopsy. In: Vauthey J-N, et al., editors. Colorectal liver metastasis. Cham: Springer Nature; 2022.
7. Zhou H, Zhu L, Song J, Wang G, Li P, et al. Liquid biopsy at the frontier of detection, prognosis and progression monitoring in colorectal cancer. Mol Cancer. 2022;21:86.
8. Ceri A, Somborac-Bačura A, Fabijanec M, Hulina-Tomašković A, et al. Establishment of liquid biopsy procedure for the analysis of circulating cell free DNA, exosomes, RNA and proteins in colorectal cancer and adenoma patients. Sci Rep. 2024;14:26925.
9. Stetson D, Labrousse P, Russell P, Shera D, Dougherty B, et al. Next-generation molecular residual disease assays: do we have the tools to evaluate them properly? J Clin Oncol. 2024;42:23.
10. Huffman BM, Aushev VN, Budde GL, Chao J, Dayyani F. Analysis of circulating tumor DNA to predict risk of recurrence in patients with esophageal and gastric cancers. JCO Precis Oncol. 2022;6
11. Marmorino F, Prisciandaro M, Giordano M, Ortolan E, Crucitta S. Circulating tumor DNA as a marker of minimal residual disease after radical resection of colorectal liver metastases. JCO Precis Oncol. 2022;6
12. Gouda MA, Huang HJ, Piha-Paul SA, Call SG, Karp DD, et al. Longitudinal monitoring of circulating tumor DNA to predict treatment outcomes in advanced cancers. JCO Precis Oncol. 2022;6
13. Chapin WJ, Till JE, Hwang W-T, Eads JR, Karasic TB, et al. Multianalyte prognostic signature including circulating tumor DNA and circulating tumor cells in patients with advanced pancreatic adenocarcinoma. JCO Precis Oncol. 2022;6:e2200060.

14. Akaike T, Thakuria M, Silk AW, Hippe DS, Park SY, et al. Circulating tumor DNA assay detects Merkel cell carcinoma recurrence, disease progression, and minimal residual disease: surveillance and prognostic implications. J Clin Oncol. 2024;42:3151.
15. Thein KZ, Biter AB, Banks KB, Duda AW, Saam J, et al. Identification of KRAS(G12C) mutations in circulating tumor DNA in patients with cancer. JCO Precis Oncol. 2022;6
16. Nakamura Y, Okamoto W, Denda T, Nishina T, Komatsu Y, et al. Clinical validity of plasma-based genotyping for microsatellite instability assessment in advanced GI cancers: SCRUM-Japan Gozila substudy. JCO Precis Oncol. 2022;6:e2100383.
17. Bando H, Nakamura Y, Taniguchi H, Shiozawa N, Yasui H. Effects of metastatic sites on circulating tumor DNA in patients with metastatic colorectal cancer. JCO Precis Oncol. 2022;6
18. Coto-Llerena M, Benjak A, Gallon J, Meier M-A, Boldanova T, et al. Circulating cell-free DNA captures the intratumor heterogeneity in multinodular hepatocellular carcinoma. JCO Precis Oncol. 2022;6:e2100335.
19. Kotecha RR, Gedvilaite E, Ptashkin R, Knezevic A, Murray S, et al. Matched molecular profiling of cell-free DNA and tumor tissue in patients with advanced clear cell renal cell carcinoma. JCO Precis Oncol. 2022;6
20. Gerratana L, Movarek M, Wehbe F, Katam N, Mahalingam D, et al. Genomic landscape of advanced solid tumors in circulating tumor DNA and correlation with tissue sequencing: a single institution's experience. JCO Precis Oncol. 2022;6
21. Kasi PM, Fehringer G, Taniguchi H, Starling N, Nakamura Y. Impact of circulating tumor DNA–based detection of molecular residual disease on the conduct and design of clinical trials for solid tumors. JCO Precis Oncol. 2022;6
22. Napolitano S, Parikh AR, Henry J, Parseghian CM, Willis J, et al. Novel clinical tool to estimate risk of false-negative KRAS mutations in circulating tumor DNA testing. JCO Precis Oncol. 2023;7
23. Cowzer D, White J, Chou JF, Chen P-J, Kim T-H, et al. Argeted molecular profiling of circulating cell-free DNA in patients with advanced hepatocellular carcinoma. JCO Precis Oncol. 2023;7
24. Kim R, Chalandon Y, Rousselot P, Cayuela JM, Huguet F, et al. Significance of measurable residual disease in adult Philadelphia chromosome-positive ALL: a GRAAPH-2014 study. J Clin Oncol. 2024;42:3140.
25. Nanou A, Miao J, Coumans FAW, Dolce EM, Darga E, et al. Tumor-derived extracellular vesicles as complementary prognostic factors to circulating tumor cells in metastatic breast cancer. JCO Precis Oncol. 2023;7
26. Urbini M, Marisi G, Azzali I, Bartolini G, Chiadini E, et al. Dynamic monitoring of circulating tumor DNA in patients with metastatic colorectal cancer. JCO Precis Oncol. 2023;7
27. Gadade DD, Jha H, Kumar C, Khan F. unlocking the power of precision medicine: exploring the role of biomarkers in cancer management. Future J Pharm Sci. 2024;
28. Bettaieb A, Paul C, Plenchette S, Shan J, Chouchane L, Ghiringhelli F. Precision medicine in breast cancer: reality or utopia? J Transl Med. 2017;15:139.
29. Bragadin AB, Dei Bianco P, Zulato E, Attili I, Pavan A, et al. Longitudinal liquid biopsy predicts clinical benefit from immunotherapy in advanced non-small cell lung cancer. NPJ Precis Oncol. 2024;8:34.
30. Lin LH, Allison DHR, Feng Y, Jour G, Park K, et al. Comparison of solid tissue sequencing and liquid biopsy accuracy in identification of clinically relevant gene mutations and rearrangements in lung adenocarcinomas. Nature. 2021;34:2168.
31. Sivakumar S, Jin DX, Tuchachinsky H, Murugesan K, McGregor K, et al. Tissue and liquid biopsy profiling reveal convergent tumor evolution and therapy evasion in breast cancer. Nat Commun. 2022;
32. Pantel K, Alix-Panabières C. Minimal residual disease as a target for liquid biopsy in patients with solid tumors. Nat Rev Clin Oncol. 22(1):65–77.
33. Klocker EV, Suppan C. Liquid biopsy in breast cancer. Memo. 2024;17:194–7.

34. Giunta EF, Malapelle U, Russo A, Giorgi UD. Blood-based liquid biopsy in advanced prostate cancer. Crit Rev Oncol Hematol. 2024;194:104241.
35. Gruen L, Schalken J. Liquid biopsy for prostate and bladder cancer: progress and pitfalls. Eur Urol Focus. 2022:904–6.
36. Yan T-B, Huang J-Q, Huang S-Y, Ahir BK, Li L-M, et al. Advances in the detection of pancreatic cancer through liquid biopsy. Front Oncol. 11:801173.
37. Ye Q, Ling S, Zheng S, Xu X. Liquid biopsy in hepatocellular carcinoma: circulating tumor cells and circulating tumor DNA. Mol Cancer. 2019;18

Chapter 4
Targeted Therapies for Solid Tumors

4.1 Personalized Cancer Medicines for Solid Tumors

Solid tumors fall generally among the categories of breast cancer, melanoma, colorectal cancer, non–small cell lung cancer (NSCLC), glioblastoma, prostate cancer (PCa), pancreatic cancer, renal cell carcinoma (RCC), and hepatocellular carcinoma (HCC), which are some of the most prevalent tumor types. Other solid tumors include gastroesophageal cancers, biliary tract cancer, and cholangiocarcinoma. In cancer treatment, basic, clinical, and translational research has led to breakthroughs in the development and implementation of targeted therapies. Targeted therapy strategies include small molecule inhibitors and biologics (Fig. 4.1 and Table 4.1), which are molecularly designed approaches that utilize the genetic basis of cancer for the discovery of novel therapeutic targets. Biomarker-guided therapy for optimizing treatment outcomes is derived from precision oncology, which is transforming cancer care. As Rai et al. state, "targeted therapies have emerged as a [frontier] in cancer treatment, revolutionizing the way we approach the disease" [1]. These therapies have a mechanism of action that disrupts cancer cell growth and survival by interfering with their signaling pathways and aims to halt or slow down the progression of cancer while being tailored to the genetic makeup of an individual's tumor. As explained in previous chapters, the molecular basis consists of either oncogene activation (ERBB2, EGFR) or tumor suppressor gene inactivation (TP53, BRCA) and dysregulated cell signaling pathways (MAPK, PI3K). In summary, biomarkers such as ERBB2, ALK fusion, and BRAFV600E guide are examples that determine targeted therapies such as trastuzuamb, crizotinib, and vermurafenib. Examples of solid tumors and targeted therapy include breast cancer treated with trastuzumab and pertuzumab; lung cancer/EGFR inhibitors treated with gefitinib and Osimertinib; colorectal cancer/anti–vascular endothelial growth factor (VEGF) antibody treated with bevacizumab; and melanoma/BRAF inhibitor treated with vemurafenib [1]. Like many other precision medicine approaches, several

P. Hays, *Personalized Medicine in Oncology*,
https://doi.org/10.1007/978-3-032-14437-9_4

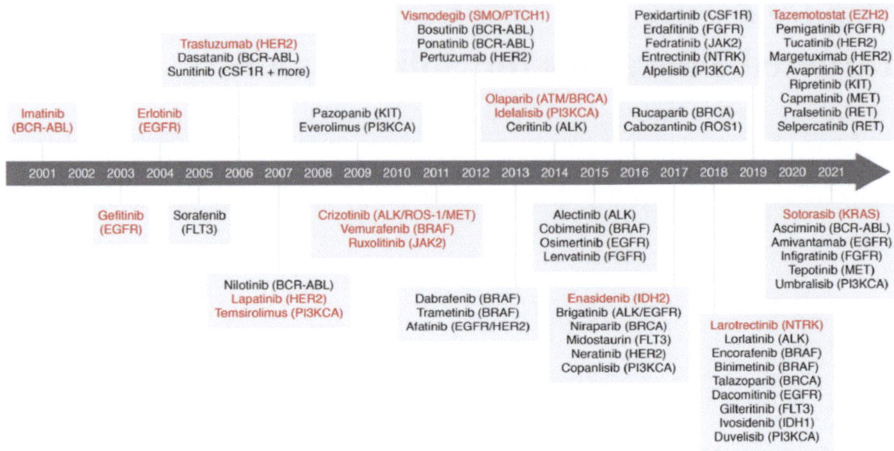

Fig. 4.1 Timeline of approval for FDA-approved therapies in oncology harboring mutation-specific indications. (Adapted from Waarts) [5]

Table 4.1 Mutation-specific treatments

Mutated gene	Common genetic alterations	Tumors implicated	Drugs
ALK	Mutation, fusion	Non–small cell lung cancer	Alectinib, brigatinib, ceritinib, crizotinib, lorlatinib
ATM	Mutation	Breast	Olaparib
BCR-ABL	Fusion	Chronic lymphocytic leukemia, acute lymphocytic leukemia	Bosutinib, dasatanib, imatinib, nilotinib, ponatinib, asciminib
BRAF	Mutation	Melanoma, colorectal, hairy cell leukemia, thyroid	Dabrafenib, encorafenib, vemurafenib, binimetinib, cobimetinib, trametinib
BRCA1/2	Mutation	Breast, ovarian, prostate	Olaparib, niraparib, rucaparib, talazoparib
CHEK2	Mutation	Breast, ovarian	Olaparib
LSF1R	Mutation, fusion	Giant cell tumor	Pexidartinib, sunitinib[A]
ECFR	Mutation, fusion, amplification	Non–small cell lung cancer	Afatinib, dacomitinib, erlotinib, gefitinib, osimertinib, brigatinib[A], amivantamab
ERBB2/3/4	Amplification, mutation	Breast	Afatinib[A], lapatinib, neratinib, tucatinib, trastuzumab[B], pertuzumab[B], margetuximab
EZH2	Mutation	Lymphoma	Tazemetostat
FGFR1/2/3	Mutation, fusion	Cholangiocarcinoma	Erdafitinib, lenvatinib[A], pemigatinib, infigratinib
FLT3	Mutation	Myeloid leukemia	Gilteritinib, midostaurin, sorafenib[A]

(continued)

Table 4.1 (continued)

Mutated gene	Common genetic alterations	Tumors implicated	Drugs
IDH1/2	Mutation	Myeloid leukemia, cholangiocarcinoma, glioblastoma	Ivosidenib, enasidenib
JAK2	Mutation	Myeloproliferative syndrome	Fedratinib, ruxolitinib
KIT	Mutation, fusion	Gastrointestinal stromal tumor, mastocytosis, melanoma	Avapritinib, imatinib, pazopanib^{A}, pexidartinib^{A}, ripretinib, sorafenib, nilotinibr, sunitinib
KRAS	Mutation	Non–small cell lung cancer	Sotorasib
MET	Mutation, fusion	Non–small cell lung cancer	Cabozantinib^{A}, capmatinib, crizotinib^{A}, tepotinib
NTRK	Fusion	Many solid tumors at low frequency	Larotrectinib, entrectinib
PDGFRA/B	Mutation, fusion	Gastrointestinal stromal tumor, mastocytosis, hypereosinophilic syndrome	Avapritinib, imatinib^{A}, sorafenib^{A}, sunitinib^{A}, lenvatinib ^{A}, pazopanib^{A}, ripretinib^{A}
PIK3CA	Mutation	Breast	Umbralisib^{A}, duvelisib^{A}, idelalisib^{A}, copanlisib^{A}, alpelisib, temsirolimus^{A}, everolimus^{A}
PML-RARA	Fusion	Myeloid leukemia	Arsenic trioxide, retinoic acid
RET	Mutation, fusion	Renal, thyroid, non–small cell lung cancer	Pralsetinib, selpercatinib, cabozantinib^{A}
ROS1	Fusion	Non–small cell lung cancer	Entrectinib, crizotinib
SMO/ PTCH1	Mutation	Medulloblastoma, basal cell carcinoma	Vismodegib

Adapted from Waarts [5]

challenges and limitations are posed by drug resistance (which can be overcome by using combination approaches), tumor heterogeneity, and side effects.

As Kulasegaran discuss, the discovery of clinically actionable genomic mutations and the consequent comprehensive genomic profiling of tumors is the foundation of precision oncology and personalized medicine in oncology and has become integrated into clinical decision workflows. The emergence of minimally invasive liquid biopsy is also playing newfound roles in innovatively providing quantitative measures of prognostic and predictive value and is also being incorporated into clinical studies and clinical practice. The treatment landscape for cancer has undoubtedly been impacted by personalized medicine for tracking acquired mutations and characterizing tumor heterogeneity [2].

The ability of broad gene and limited gene panels to identify molecularly based treatments was evaluated in a report published in *Nature Medicine*, where a panel of 324 cancer-related genes, as identified by using FoundationOneCDX, was compared to a limited panel (cytotoxic lymphocyte

(CTL)) of 87 indel genes, SNVs or genome-wide copy number variations (CNVs) to determine molecular-based recommended therapies (MBRTs). The primary endpoint was patients, or the proportion thereof, with MBRT identified. The proportion of patients with an MBRT identified was the first endpoint, whereas patients who had an MBRT initiated versus those who did not was the secondary endpoint. In this report, 741 patients were screened, of which 45.7% had tumor samples, of which 175 had MBRTs identified by the FoundationCDx panel (51.6%) and 125 had MBRTs identified by the limited panel (36.9%), marking a 14.8% increase. The authors concluded that the study's primary endpoint had been met. Among the 339 patients, 192, or 56.6%, had one actionable alteration identified that led to an MBRT match, of which the PI3K-AKT-mTOR pathway (45;22;14), homologous recombination deficiency (HRD) (21;12;5), the BRAF pathway (7;3;0), and the HER2 pathway (6;5;2) were found to be targetable. Alterations in tumor mutational burden (TMB) ($n = 36$), BAP1 ($n = 6$), and gene rearrangements ($n = 10$) served as the bases for identification when only interrogated with the F1CDX panel. A total of 89 patients (48; 41) had MBRTs identified but not initiated. Five patients receiving differing targeted therapies, immunotherapies, or a combination had a duration of response (erdafitinib: 9 months (early discontinuation due to toxicity), rucaparib–atezolizumab: 4 months (CTL; F1CDX), durvalumab–tremelimumab: 4 months (F1CDX), olaparib: 18 months (CTL), and encorafenib–binimetinib: 15.6 months (CTL)). Although the authors state that the PI3K-mTOR signaling pathway may pose challenges in intrinsic and acquired resistance, the molecular alterations identified would conceivably lead to the administration of targeted therapies with clinical efficacy. The study showed that the primary endpoint had been met and that an increase in treatment recommendations of 10 percentage points occurred that did not require predictive biomarkers when they were commercially available, such as the FoundationOneCdX when compared to the homemade control gene panel (i.e., CTL) [3]. Forrest et al. conducted a genome-sequencing analysis of 888 pediatric solid tumors as well and also found opportunities for targeted therapy administration through the identification of molecular alterations [4].

4.2 Mechanisms of Drug Action

Kinases, which constitute a targeted therapy class, include downstream tyrosine kinases, which respond to cellular cues that are grouped into serine/threonine kinases (TKs) and that serve as growth factor receptors. They exist in either type I or type II conformation, are active or inactive, and compete in the ATP-binding pocket of the kinase for adenosine triphosphate (ATP). They can also be allosterically inhibited. One of the most common types of tyrosine kinases is receptor tyrosine kinase, which causes the autophosphorylation of intracellular tyrosine kinase domains through the dimerization of receptors of activating downstream effectors that target EGFR and bind extracellular domains of human epidermal growth factor receptor (HER) receptor tyrosine kinases (RTKs) under normal physiologic conditions. When mutated, the result is constitutive downstream pathway signaling that is characteristic of multiple cancers, including EFGR-activating mutations in HER2 amplifications/activating mutations in breast cancer and NSCLC [5].

Monoclonal antibodies lead to RTK inhibition, and both RTK internalization/degradation and antibody-dependent cellular cytotoxicity form another class of targeted therapies with a distinct mechanism of action dependent on binding to the RTKs in the juxtamembrane part of the extracellular (EXC) domain of receptor tyrosine kinases (Fig. 4.2). Other therapies include erdaitinib, infiigratinib, and pemigatinib, which fall under the FGFR/PDGFR/VEGFR family of mutations whose downstream effect is increased angiogenesis. Downstream signaling effectors also include Rat sarcoma (RAS) GTPases—discussed later—of RAF/MEK/ERK serine/threonine kinases, the MAPK signaling pathway, and the RAS protein that initiates a signaling cascade as a plasma membrane protein that moves between its GTP-bound active state and the GDP-bound inactive state in a cyclical fashion, which upon ligand binding activates itself through autophosphorylation. A signaling cascade is initiated through the activation and phosphorylation of RAF, MEK ½, and ERK1/2. ERK1/2 phosphorylates a collection of molecules found after translocating to the nucleus, with gene expression and cellular function changes resulting. Vemurafenib, dabrafenib, and encorafenib fall under the category of RAF inhibitors and lead to signal inhibition through the V600E mutant BRAF protein. After the addition of MEK inhibitors, RAF inhibitor therapy leads to the inhibition of the adverse events of RAF therapy, such as cutaneous lesions that can increase the suppression of MAPK while prolonging responses in melanoma [5].

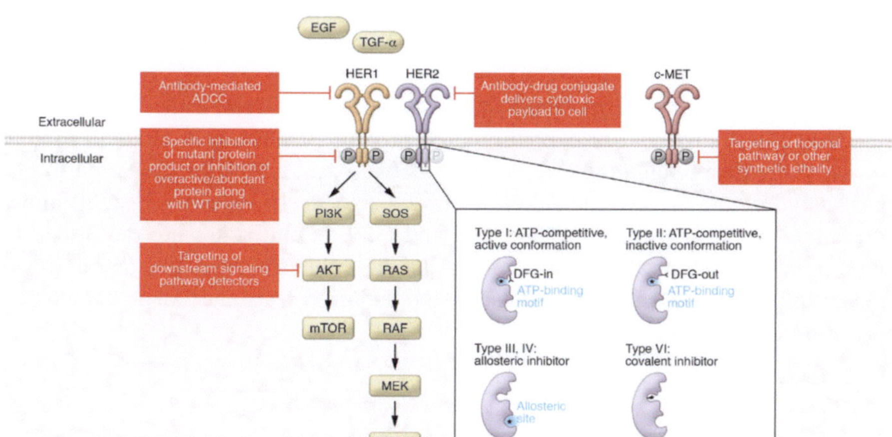

Fig. 4.2 An example of the HER2 RTK. (Adapted from Waarts) [5]

PI3K/AKT/mTOR pathways are frequently implicated in cancers of RTKs. Under normal physiology, PI3K has a catalytic subunit that is activated by RTKs' ligand binding, of which the cytoplasmic domain of RTKs is targeting by PI3K. The mechanism of action is the phosphorylation of the precision medicine (PM) lipid substrate PIP2 by PI3K, which then becomes PIP3. AKT is then activated, which then leads to the phosphorylation of downstream regulators such as the mechanistic target of rapamycin (mTOR). PTEN negatively regulates this pathway through PIP3 phosphorylation. Idelalisib, copanlisib, duvelisib, umbralisib, and alpelisib fall under the category of PI3K inhibitors, of which alpelisib is undergoing clinical evaluation in breast cancer. This pathway is also considered mutation agnostic. Capivasertib is an AKT inhibitor evaluated in phase II trials, and FDA-approved mTOR inhibitors include everolimus and temsirolimus [5].

Tumor suppressors BRCA and TP53 also have unique mechanisms of action, and when their function is restored, antitumor activity results. BRCA1 and BRCA2 repair homologous recombination double-stranded breaks while maintaining genome integrity. PARP inhibitors are active in BRCA mutated cancers. PARP1 falls under the category of being a DNA damage sensor. It recruits DNA repair proteins by binding ssDNA breaks and synthesizing poly(ADP-ribose) chains. By competing with cofactor NAD+, PARP inhibitors inhibit PARP catalytic activity, trapping damaged DNA, leading to DSBs, and stalling the replication fork. HR proteins recruit BRCA1/2 for DNA repair in HR-competent cells. However, DNA fragmentation and apoptosis result from error-prone, nonhomologous end joining in BRCA1/2 mutant cells. PARPi veliparib, niraparib, talazoparib, olaparib, and rucaparib derive benefits from trapping PARP rather than inhibiting the catalytic subunit.

TP53 mutations fall under the category of missense mutations, which derive from the protein's DNA-binding domain that leads to a loss or gain of function and later the conformation of p53, leading to its unfolding. Many compounds under investigation attempt to stabilize the native p53 conformation, thereby restoring its function.

In Figure 4.2, a small molecule inhibitor binds its target, either an inhibited mutated protein product, an overstimulated protein product, or a mutated protein whose downstream signaling effector is affected. Also, mAbs are delivered to targeted cells' cytotoxic payloads after activating ADCC. In Figure 4.3, small molecule inhibitors in both their GTP-bound and GDP-bound states are developed to target mutated RAS proteins, for combination and other therapies that target downstream and upstream. Intrinsic resistance and acquired resistance also characterize RAS inhibitors.

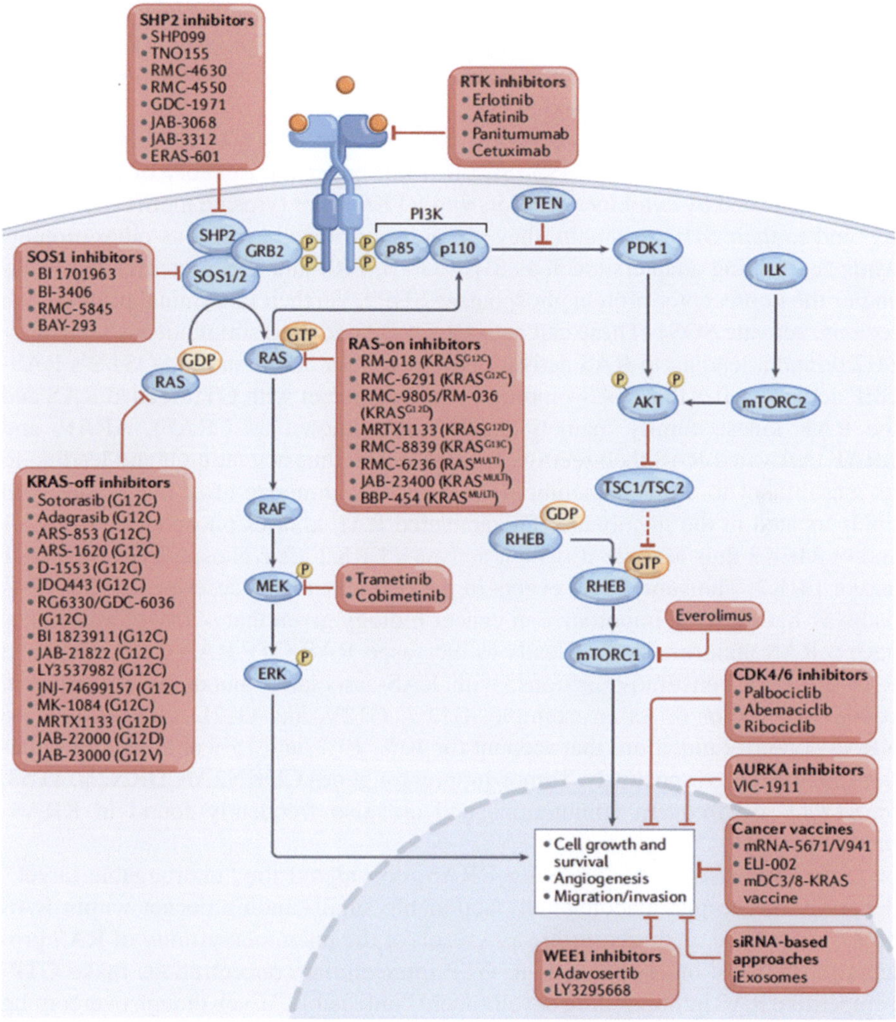

Fig. 4.3 The RAS signaling pathway. (Adapted from Punekar) [6]

4.3 The KRAS Target (Fig. 4.3)

The oncogenic RAS target has been extensively characterized in the literature, which has described the difficulty posed by the undruggable KRAS target, breakthroughs in targeted therapies of the RAS pathway, and primary, acquired, and adaptive resistance mechanisms to KRAS inhibition ensuing from treatment, along with mechanisms of action and resistance. The most prominent RAS malignancies are NSCLC and colorectal cancer (CRC). The RAS protein, as described earlier, belongs to the GTPase class of proteins and cycles between the GDP-loaded off and the GTP-loaded on cell membrane that involve RAS–guanine nucleotide exchange factor (RAS-GEF) action and RAS–GTPase-activating proteins (RAS-GAPs). RAS-GEFs cellularly catalyze the GDP to GTP. The primary RAS-GEFs that are activated by RTKs are SOS1 and SOS2.

The mechanism of action is described next. Activated by both cytokine receptors and RTKs, both SOS1 and SOS2 (SOS1/2) fall under the category of RAS-GEFs that are activated by cytokine receptors and RTKs. After tyrosine motifs (pY- X- N-X) bind to their SHF-2 domain, they are phosphorylated in various other proteins while scaffolding adapters (such as SHC, GAB, FRS and IRS proteins) and RTKs and/or the nonreceptor protein phosphatase SHP2, via their C-terminal proline–rich regions, activate SOS1. These can activate GRB2 and bind simultaneously via their SH2 domain, leading to RAS activation by precisely coordinating SOS1/2's RAS-GEF activity. After this, RAS-binding domains interact with GTP-loaded RAS and the RAF kinase family, namely RAF1 (also known as CRAF), ARAF, and BRAF. Activated RAS then recruits RAF proteins, thus activating it and leading to its recruitment to the cell membrane, where they dimerize after interacting with lipids located in the membrane. The activated RAF kinases phosphorylate MEK1 and/or MEK2 thus activate it, which activates ERK2 after phosphorylating ERK1 and/or ERK2. The subsequent events in the pathway are as described earlier. This pathway has extreme importance in cancer biology given that ~20% of all cancers have a RAS abnormality that leads to increased RAS-GTP:RAS-GDP ratios and RAS effective constitutive actions, with RAS-associated mutations occurring in codons 12, 13, or 6. As an example, G12C, G12V, and G12D substitutions are KRAS codon 12 mutations that account for 40%, 19%, and 15% of all KRAS mutations in NSCLC, respectively. Tumor suppressor genes CDKN2A/CDKN2B, TP53, or STK11 are frequent comutations and are also frequently found in KRAS-mutant tumors.

Difficulty exists in the targeting KRAS, considered the "undruggable target," denoting that no pharmacologically actionable small-binding pocket within RAS proteins could be made accessible as a result of the picomolar affinity of RAS proteins for GTP. In other words, high GTP intracellular concentrations make GTP-competitive RAS inhibitor drug development "unfeasible." Even though overcoming ATP binding to protein kinases is possible, their development necessitates significant binding properties for these small molecule inhibitors to overcome the picomolar affinity of RAS for GTP [6].

4.4 KRASG12C Inhibitors in the Clinic

The phase I/II CodeBreak 100 FIH study evaluated sotorasib in KRAS G12C mutant solid tumors ($n = 22$), which revealed a PR in 1/6 NSCLC patients. An ORR of 32.2% and a disease control rate (DCR) of 88.1% were demonstrated in 129 patients, and an mPFS of 6.3 months was demonstrated in 59 patients who developed advanced-stage NSCLC. In addition, 42 CRC patients had an ORR of 7.1%, a DCR of 73.8%, and an mPFS of 4.0 months. In the phase II portion, 124 evaluable advanced pretreated KRASG12C-mutant NSCLC patients had an mPFS of 6.8 months, an ORR of 37.1%, and an mOS of 12.5 months. These impressive results led to sotorasib's approval in 2021 for this patient population. The PDAC cohort in this study revealed an ORR of 21.1% and a DCR of 9.7%. In the phase III CodeBreaK 200 trial, the combination of sotorasib with docetaxel was evaluated in second-line KRASG12C-mutated NSCLC, and PFS served as the primary endpoint. Based on results from the phase I/II KRYSTAL trial, adagrasib was the second KRASG12C target to receive approval, revealing a PFS of 11.1 months in 16 patients in the phase 1/Ib part [6]. Another cohort within the phase II KRYSTAL-1, KRASG12C PDAC patients had an ORR of 50% and an mPFS of 6.6 months, and KRASG12C GI cancers had an ORR of 35%. Also, 45 CRC patients with the same mutation who were enrolled in the KRYSTAL-1 trial had a DCR of 87%, an ORR of 22%, and an mPFS of 5.6 months with adagrasib monotherapy.

- Entering clinical development are several other KRASG12C inhibitors that have similar mechanisms of action. Patients with advanced-stage KRASG12C solid tumors were enrolled in a phase I trial evaluating GDC-6036 (also known as RG6330)–kinase inhibitor) combinations in addition to the SHP2 inhibitor GDC-1971 and other monoclonal antibodies.
- JDQ443 is undergoing phase I/II trial evaluation as both monotherapy and in combination with TNO155 and is another covalent irreversible KRASG12C- off inhibitor that has demonstrated a favorable pharmacokinetic profile and potential antitumor activity in preclinical models.
- A phase III trial confirming the antitumor activity of JDQ443 is also underway featuring NSCLC patients treated with docetaxel who had prior treatment with KRASG12C-mutant inhibitors (and also in combination with KontRASt-02). Additionally, other JDQ443-based combination therapies are being tested in phase I/II platform studies for other tumor types.
- LY3537982, a selective KRASG12C inhibitor, is in development for KRASG12C-mutant tumors as monotherapy and in combination with other agents in phase I clinical studies.
- JNJ-74699157, D-1553, JAB-21822, BI 1823911, MK-1084, and numerous other inhibitors of KRASG12C fall under the category of KRASG12C- targeted compounds that are in phase I/II trials and includes other KRAS-mutant inhibitors that are in preclinical development [6].

4.5 Mechanisms of Resistance for KRAS Inhibitors and Overcoming Them

Considerable resistance to KRAS12GC inhibitors takes the form of primary, acquired, and adaptive resistance. Primary resistance, the least well understood, is postulated to result from mutational heterogeneity and comutations. Acquired resistance is also called de novo resistance, being undetectable before therapy. Amino acid residues in the 12, 68, 95, and 96 positions are implicated in acquired resistance, examples being Y96D mutations that lead to clinical resistance to adagrasib by interfering with its binding thanks to switch 2 pocket alterations. Liquid biopsy analysis at baseline and the time of disease progression in NSCLC and CRC revealed acquired molecular mutations in 19 out of 67 patients, or 28% of patients, and 33 out of 45 patients, or 73% of patients, respectively. Patients who were resistant to adagrasib were analyzed for secondary KRAS mutations, and the study investigators found the mutations H95D/Q/R, G13D, Y96C, G12D/R/V/W, Q61H, or R68S in nine patients, or 23% of patients, or that they existed with loss-of-function mutations in PTEN and NF1, MET and KRASG12C, and amplifications; with oncogenic fusions involving RET, FGFR3, ALK, RAAF1, and BRAF; and with activating mutations in NRAS, BRAF, MAP2K1, and RET. As the review authors note, the switch 2 pocket of KRASG12C implicated in adagrasib resistance was shown through in vitro validation studies to confirm R68S, Y96C, and H95D/Q/R second-site mutations.

In contrast, in patients resistant to adagrasib, sotorasib-sensitive double mutants with G12C/H95R, G12C/H95D, and G12C/H95Q double mutants are still sensitive to treatment, leading to benefits from this agent, even when factoring in considerations of common cross-resistance mechanisms. Secondary mutations strongly associated with resistance to KRAS inhibitors include the R68S, C12F, Y96C, and H95D/R mutations that were found after a mutagenesis screen of greater than 3500 mutations in KRASG12C was performed in an H358 cell line that contained KRASG12C in one allele and KRASWT in the other allele [6].

Adaptive resistance involves RAS-MAPk pathway reactivation due to the derepression of the MYC target. An example is the activation of wild-type HRAS and NRAS in KRASG12C-mutated solid tumor cell lines, which leads to the adaptive resistance to sotorasib. According to Punekar et al., BRAF and MEK inhibitor combinations for melanoma are representative of vertical inhibition with promising survival outcomes; however, they incur resistance. In turn, horizontal combinations are shown through targeting parallel pathways, and these also lead to resistance and to unacceptable toxicity [6]. Vertical combinations include sotorasib combined with EGFR TKIs such as afatinib or the anti-EGFR monoclonal antibody panitumumab. The former combination was evaluated in the CodeBreaK 101 trial and presented with a favorable safety profile, with only diarrhea and nausea reported as treatment-related adverse events (TRAEs) in 69.7% and 21.2% of patients (grade 3 or greater in 21.2% and 0%), respectively. An ORR of 20.0% and a DCR of 79.0% were observed in the one-dose cohort, with stable disease (SD) in three of five patients with prior sotorasib monotherapy. Another vertical therapy approach is seen in KRYSTAL-1 and KRYSTAl-10, where adagrasib is combined with cetuximab and adagrasib is combined with afatinib in NSCLC patients. Also, some have suggested that KRAS-mutant cancers could be served by using SHP2 inhibition as a result of its effects on JAK-STAT signaling in KRAS-independent pathways.

After many years of preclinical development, potent, highly selective, and bioavailable inhibitors of SHP2 are now undergoing clinical testing. On the basis of this evaluation, the KRYSTAL-2 trial is underway evaluating TNO155 in combination with adagrasib, and sotorasib was investigated in CodeBreak 101 with KontRASt-01 andn JDQ443. CodeBreaK 101 is also investigating sototasib as a combination therapy with RMC-4360 (a SHP2 inhibitor similar to RMC-4550) and various other KRASG12C and SHP2 inhibitors as well as trametinib with or without panitumumab in KRASG12C-mutant solid tumors. Inhibiting mTOR with KRAS inhibition is an example of a horizontal combination approach to overcome adaptive resistance. In pre-clinical models of PDAC, bypass signaling via integrin-linked kinase-mediated phosphorylation, which has been linked to KRAS inhibition through Rictor, a component of the mTOR complex 2 (mTORC2), entails the mTORC2-mediated phosphorylation of AKT.

The identification of KRAS mutations in lung cancer has led to the discovery of targeted therapy approaches, both as monotherapies and in combination, and further development through clinical investigation. Obstacles remain, though, in addressing the resistant, undruggable KRASG12C alteration, and the development of effective inhibitors remain ongoing. Resistance has led to modest outcomes for single-agent treatment, and many researchers advocate a reductionist approach to assess resistance effectively [6].

4.6 Breast Cancer

Early studies in precision medicine focused on the validity of using personalized medicine approaches for breast cancer. One review highlighted the complexity (terming it utopia or reality) and heterogeneity of breast cancer and the lack of determinacy in the clinical actionability of genomic testing for inherited mutations. Key findings indicate that tumor heterogeneity complicates treatment success, with variability in gene mutations affecting therapy outcomes. The study concludes that molecular subtyping and genomic analysis have revolutionized breast cancer management, offering new therapeutic targets and improving treatment strategies. Implications include the potential for personalized medicine to enhance patient outcomes by identifying specific biomarkers and developing targeted therapies, despite challenges posed by tumor heterogeneity (Fig. 4.4).

Data from this review showed that PARP inhibitors could be targeted therapies for TNBC, where clinical trials showed an RR of 54% in a cohort of patients on 400 mg of olaparib and 25% in a cohort of patients on 100 mg of olaparib. Additionally, the use of tumor-infiltrating lymphocytes (TILs) for breast cancer, currently the standard of care for advanced melanoma, was highlighted in which a TIL-rich tumors had a predictive effect for superior overall survival regardless of disease type, especially so in early TNBC, through a meta-analysis study that was conducted that analyzed data from 2987 patients with early-stage BC, which showed that TIL-rich tumors had associations with distant recurrence, a risk of recurrence, and death at 22%, 30%, and 34%, respectively [7].

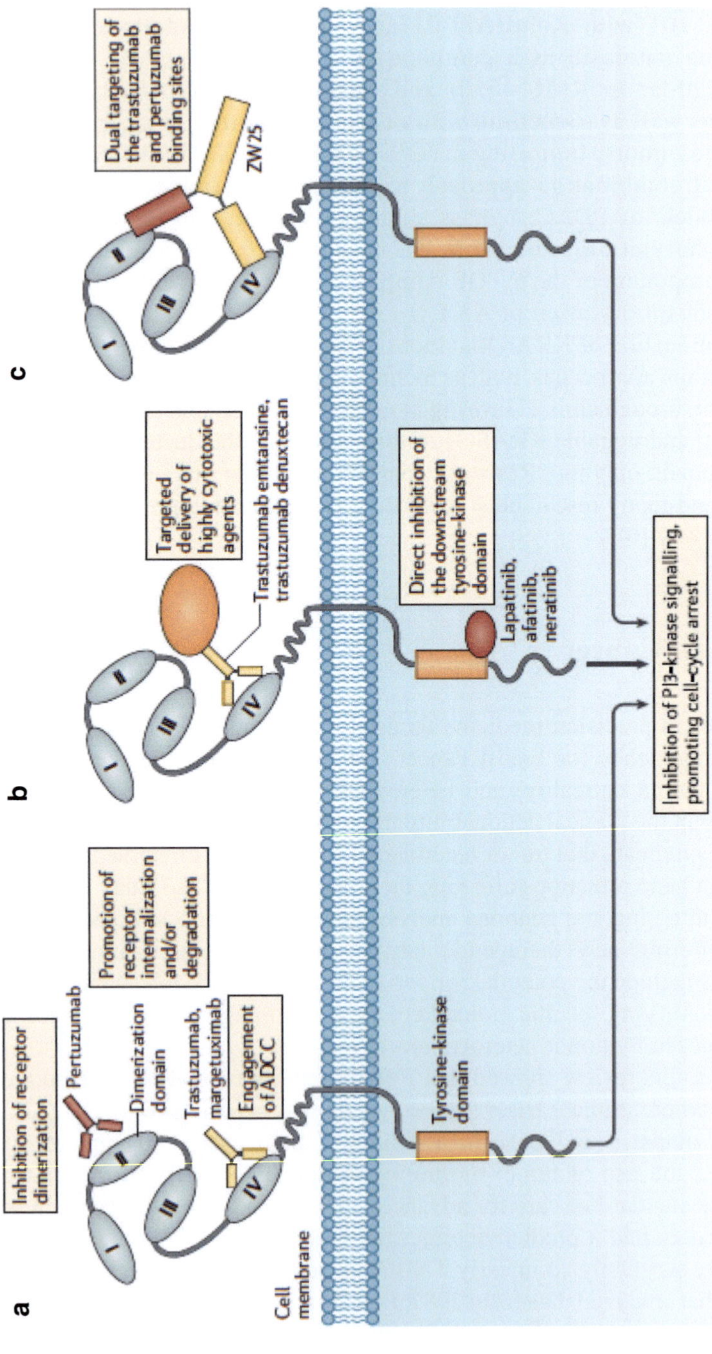

Fig. 4.4 Mechanism of action for HER2 targeted agents. (Adapted from Oh) [79]

The multicenter randomized phase II PACE trial did not lead to improved PFS in HR+/HER2 mBC patients who had disease progression on CDK4/6i with AI treatment when evaluating them while adding palbociclib to fulvestrant and avelumab after endocrine therapy with CDK4/6 inhibitor administration. Although CDK4/6 inhibitors are considered the standard of care, this study intended to determine whether "patients might derive benefit beyond initial progression to continue on therapy with treatment with CDK4/6." Kaplan–Meier curves showed an mPFS of 4.8 months on F, 4.6 months on F + P, and 8.1 months on F + P + A, with patients who had baseline ESR1 and PIK3CA mutations demonstrating a greater difference in PFS in F + P and F + P + A vs. F alone. The investigators concluded that no improvement in PFS was seen with the additive treatment of palbociclib to fulvestrant versus endocrine treatment in this patient population who had progressed on CDK4/6 inhibitors [8].

Updated results from the monarchE trial for HR+/HER2- high-risk early breast cancer (EBC) showed that adjuvant abemaciclib plus endocrine therapy (ET) resulted in persistent disease-free and invasive disease-free survival in patients beyond a 2-year treatment period. Of the 5637 patients, the intention-to-treat (ITT) population showed a sustained abemaciclib benefit for distant relapse-free survival (DRFS), as was demonstrated in sustained hazard ratios (HRs) of 0.680 (95% CI 0.599–0.772) and 0.675 (95% CI 0.588–0.774). The persistent benefit of abemaciclib translated into the consistent separation of survival curves with deep improvement in DRFS and IDFS rates, namely 6.7% and 7.6%, respectively, with fewer deaths in the abemaciclib plus ET arm when compared with ET monotherapy (208 vs. 234) and with no statistical significance being reached in overall survival (OS). The investigators concluded that the benefit of further administration of abemaciclib in high-risk EBC patients was seen for patients treated with abemaciclib and ET, with decreased risk of treatment in terms of a reduced risk of invasive and distant disease recurrence [9].

FDA approval was recently announced for the PARP inhibitor talazoparib, approved for advanced breast cancer, and was evaluated in the double-blind randomized trial TALAPRO-2 for treating homologous recombination repair (HRR)–mutated metastatic castration-resistant prostate cancer (mCRPC) in combination with enzalutamide. Furthermore, mCRPC patients ($n = 1035$) stratified according to mHRR were randomized into two cohorts to be administered enzalutamide with talazoparib or placebo. The primary endpoint in cohort 1 was rPFS, consisting of all comers and all homologous recombination repair mutation gene (HRRm) patients in cohorts 1 and 2 or the combined HRRm population. OS served as the secondary endpoint. Even though a statistically significant improvement was seen (HR = 0.53 (95% CI 0.51–0.78)), the FDA did not consider the radiographic progression free survival (rPFS) improvement clinically meaningful, although approval was limited to HRRm with rPFS improvements and favorable OS results. The authors state that this was the "first approval for the first-line treatment of HRRm mCRPC patients" [10].

An ASCO guideline recommendation update was issued in 2024 on CDK4/6 inhibitors and optimal adjuvant chemotherapy for early breast cancer. These recommendations put forth that abemaciclib with endocrine therapy served as the preferred strategy in the treatment of high-risk EBC, whereas ribociclib with ET treatment was recommended in EBC. The monarchE and NATALEE trial provided evidence for these regimens, which have been met with FDA approval. In the ITT monarchE population for HR+/HER2- early breast cancer, treatment for 2 years with abemaciclib plus ET may be provided for patients meeting the eligibility criteria of having a high risk of recurrence and positive axillary lymph node. ASCO also recommended for patients with stage II and III breast cancer that have a high risk of recurrence that "adjuvant ribociclib (400 mg once daily, 3 weeks on, followed by 1 week off) for 3 years with ET be administered on the basis of the phase III NATALEE trial" [11].

ET with or without the mTOR inhibitor everolimus had efficacy in high-risk HR+ early-stage BC in a phase III randomized study, resulting in improvements in PFS when combined with ET. TAMRAD investigated the combination treatment of tamoxifen with everolimus, showing improvement in PFS and OS. BOLERO-2 evaluated exemestane + everolimus among patients previously treated with aromatase inhibitor (AI), demonstrating improvement in PFS. In that study, 1939 patients, with 1792 eligible for analysis, were randomly assigned 1:1 and were stratified according to risk group, with invasive disease-free survival being the primary endpoint. The secondary endpoints were OS and safety. The study showed that when everolimus was added to ET, it did not result in improvements in iDFS or OS. No difference was seen in iDFS (HR 1.08 (95% CI 0.86–1.36)), or OS (HR 1.19 (95% CI 0.89–1.6)) among postmenopausal patients (n = 1221). Among 571 premenopausal patients, everolimus improved both OS (HR 0.49 (95% CI 0.28–0.86)) and IDFS (HR 0.64 (95% CI 0.44–0.94)), although higher grade 3 and 4 events were seen as outcomes. The authors concluded that adjuvant everolimus + ET treatment for 1 year did not improve overall outcomes but suggested that treatment in patients who are still premenopausal after chemotherapy could receive mTOR inhibition [12].

YES1 has transformative qualities in lung and breast epithelia, as shown in in vitro assays such as analysis by Western blot, which demonstrated that when overexpression was induced in YES1, it led to tyrosine (Y357) phosphorylation, but not on serine 127 on the YAP1 protein, thereby indicating that YAP1 was not turned on. YES1 overexpression was induced, and this led to the promotion of the YAP1 translocating to the nucleus. The knockdown of YAP1 in YES-1 overexpressing cells through si-RNA-mediated mechanisms led to YAP1 depletion with no effect on the phosphorylation status of SRC family of kinases (SFK)s, but eliminated EGF-independent growth in YES1-overexpressing MCF10A and human bronchial epithelial cells (HBECs) and led to increased sensitivity to dasatinib, suggesting that the amplification of YES1 functions is a primary oncogenic driver in breast and lung cancer in a YAP1-dependent manner. Also, in vitro assays, AP1 plays a factor in YES-1 mediated resistance to EGFR and ALK TKIs. Sensitivity to ALK and EGFR TKIs was fully restored in YAP1-overexpressing cells, which in turn abrogated Y357 phosphorylation. A Y357 mutant of YAP1 was also generated, leading to the elimination of the YES1 phosphorylation site, and as the investigators concluded, Y357F mutant expression observed in cells led to the detection of decreased YAP1 phosphorylation on Y357. One of the more important points is that the overexpression of YAP1 leads to phosphorylation by YES1 of Y357 and full resistance.

The following set of experiments focused on how SFKs and primary drivers could overcome resistance to anaplastic lymphoma kinase (LK) TKIs and EGFR mediated by YES1 or the overexpression of YAP1 through dual pharmacological inhibition. Dasatinib is an FDA-approved inhibitor of c-KIT, ABL, and SRC and has considerable potent activity against mutant EGFR, and it was selected for evaluation in EGFRm cell lines. Repotrectinib was evaluated in ALK+ cell lines as an inhibitor that has activity against many SFKs, including YES1, and was developed to overcome ROS1, ALK, and TRK solvent front mutations.

- EGFRm cell lines with either YAP1 or YES1 overexpression showed equal sensitivity to dasatinib when compared to parental cell lines.
- In parental H3122 cells, YES1-overexpressing or YAP1-overexpressing ALK+ showed equal sensitivity to alectinib.
- YES1/YAP1/HIPPO signaling drives acquired resistance (AR) and ARSFK inhibition may be exploited for targeted therapy-driven treatment for primary tumorigenesis.
- Results demonstrate that SFK inhibition in AR driven by YES1/YAP1 signaling while targeting primary tumorigenesis has therapeutic potential [13].

In the AMEERA-5 trial, a randomized phase III study, the oral ER1 degrader amcenestrant inhibits ER pathway signaling (the other approved agents in this class being fulvestrant and elacestrant). Amcenestrant plus palbociclib was evaluated vs. palbociclib and letrozole in ER+/HER2- patients with advanced BC. Preliminary results revealed in patients assigned in a 1:1 ratio to the amcenetrant "(200 mg once daily) + standard palbociclib" dosage (125 mg/once daily) or letrozole 2.5 mg daily + standard palbociclib that PFS was 82.7% (6 month) in the A+P+L cohort versus 86.9% in the L+P cohort without A. TEAEs occurred in 85.6% vs. 85.4% of patients, with 46.3% vs. 60.8% being grade 3 or higher. The authors explain that the drug–drug interaction of A+P may have contributed to the findings as a result of decreased exposure to the CDK4/6 agent [14].

The RIGHT choice trial conducted in 13 countries was an open-label phase II study that revealed a set of results for advanced HR+/HER2- BC that manifested with clinical aggression in premenopausal women versus combination chemotherapy (CT) rates (capecitabine plus vinorelbine, paclitaxel plus gemcitabine, and docetaxel plus capecitabine). In the ribocliclib arm where patients received 600 mg once per day on a 3-week-on, 1-week-off schedule, the ORR was 66.1% and 61.8% and the median time to response was 4.9 months and 3.2 months, respectively [15].

Batalini et al. conducted a real-world analysis of breast cancer tumor samples through comprehensive genomic profiling; gPALB2, gBRCA, and sBRCA testing; and HRD biomarker testing on these samples. The study found that HRD was detected in 21% of patients with mBC.

Key Results

- "177 patients on PARPi were assessed for outcomes, with similarity in gBRCA and sBRCA/gPALB2 cohorts: gBRCA versus sBRCA/gPALB2
- rwPFS: 6.3 vs. 5.4 months (hazard ratio [HR], 1.37 [0.77–2.43])
- rwOS: 16.2 vs. 21.2 months (HR, 1.45 [0.74–2.86])
- patients with HRDsig+ vs. HRDsig–:
  longer rwPFS (6.3 vs. 2.8 months; HR, 0.62 [0.42–0.92]),
  numerically longer rwOS (17.8 vs. 13.0 months; HR, 0.72 [0.46–1.14])."

The results showed the improved survival outcomes of PARP inhibitors for mBC patients, and significantly, patients with gPALB2 and sBRCA derive comparable benefit from PARPi as those with gBRCA mutations, with the implication that testing for the presence of HRD signature biomarkers (in the context of a complex HRD gene alteration landscape) would benefit a larger cohort [16].

CDK4/6 inhibitors were evaluated in a study with the status of beyond progression (BP) against HR+/HER2- mBC patients receiving upfront CDK4/6 inhibitors in an analysis of real-world biomarkers through this retrospective study (Fig. 4.5). The ESR1 alteration that was detected through ctDNA was found to be predictive of negative clinical outcomes, measured according to HR, PFS, and mPFS.

Key Results

- "The significance of CDK4/6i BP was retained (HR, 0.54; 95% CI 0.35–0.83; $p = 0.005$) along with
- ESR1 SNVs (HR, 1.48; 95% CI 1.05–2.09; $p = 0.024$)
- TP53 SNVs (HR, 2.15; 95% CI 1.51–3.08; $p < 0.001$)
- For CDK4/6i BP, PFS was significantly worse (HR, 1.99; 95% CI 1.34–2.97; $p = 0.001$; log-rank test; $P = 0.0005$)
- Upfront CDK4.6i mPFS was 15.9 months (vs. 10.23 months for CDK4/6i BP)
  - PFS rates at 6 and 12 months were 79% and 61%, respectively."

The investigators concluded that PFS and OS rates play integral parts in the approach of CDK4/6i BP for positive progression-free survival and overall survival for patients harboring ESR1 mutations and that the characterization of biomarkers will be important for constructing and guiding clinical decision algorithms and designing sequence strategies [17].

Brett et al. identified in patients with ESR1-mutated breast cancer who had progressed on prior CDK4/6i the utility of abemaciclib through a gene panel. ESR1-mutated tumors are associated with resistance after progressive disease on abemaciclib and CDK4/6 therapies. Questions surrounding post-administration therapy after this resistance are ongoing. A retrospective multicenter cohort study was conducted on mBC patients with ESR1 mutations who received abemaciblib after progressing disease on ET plus palbociclib.

Key Methods The following retrospective multicenter study enrolled a cohort of patients with ESR1-MUT MBC who were receiving abemaciclib and who had disease progression after treatment on ET plus palbociclib:

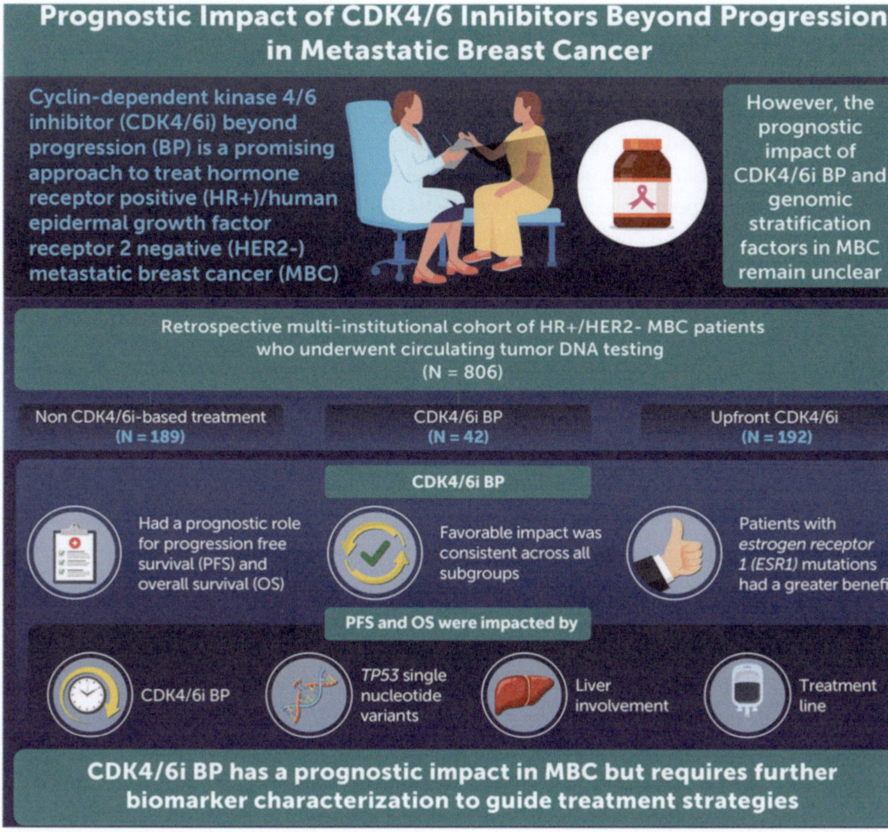

Fig. 4.5 Prognostic impact of CDK4/6 inhibitors. (Adapted from Gerratana) [17]

- "After comparing abemaciclib PFS in patients with mutations (CDKi-R[–] vs. CDKi-R[+]), investigators generated a panel of CDK4/6i resistance genes.
- Using patient-derived circulating tumor cell lines, they showed that ESR1-MUT and CDKi-R mutations affected sensitivity to abemaciclib."

Key Results

- PD on ET plus palbociclib in ESR1-MUT mBC:
- For mPFS, CDKi-R(−) ($n = 17$) was 7.0 months vs. CDKi-R(+) ($n = 11$), which was 3.5 months; HR 2.8.
- CDKi-R mutations induced resistance to abemaciclib, but were not associated with resistance to CTCs invitro in immortalized breast cancer cell; however, ESR1-MUT was not implicated.
- Longer PFS is associated with abemaciclib; CDKi-R(−) is associated with abemaciclib resistance, whereas ESR1-MUT mBC after receiving palbociclib did not cause abemaciclib resistance.

One of factors motivating the study was that even though abemaciclib is also validated as a monotherapy, palbociclib and ribociclib differ from each other both pharmacokinetically and pharmacodynamically, leading to potential therapeutic activity in the setting of abemaciclib resistance.

The authors found that the CDK4/6i resistance alterations in a multigene panel generated a prognostic signature for PFS in abemaciclib-treated HR+/HER2- MBC patients in a retrospective cohort in the post-CDK4/6i treatment setting with ESR1 mutations, showing the significance of a multigene approach over the use of a single gene marker. The panel consisted of genes involved in cell-cycle regulation, such as CCNE2, RB1, CCNE1, and AURKA, and signaling pathways involving growth factors (FGFR1, FGFR2, ERBB2, PTEN, AKT1, and FAT1) [18].

4.7 Lung Cancer

Osimertinib had CNS efficacy with or without chemotherapy that was determined for EGFR mutant advanced NSCLC (aNSCLC). Results were reported from the phase III FLAURA2 trial. In that trial, 30–50% of advanced NSCLC patients develop metastatic CNS disease within 5 years of diagnosis, and their detection rates are improving with survival and enhanced detection. Osimertinib is a third-generation irreversible oral EGFR TKI that targets the T790M mutation. Randomly assigned patients with at least one CNS lesion and patients with baseline CNS metastasis or CNS progression or death had an HR of 0.67 (95% CI 0.43–1.04). CNS ORRs were 69% monotherapy (Osimertinib alone) and 73% in the combination group (Osimertinib plus platinum-pemetrexed); CNS complete response was seen in 59% versus 43% of patients, respectively. The study authors concluded that the CNS combination therapy, regardless of baseline CNS metastasis, delayed CNS progression [19].

The phase II EORTC LCG-1613 APPLE trial reported on OS results for advanced EGFR mutant NSCLC patients receiving Osimertinib versus gefitinib followed by Osimertinib, which is considered the standard of care; however, this sequential approach has not been evaluated at the time of progression. In that trial, 73% of patients crossed over to Osimertinib; upfront treatment versus the sequential treatment was associated with a lower risk of brain progression, with comparable OS demonstrated between both groups (HR, 1.01 (90% CI 0.61–1.68)). The study authors concluded that sequential treatment in advanced EGFR mutant NSCLC patients is associated with more-frequent brain progression [20].

KRASG12C mutated NSCLC tumors demonstrated targetability to sotorasib in a real-world study that identified the KEAP mutation as a comutation associated with resistance as a result of shorter real-world overall survival (rwOS) and OS in a patient cohort previously treated with anti-PD-L1 therapy that also experienced grade 3 adverse events, as revealed in a fascinating study in *JCO PO* by Thummapalli et al. Results include a 12.6-month median OS, a 5.3-month median rwPFS, and a 28% real-world response rate with manageable toxicity profiles. Clinical data, including NGS results, were reported, and genomic data presenting the occurrence of STK11, KEAP11, and TP53 comutations were identified though tissue ctDNA and NGS analysis as well as TMB biomarkers, along with the immunohistochemistry (IHC) results of PD-L1 expression when available. A fascinating part of this study is that toxicity to prior PD-L1 therapy was observed, and aspects of this were identified. In specific, 25 patients, or 29% of patients, who had prior anti-PD-L1 exposure experienced an immune related adverse event (iRAE); however, the investigators noted an association between the sotorasib initiation and proximity of the last dose of anti-PD-L1 treatment and adverse event development after sotorasib treatment. 13 of 14 cases of sotorasib TRAE-related treatment discontinuation and 15 of 16 cases of G3+ sotorasib TRAEs were seen among patients with prior exposure to anti-PD-L1 treatment within 12 weeks of sotorasib treatment initiation. Hepatoxicity was an adverse event treated with systemic steroids. This led to how the sequencing of sotorasib initiation would be managed in the clinical setting in KRASG12C mutated tumors. The KEAP coalteration was a marker of resistance, which would lead to the development of stratification factors in "future randomized clinical trials" [21].

Selpercatinib has been approved for RET-fusion-positive NSCLC and serves as a potent RET kinase inhibitor. Serial CNS scans derived from the randomized phase III trial LIBRETTO-431 were analyzed, which tested the treatment versus pemetrexed with or without pembrolizumab. The incidence of CNS metastasis was reduced with this agent and chemotherapy, with an HR of 0.17 (95% CI 0.04–0.69), demonstrating a protective effect while delaying CNS metastasis. The median time to intracranial response was 1.4 months, whereas DOR had not yet been reached. Patients without previous CNS radiotherapy had an IRR of 93.3% (14/15) with the agent vs. 64.3% (9/14) without, and a more common intracranial response (93%) was observed in those without prior therapy than in those with prior therapy (50%) [22].

Taletrectinib, a CNS-active TKI with activity against the ROS1 mutation, demonstrated positive prolonged PFS and overall responses, activity in intracranial lesions and also against acquired resistance mutations, and a tolerable safety profile, as reported in the recent TRUST-1 study in *JCO*. With DOR, cORR was the primary endpoint, and PFS and safety were the secondary endpoints. Furthermore, 173 patients were enrolled (TKI naive (n = 106)): 73% had never smoked, and 67 had prior crizotinib pretreatment. Also, cORR and intracranial cORR were 91% and 88%, respectively, in TKI patients and 52% and 73%, respectively, in patients who were treated with crizotinib. In TKI-naive patients, mDOR and mPFS were not reached. Also, mPFS was 7.6 months (95% CI 5.5–12.0 months), and median DOR was 10.6 months (95% CI 6.3 months to NR) in crizotinib-treated patients. Eight of 12 patients, or 67% of them, with G2032R mutations responded. TEAEs included increased ALT (68%), increased aspartate aminotransferase (AST) (76%), and diarrhea (70%), which were mostly grade 1. The study authors concluded that taletrectinib showed tolerable safety and durable efficacy in Chinese patients with ROS1+ NSCLC with prolonged PFS and activity against intracranial lesions [23].

In a phase I study, neoadjuvant therapy targeting the EGFR exon 21 p.L858R mutation was evaluated. The targeted treatment Osimertinib is an EGFR TKI and is the standard of care for mNSCLC. Numerous benefits and risks come with neoadjuvant therapy, including the potential for a shorter duration of therapy, the opportunity for prior exposure to treating micrometastasis, and the risk incurring treatment-related AEs and tumor progression. A total of 27 patients entered a multi-institutional phase II trial prior to surgical resection. Major pathologic response was the primary endpoint and was 14.8% (95% CI 4.2–33.7). CPR was not observed. Patients did not have AEs or experience surgical delays. TP53 (42%) and RBM10 (21%) were the tumor genomic alterations that were stipulated as being factors in limiting PR to neoadjuvant treatment, which were observed to not occur on the basis of tumor stage and mutation subtype. The investigators also assessed changes in transcription within tumors at residual disease and found an increase in WNT/beta-catenin activity. YAP upregulation was also observed, whereas other studies showed that RELA, a NF-kappaB transcription factor, and ILS were also upregulated, which drove EGFR persistence. Despite the positive results in transcriptional activity mediating EGFR persistence with no real safety concerns, the trial was determined to be negative, not achieving a major pathologic response (MPR) rate of 50% with the administration of neoadjuvant Osimertinib treatment, and would not necessarily validate the use of treatment in the neoadjuvant treatment, unlike the positive responses seen in the FLAURA trial, where neoadjuvant treatment was correlated with ameliorated disease free survival (DFS), event free survival (EFS), and OS in patients not achieving a greater than 50% MPR [24].

The phase III CROWN study evaluating treatment for ALK-positive NSCLC found that lorlatinib improved PFS and intracranial activity in previously untreated patients. In a study reported in *JCO*, long-term outcomes were reported in a follow-up study. ALK TKIs are considered standard therapy in first-line settings, and lorlatinib, a brain-penetrant third-generation ALK -TKI, is superior to second-generation ALK inhibitors for ALK-resistant tumors. PFS by Response Evaluation Criteria in Solid Tumors (RECIST) served as the primary endpoint, and OS served as the secondary endpoint. Molecular profiling was conducted through a 74-gene ctDNA NGS assay. Here, 296 patients received either crizotinib ($n = 147$) or lorlatinib ($n = 149$). The efficacy results were as follows: mPFS was NR in the lorlatinib cohort (95% CI 64.1 to NR) and 9.1 months in the crizotinib group (95% CI 7.4–64.3). HR was 0.08 for disease progression or death for lorlatinib vs. crizotinib in baseline brain metastatic patients. Also, mPFS in lorlatinib vs. crizotinib was NR (95% CI 32.9 to NR) vs. 6.0 months (95% CI 3.7–7.6). According to an investigator assessment, the time to intracranial progression reported an HR of 0.06 (95% CI 0.03–0.12) (longer with lorlatinib vs. crizotinib). Weight gain (23% vs. 2%), hypertriglyceridemia (25% vs. 0%), hypertension (12% vs. 1%), and any-grade CV AE was reported in 42 of 149 patients (28% in the lorlatinib cohort vs. 40 out of 142 (28%) in the crizotinib cohort). The study investigators concluded that these results signaled an "unprecedented outcome for patients with advanced ALK-positive NSCLC," showing prolonged intracranial efficacy without any new safety signals [25].

CNS-penetrant TKIs were evaluated in NSCLC patients with ALK and EGFR mutations with and without stereotactic radiosurgery in TURBO-NSCLC, a multi-institutional retrospective analysis. Out of 317 patients identified there were 200 receiving TKI (Osimertinib and alectinib) only and 117 receiving TKI + SRS. Patients in the latter group were more likely to have brain metastasis (BM) ($p < 0.001$) and neurologic symptoms, suggesting that this subgroup may benefit from upfront SRS ($p < 0.001$) with similar median OS. The cumulative incidence curves of local CNS progression were 12 mo for the TKI cohort versus 24 mo for the TKI + SRS cohort. Local CNS control was significantly improved with TKI + SRS (HR 0.30 (95% CI (0.16–0.55)). The study authors proposed that this may be the only large study comparing these two treatment modalities that leads to improved CNS progression and local control in treatment-naive CNS-penetrant EGFR and ALK-driven NSCLC with the addition of upfront SRS [26].

Resistance to EGFR-driven mutations in targeted therapies was reported by Giustini et al. EGFR mutations, which occur in exon 19 deletions and the mutated L858R, are some of the most targetable alterations in NSCLC, with relapse after Osimertinib first-line therapy, and known mechanisms include secondary EGFR mutation, MET amplification, cell-cycle gene alterations, and PIK-3 pathway activations.

The reasons underlying the resistance to therapy to an established first-line agent such as Osimertinib for EGFR-mutated NSCLC may lie within how these acquired drivers of oncogenesis lead to tumor heterogeneity. The study authors posit that the "subclones of resistance mechanisms" arise from selective pressure leading to the administration of combination therapies that would be indicated by postprogression biopsies [27] (Table 4.2).

According to another report on Osimertinib resistance, the underlying mutation is the intergenic ANK3-RET fusion, as evidenced by acquired RET fusions that drive further oncogenesis. However, this mutation is targetable given that the patient harboring the mutation has shown durable responses to a Osimertinib (40 mg once

Table 4.2 The initial treatment of resistant patients and response

Patient	Resistant mutation	Therapy with progression	Post-resistant therapy	Clinical Response after post-resistant therapy
D: 65-year-old man	Developed BRAF V600E mutations	Progression on Osimertinib	Combination of Osimertinib, dabrafenib, and trametinib	Remained on treatment for 23 months while using oligoprogression therapy
E: 56-year-old man	Developed BRAFV600E mutations	Progression on Osimertinib	Combination of Osimertinib, dabrafenib, and trametinib	Clinical deterioration
G: 57-year-old woman	Developed BRAF V600E, N581S mutations	Progression on Osimertinib	Combination of Osimertinib, dabrafenib, and trametinib	PR ongoing

Adapted from Guistini et al. [27]

daily) and pralsetinib (200 mg once daily) combination (12 months, SD after 5 months of treatment), with primary tumor regression and the disappearance of liver metastasis. Two of the unique aspects of this case report are the use of RNA-NGS for detecting the gene fusions and the fact that the complementary RNA-NGS delivered clinically actionable targets such as METex14 after the prospective genomic profiling of 2522 lung adenocarcinomas, which were undetectable through DNA-NGS [28].

A study by Ambrosini showed that the ALK mutation, commonly found in NSCLC, has shown clinical potential in GI cancers through analysis of a molecular case series and an international dataset. ALK rearrangements were detected through NGS, IHC, and fluorescence in situ hybridization (FISH). Tumor samples were stratified according to histology with PFS and evidence of SD as primary endpoints. ORR was determined to be the total of complete and partial responders divided by the number of evaluable patients. DCR was the sum of ORR plus the ratio of between disease stabilizations and the total number of evaluable patients. First-line ALK agents alectinib, crizotinib, and entrectinib were the selected targeted agents, with lorlatinib as the further line agent. Response dynamics and best response were determined according to the primary tumor site and targeted agent. The median follow-up time was 39.6 months. At the time of data cutoff date, all patients experienced progressive disease to first-line ALKi or death, whereas 11 (85%) died. Moreover, mPFS and mOS were 5.0 months (95% CI 3.68 to no response) and 9.3 months (95% CI 5.46 to no response), respectively. The authors suggested that NGS and comprehensive genomic profiling would be implemented for the treatment of GI cancers. Despite being rare in other nonlung solid tumors and GI, "ALK translocations represent an important therapeutic target." The study authors concluded that patients "with GI malignancies harboring ALK translocations are at risk of being neglected and excluded from a personalized treatment that could have significant impact on their cancer" [29].

Genetic testing for the NTRK fusion was suggested by one study in lung cancer patients. One such agent targeting NTRK fusions, larotrectinib, was shown to extend survival benefit, have rapid and durable responses, be highly active, and have favorable long-term safety profiles. In a cohort of 20 patients, of which 15 were evaluable, ORR results included "73% (95% CI 45–92); one (7%) patient had a CR, 10 (67%) had a PR three (20%) had SD, and one (7%) had PD as best response. The median DOR, PFS, and OS were 33.9 months (95% CI 5.6–33.9), 35.4 months (95% CI 5.3–35.4), and 40.7 months (95% CI 17.2 to not estimable), respectively."

- The ORR was as follows among patients with baseline CNS metastasis: 63% (95% CI 25–91).
- Waterfall plots revealed tumor regression, with a 70–100% change in target lesions ($n = 4$). Swimmer plots revealed durable response between 27–54 months among five patients.
- At a median follow-up of 17.4 months, mDoR was 33.9 months (95% CI 5.6–33.9).

- At 12 and 24 months, the DoR rates were 81% and 65%, respectively.
- The mPFS was 35.4 months (95% CI 5.3–35.4), at a median follow-up of 16.6 months.
- At a median follow-up of 16.2 months, the mOS was 40.7 months (95% CI 17.2 to not estimable).
- The OS rates at 12 months and 24 months were 86% and 75%, respectively. The study also revealed CNS benefit with lower rates of brain metastasis and CNS disease control and efficacy among the treatment population, with or without prior systemic therapy [30].

Advanced lung cancer patients also underwent a similar combination therapy regimen with pertuzumab and trastuzumab with ERBB2 amplification (13 ERBB2 oncogenic mutations, insertions, or deletions: S310F, D769H, D769Y, G309A, G309E, L755S, V777L, V842I, E321G, R896C, R678Q, P780ins, and del L755-T759) in reporting results from the TAPUR study. Patients were treated with "pertuzumab once every 3 weeks with an initial dose of 840 mg intravenous (IV) infusion over 60 minutes followed by additional doses of 420 mg IV infusion over 30–60 minutes; and trastuzumab once every 3 weeks with an initial dose of 8 mg/kg IV infusion over 90 minutes followed by additional doses of 6 mg/kg IV infusion over 30–60 minutes." OR per RECIST vs. 1.1 or SD at least 16+ weeks of duration served as the primary endpoint of disease control (DC). PFS, OS, DoR, and SD duration served as secondary endpoints [31].

Key Results
From November 2016 to July 2020, 28 patients with NSCLC ($n = 27$) and SCLC ($n = 1$) with ERBB amplification ($n = 12$) were enrolled, and all patients were evaluable for efficacy and toxicity.

- The OR rate of 11% (95% CI 2–28) and the DR rate of 37% (95% CI 21–50) were observed in three patients with PR (two ERBB2 mutation; one both amplification and mutation) and seven patients with SD16+ (two amplifications, five ERBB2 mutations).
- Five patients experienced grade 3 or 4 A or serious AEs that were possibly related to the pertuzumab and trastuzumab regimen.

The investigators concluded that in advanced lung cancer with ERBB2 amplification and exon 20 insertion mutation, the combination therapy showed evidence of antitumor activity [32].

In the HER2CLIMB randomized clinical trial, tucatinib was evaluated versus placebo in previously treated ERBB2-positive mBC with brain metastases. Highly specific for ERBB2, tucatinib is a small molecule inhibitor with a 1000-fold specificity for EGFR. When combined with capecitabine and trastuzumab, tucatinib has favorable efficacy and safety profiles. ERBB2-positive BC is frequently associated with poor prognosis, with more than 50% of patients developing brain metastases (BMs). This combination has reported positive intracranial outcomes, however.

According to the report, HER2CLIMB is a double-blind, randomized, placebo-controlled clinical trial in an international and multicenter setting that is evaluating tucatinib in combination with capecitabine and trastuzumab. Clinical endpoints include DOR-IC and ORR-IC in patients that at baseline have measurable intracranial disease. In the subgroup analysis, at 29.6 months of median follow-up, the mOS was 21.6 months (95% CI 18.1–28.5) in the tucatinib-combination group and 12.5 months (95% CI 11.2–16.9) in the placebo-combination group, where the former was 9.1 months longer. The combination arm showed improvement. A risk reduction of developing new brain lesions was also observed in those with BM, with improved OS. The DOR-IC was 8.6 months (95% CI 5.5–10.3 months) 3.0 months (95% CI 3.0–10.3 months) in the tucatinib-combination group and in the placebo-combination group, respectively.

Key Results

- Patients with active BM at baseline
- mOS:
  21.4 months in the tucatinib-combination group
  11.8 months (95% CI 18.1–28.9 vs. 10.3–15.2 months) in the placebo-combination group
- In the tucatinib-combination group, the mOS was reported as being 9.6 months longer.
- Estimated 1-year OS:
  Tucatinib-combination group: 70.7% (95% CI 61.5%–78.1%)
  Placebo-combination group and: 46.4% (95% CI 33.1%–58.8%)
- Estimated 2-year OS was for two groups.
  Tucatinib-combination group: 48.9%
  Placebo-combination group: 21.4% (95% CI 39.4%–57.8%; 95% CI 11.8%–32.9%)
- A 47.6% risk of reduction in death was observed in the tucatinib-combination cohort versus the placebo-combination cohort (HR 0.52 (95% CI 0.36–0.77)).
- Intracranial responses CNS-PFS
  - In patients with brain metastases, tucatinib led to maintained CNS-PFS benefit with a longer follow-up.
  - In the tucatinib-combination group, mCNS-PFS was 5.7 months longer than in the placebo-combination cohort for all patients.
  - The mCNS-PFS for patients with active BMs was as follows:
    9.6 months for the tucatinib-combination cohort
    4.0 months for the placebo-combination cohort

The study reported that intracranial responses CNS-PFS were 5.6 months longer in the tucatinib-combination cohort.

Among the entire ITT cohort, the tucatinib-combination group had a median new brain lesion-free survival of 11.1 months longer than the placebo group: 24.9 months to 13.8 months, respectively. The study authors also observed that the tucatinib arm was associated with a lower risk of deteriorating quality of life and was also well tolerated. They concluded that the combination treatment of tucatinib and capecitabine remains a viable treatment option for previously treated ERBB2-positive mBC patients developing BMs [33].

In a study titled "Efficacy of Endocrine Therapy Plus Trastuzumab and Pertuzumab vs. De-escalated Chemotherapy in Patients with Hormone Receptor–Positive/ERBB2-Positive Early Breast Cancer: The NeoadjuvantWSG-TP-II Randomized Clinical Trial," Gluz et al. performed a comparison of neoadjuvant ERBB2 blockade (pertuzumab and trastuzumab) with chemotherapy versus in combination with ET in a de-escalated dosing in HR+/ERBB2+ EBC patients. In this trial, the authors pointed out that two neoadjuvant treatments were compared and that the chemotherapy combination arm ($n = 92$) was clearly superior in terms of pCR rate when compared to the ET combination arm ($n = 93$), with the objective being to confirm this. Secondary endpoints included changes in tumor size, radiographic response through ultrasound and mammography, and OS and HRQOL assessed through questionnaires, PAM50 subtype, and early response.

Key Results

- Clinically node-positive EBC was seen 58 patients, or 28% of them, and 121 patients, or "58% [of them] had cT2 to cT4 tumors (median [range] age, 53 [25–83] years)."
- The pCR rates were as follows:
  - For, ET plus trastuzumab and pertuzumab arm, it was 23.7% (95% CI 15.7%–33.4%), compared to paclitaxel plus trastuzumab and pertuzumab arm, which was 56.4% (95% CI 46.2%–66.3%) (odds ratio, 0.24; 95% CI 0.12–0.46; $p < 0.001$).
- The pCR rates (ypT0/is, ypN0) were as follows:
  - ET plus trastuzumab and pertuzumab arm was 23.7% (95% CI 15.7%–33.4%), which was clearly inferior to the paclitaxel plus trastuzumab and pertuzumab arm, which was 56.4% (95% CI 46.2%–66.3%) (OR, 0.24; 95% CI 0.12–0.46).

The report demonstrated that ERBB2+ EBC is a "highly chemotherapy-sensitive disease" with a pCR rate of 72% after 12 weeks of treatment in this intermediate-risk, stage II population. The study authors concluded that the "phase 2, multicenter WSG-TP-II randomized clinical trial shows an excellent pCR rate after de-escalated 12-week paclitaxel plus trastuzumab and pertuzumab (and clearly superior to ET plus trastuzumab and pertuzumab) as a universally applicable, efficacious, and well-tolerated standard regimen in intermediate- to high-risk ERBB2-positive disease" [34].

A negative result was reported by Mouabbi et al. on the nonprognostic value of ERBB2 expression, wherein IHC analysis showed that low ERBB2 expression (1+ or 2+) and negative ERBB2 expression had equal survival outcomes when treated with targeted therapies plus ET. In this report, 1585 women were randomized to CDK4/6i ($n = 912$, first line; $n = 172$, second line), everolimus ($n = 475$) and alpelisib ($n = 26$). PFS and OS were not found to be statistically significant between both groups. Previous reports have been inconsistent, with some reporting that poor prognosis was associated with low ERBB2 expression in HR+ mBC patients, whereas others reported that response to CDK4/6is was not affected and that "more data are needed to better understand whether low ERBB2 expression is truly prognostic."

Key Results

- Treatment with TT and ET in patients with no ERBB2 had a similar mPFS of 9.1 months and mOS of 28.1 versus 26.4 months (HR, 1.05; 95% CI 0.92–1.21), with no statistically significant difference.
- "Outcomes in patients treated with first-line CDK4/6is and ET
  - In a median follow-up time of 17.5 months, patients treated with CDK4/6is plus ET having low versus no ERBB2 expression, ranging from 1 to 110 months, demonstrated no statistically significant difference in mPFS (13.0 vs. 11.6 months ((HR, 1.09; 95% CI 0.92–1.29)) and mOS (32.4 vs. 31.2 months ((HR, 1.14; 95% CI 0.92–1.39))."

    "Outcomes in patients treated with second-line CDK4/6is, everolimus, or alpelisib and ET"
  - In patients with low versus no ERBB2 expression, with a median follow-up time of 12.4 months, treated in the second-line setting with "CDK4/6is and ET, there was no statistically significant difference in mPFS (7.3 vs. 7.1 months; HR, 1.20; 95% CI 0.83–1.72) and mOS (31.5 vs. 24.9 months; HR, 1.24; 95% CI 0.80–1.92)."

Patients with low versus no ERBB2 expression when administered a combination with second-line everolimus, alpelsib, and ET showed no differences in mPFS (6.5 vs. 6.0 months; HR, 1.08; 95% CI 0.87–1.33) and mOS (21.3 vs. 19.0 months; HR, 1.01; 95% CI 0.82–1.25) as well as when administered with second-line everolimus and alpelsib in combination with ET, refuting claims that ERBB2 expression can serve as a biomarker for the efficacy of CDK4/6i. This study suggests that in HR-positive metastatic breast cancer patients with no expression of ERBB2 treated with TT and ET, low ERBB2 expression is not associated with any distinctive clinicopathologic features and has no prognostic value. The authors surmise that variability as a result of testing methods and pathologic interpretation may be the reason for this result. They conclude that in patients with HR+ metastatic breast cancer treated with TT plus endocrine therapy, a low expression of ERBB2 was not associated with survival outcomes, with results supporting the standard of care in low ERBB2 expression endocrine-based therapy decision-making [35].

4.8 Melanoma

Other studies have confirmed that alternate BRAF mutations in advanced melanoma are not trivial, including rare, non-V600E/K mutations. One was a study evaluating the molecular profiles, frequency, and clinical efficacy of targeted therapies for these mutations in a national cohort.

"2227 patients included in MelBase,

- BRAF mutation: 904 (40.6%)
- V600E/K BRAF mutation 805, (subset B1, 89%) and
- Non-V600E/K BRAF mutation (51):
  - Non-E/K V600 BRAF mutation: 24 (subset B2, 2.6% of BRAF mutations overall)
    47% of all non-V600E/K BRAF mutations and non-V600 BRAF mutation: 27 (subset B3, 3% of BRAF mutations overall and
    53% of all non-V600E/K BRAF mutations)
  - Overall frequency of almost 6% for all non-V600E/K mutations (B2/B3) results."

For the following, MAPKis were used at least once:

- In patients in B1 or G1 (therapeutic group 1), it was used in 78.3%, 79.2%, and 33.3% of cases.
- "75.9% of G1, 89.5% of G2, and 22.2% of G3 patients [served] as first-line therapy for B2 (therapeutic group 2 = G2), and B3 (therapeutic group 3 = G3) mutational subsets."
- "In all groups, BRAFi was mainly used in combination with MEKi for all groups in a frequency significantly lower in the latter subset than in G1 and G2."

Key Results

- ORR
  - G1: 56%, 353 of 631
  - G2: 58%, 11 of 19
  - G3: subset with an ORR of only 22% (2 of 9) (much lower)
- CR
  - G1: 20% (124 of 361)
  - G2: 16% (3 of 16)
  - G3: 11% (1 of 11)
- PR
  - G1: 36% (229 of 631)
  - G2: 42% (8 of 19)
  - G3: 11% (1 of 11)
- DCR
  - G1: 86% (541 of 631)
  - G2: 100%
  - G3: 4% (4 of 11)

There were significant improvements in mOS, mPFS, and ORR in metastatic melanoma patients harboring V600E/K BRAF alterations in registration trials, particularly when using BRAFi and MEKi combinations with an ORR of 64%–70%, an mPFS of 11.1–14.9 months, and an mOS of 22.3–33.6 months) [36].

4.9 Colorectal Cancer and Gastric Cancers

As reported in *JCO*, in second-line settings of advanced gastric cancer treatment, a biomarker-integrated umbrella trial (for advanced gastric cancer (AGC)) screened targeted agents for this disease. In total, 318 patients with HER2-negative disease were randomized in a 4:1 ratio to biomarker versus control, and by using IHC and in situ hybridization, they were screened for druggable targets. In the biomarker group, patients ($n = 254$) were administered with a targeted therapeutic agent and paclitaxel combination (afatinib, EGFR cohort; $n = 67$); PIK3CBeta inhibitor was used for the PTEN cohort ($n = 37$); for PD-L1+, anti-PD-1 inhibitor was administered; and NIVO was administered for the dMMR/MSIh cohort ($n = 48$). The control group received standard-of-care treatment: paclitaxel with or without ramucirumab (NONE; $n = 102$). The mPFS and mOS values were 3.7 months (95% CI 3.1–4.1) and 8.6 months (95% CI 7.7–9.8) in the biomarker group and 4.0 (95% CI 3.0–4.6) and 8.7 months (95% CI 7.1–9.9) in the control group. When afatinib was added, prolonged survival did not result in patients harboring the PTEN mutations and led to only marginal survival benefit; nivolumab demonstrated a durable survival benefit of mOS of 12 versus 7.6 months when added to treatment. The investigators concluded that even though there was no improved survival in comparison to the control arm, the allocation of patients with AGC were feasible for treatment under an umbrella design [37].

In the CALGB/SWOG 80405 phase III cancer and leukemia group B trial, HER2 gene expression levels had prognostic and predictive ability in patients with mCRC. No difference in OS was observed in patients receiving chemotherapy in first-line settings in combination treatment with bevacizumab and cetuximab. Through the use of NGS (FoundationCDx) and NanoString and an 800-gene panel, the prognostic and predictive potential of HER2 gene expression and amplification was profiled in 559 patients. High HER2 gene expression, independent of treatment, was associated with longer OS (32 vs. 25.3 months) and longer PFS (11.6 vs. 10 months). In the HER2 expression group, an OS benefit was observed for cetuximab versus bevacizumab. Worse PFS was observed for cetuximab in the low-expression group [38].

Domingo et al. performed a study reported in *JCO* on the prognostic and predictive value of Immunoscore (IS) in stage III CRC in a pooled analysis of cases. Immunoscore may predict the benefit of the duration (6 vs. 3 months) of adjuvant FOLFOX chemotherapy. Among 30,061 cases with tumor samples, 2643 were eligible for IS testing. Low and high immunoscore classified cases into two categories for DFS. Additionally, 877 tumors were classified as low IS in younger patients, where they were more common in the high-risk class (T4 and N2, 52.9% IS low, and 42.2% IS high; $p < 0.001$). The CAPOX, FOLFOX, and combined cohorts had significantly shorter DFS values. The prognostic value was higher in younger patients who were less than 65 years old when compared to older patients (> 65 years) in the CAPOX cohort and in DNA MMR than DNA MMD disease. The authors state that these scores merit validation and that IS is prognostic in stage III CRC patients when administered with FOLFOX [39].

PIK3CA-activated stage III colon cancer tumors were studied in the CALGB/SWOG 80702 trial for assessing improved survival with adjuvant COX inhibition. That study found that PIKCA mutational status was predictive of ameliorated response to COX inhibitor celecoxib. In this trial, 259 of 1197 tumors displayed gain-of-function mutations through WES, exhibiting ameliorated DFS (HR, 0.56 (95% CI 0.33–0.96)) compared with wild-type mutational status (HR, 0.89 (95% CI 0.70–1.14)). OS was also similarly improved (HR 0.44 (95% CI 0.22–0.85) versus 0.94 (95% CI 0.68–1.38)). As a result of the potential utility of PIK3CA, this study suggests the selective usage of COX-2 inhibitors as a standard treatment for colorectal cancer [40].

Lynch syndrome (LS) is a precursor to CRC, particularly evident in patients with mismatch repair deficiency (MMR-D). However, a portion of CRC patients are MMR proficient (MMR-P). In one study evaluating this phenomenon in 17,617 patients harboring solid tumors, 99 pooled CRCs were assessed, with 1.4% ($n = 242$) having LS and a total of 36% (86 of 242) of patients with LS having had at least one CRC that underwent NGS profiling, amounting to 99 pooled CRCs assessed. Also, 10%, or 10, of 99 total CRCs were MMR-P, with MSS status showing 100% concordance with retained MMR staining. MSH6 and PMS2 variants occurred in a total of 89% (8 of 9) of patients in the MMR-P group, which was considerably less than that for the MMR-D group (30%, or 23 of 77), wherein the study authors concluded that "MMR-P CRC was later onset and more commonly metastatic when compared with MMR-D CRC in patients with LS that remained at risk for MMR-P CRC" [41].

Lynch syndrome and its association with glioblastoma (GBM) was also investigated in the context of MMR-D; Isocitrate dehydrogenase wildtype (IDH-wt) was also tested, having "major implications for the treatment, screening and prevention" of gliomas. For 1225 treatment-naive adult gliomas, somatic NGS was performed, resulting in nine gliomas harboring MMR-D (9/1225; 0.73%) in a younger patient population, leading the authors to recommend that MMR-D and LS should be screened in glioblastoma patients under 50 years of age [42].

One study showed that in the HER2 signaling pathway, gene coamplification and ERBB2 CN were "negative and positive predictors of PFS in trastuzumab-treated HER2-positive AGC patients, respectively." NGS measured ERBB2 copy number (CN) and was shown to be a predictive biomarker for trastuzumab efficacy in HER+ advanced gastric cancer (AGC) and advanced esophagogastric cancer. This study also posited an association between response and resistance to trastuzumab and ERBB2 amplification.

Key Points

- HER2-positive AGC patients harboring a VAF of ERBB2 may require HER2 TKIs and trastuzumab deruxtecan and showed poor outcomes.
- A select number of HER2 positive AGC patients having high VAF and ERBB2 sequence variant had poor prognosis with the determination that gene coamplification and ERBB2 CN in the HER2 signaling pathway can serve as useful predictive biomarkers for determining clinical outcomes on trastuzumab treatment.

In the HER2 pathway, the median ERBB2 CN was 20 and coamplifications occurring in AKT1, BRAF, EGFR, FGFR, IGF1R, MET, PIK3CA, and KRAS and gene comutations in ERBB2, PIK3CA, PTEN, KRAS, and BRAF were detected in 13 patients, or 18% of them, and 14 patients, or 19% of them, respectively. MYC (16%) and CCNE1/CCND1/CDK6 (30%) amplifications and the commonly occurring mutations KRAS/BRAF (3%), TP53 (72%), PIK3CA/PTEN (8%), and ERBB2 (7%) genes were also detected [43].

Gupta et al. reported on the results from the TAPUR study on CRC patients treated with pertuzumab plus trastuzumab with either ERBB2 amplification or ERBB2/3 mutations, where commercially available targeted agents were evaluated for antitumor activity in advanced cancer patients in a pragmatic phase II basket trial with potentially actionable genomic alterations. Patients had ECOG scores of 0–2 and adequate organ function with no remaining standard-of-care treatment options. DC, OR, and SD16+ were the primary endpoints, and OS, PFS, and response duration served as secondary endpoints.

4.9.1 Results

CRC patients ($n = 38$) harboring ERBB2 amplifications ($n = 28$) or ERBB2/3 mutations ($n = 10$) were treated with P + T. In the ERBB2 amplification cohort, DC and OR were observed in 54% and 25% of patients, with mPFS and mOS (95% CIs) at 17.2 (11.1–27.4) weeks and 60.0 (32.1–102.3) weeks, respectively. DC and OC were seen in 10% and 0% in the ERBB2/3 mutation group, respectively; mPFS and mOS were seen at 9.6 (5.1–16.0) weeks and 28.8 (7.6–146.3) weeks, respectively. Infusion reaction, left ventricular systolic dysfunction, and decreased lymphocyte count were reported as serious and grade 3 adverse events. The study authors concluded that although in CRC patients with ERBB2/3 mutations, P + T treatment did not have any significant antitumor activity, this combination warrants further study in CRC patients with ERBB2 amplification. P + T treatment displayed antitumor activity in heavily pretreated "CRC patients with heavily pretreated colorectal cancer with ERBB2 amplification but did not demonstrate antitumor activity in patients with ERBB2 or ERBB3 mutations" [44].

The phase II RELATIVITY-060 evaluated relatlimab in patients with unresectable gastric or gastroesophageal junction (GEJ) adenocarcinoma with LAG-3 expression greater than or equal to 1% when nivolumab and chemotherapy were added. When compared with nivolumab and chemotherapy alone, the primary endpoint was not met in the trial (ORR according to a blinded independent review). Stratification was carried out according to LAG-3 expression (greater than 1% versus less than 1%) and PD-1 CPS < 1. The ORR was 48% in the N + R + C arm and 61% in the N + C arm. Also, mPFS was 7.0 versus 8.3 months; mOS was 13.5 months versus 16.0 months—HR 1.04. In all treated patients, 69% and 61% discontinued treatment in the N + R + C and N + C arms, respectively, and among all treated patients, "42% and 36% of patients discontinued because of any-grade TRAEs."

However, in patients with LAG-3 expression greater than 1%, the endpoint of improved OR was not reached when relatlimab was added to N + C when compared to N + C alone, and further "studies are needed to address whether anti-LAG3 to anti-PD-1 plus CT can benefit specific GC/GEJC patients" [45].

Another study, published in *Nature Medicine*, demonstrated that targeted therapy could be guided by using ctDNA analysis (as described in Chap. 3) in advanced gastrointestinal tumors. The investigators identified biomarker-matched therapy and efficacy was shown by "biomarker-matched therapy guided by ctDNA," as well as survival outcomes of the matched therapy according to ctDNA clonality and plasma copy number. Although CGP has become standard in precision oncology, ctDNA and its implementation are underutilized in terms of addressing clinical utility and tumor heterogeneity. In the GOZILA study, an observational, nationwide, and prospective ctDNA profiling study was conducted leading to evidence for the "clinical utility of ctDNA profiling in advanced solid tumors" with a 24% match rate for targeted therapy with improved OS when compared to unmatched therapy (HR, 0.54), showing that the value of ctDNA reflects tumor heterogeneity with adjusted plasma copy number and biomarker clonality identified to predict the efficacy of treatment. Comprehensive genomic profiling (CGP) is standard care, and ctDNA is widely used because of its rapid turnover time and minimally invasive nature, with the potential for identifying targeted therapy with clinical efficacy; however, when compared to tissue testing, ctDNA genotyping has not been universally adopted. Because ctDNA represents a "composite of DNA released from all tumor subclones," it may have genomic alterations distinguished from the original dominant tumor clone (6–8). The clonality and clones harboring nascent alterations influence their biological impact and relevance, with rarer clones having less clinical relevance than more-common ones. This knowledge gap led to the construction of the GOZILA study, which evaluated targeted therapy efficacy determined through biomarker matching detected through ctDNA in 4000 patients with advanced solid tumors. Major tumor types included CRC (n = 1820), pancreatic (n = 899), and BTC (n = 291), with metastatic sites such as the liver, lymph nodes, lung, and peritoneum.

Key Results

- Identified biomarkers were TP53 (33%), the most frequently identified alteration, with APC (19%), KRAS (13%), and EGFR (11%) following, where ctDNA genotyping identified 952 (24%) patients matched with at least one targeted therapy through biomarker analysis. Biomarker-matched therapy took place the most, with CRC at 38%, followed by pancreatic cancer (4%), esophageal cancer (8%), and neuroendocrine tumors or carcinoma (10%) as less-frequent biomarker-matched therapies.
- In first-, second-, and third-line therapies, biomarker-matched treatments were administered for 473 RAS wild-type mutations, 163 ERBB2 amplifications and mutations, and 113 BRAF mutations and alterations, primarily serving as biomarkers in guided matched therapy, followed by tumor mutation burden (n = 77) and microsatellite instability (n = 52).

- MSI high (76%) was the most targetable biomarker for matching treatment recommendations, "followed by ERBB2 (51%), KIT(48%), TMB high (28%), BRAF (22%) and MET (20%)." In summary, this study demonstrates that through ctDNA profiling, biomarker-aligned treatments can lead to treatment effectiveness that is equivalent or perhaps in some cases superior to conventional tissue-based genotyping.
- An extended mPFS of 4.7 months (95% CI 4.2–5.3 months) was similarly associated with matched therapy, "relative to unmatched (2.8 months, 95% CI 2.8–3.0 months; HR 0.65, 95% CI 0.61–0.71) as well as overall survival (OS) (18.6 months, 95% CI 17.4–20.5 months versus 9.9 months, 95% CI 9.5–10.4 months; HR 0.54, 95% CI 0.49–0.59)."

The clonality of targeted biomarkers is determined by dividing VAF by the maximum VAF detected in the sample, as influenced by observed therapeutic efficacy, which is critical to therapeutic clinical decision-making, whereas the sensitivity of the association between efficacy benefit and the clonality of the "biomarker-targeted therapies to variation in clonality threshold" is less well understood. A marked increase in radiographic response occurred at the optimal clonality of 0.4, where treatment selection was based on clonal biomarkers (26% versus 7%, $p = 0.055$) and PFS (median 3.0 months versus 1.4 months; HR 0.56, 95% CI 0.36–0.85).

As the authors state about the significance of the study, patients treated with matched targeted therapy biomarker characterization as conducted in the GOZILA study have "established a new benchmark in the field of precision oncology," as shown through ctDNA analysis, and this characterization can remarkably increase OS when compared to patients receiving unmatched therapy. The identification of eligible patients has been one of the challenges of precision oncology that was mitigated by the results of the GOZILA study, where the number of ctDNA-guided therapies was higher than recently published studies using tissue testing, which demonstrated the following clinical benefits: reducing the risk of death by more than 40% and a twofold higher response rate. Another central feature of targeted therapy administration was highlighted: ctDNA-guided treatment benefit decreases after first-line setting treatment, which may be due to the widely held theory of "cancer evolution under therapeutic selective pressure," which shifts targeted therapies to earlier lines of treatment for better survival. As the study authors conclude, ctDNA profiling across solid tumors leads to therapeutic agents and interventions that show both the method's survival benefit and relevance and the predictive value of clonality and "describes an effective, data-driven rubric [according to] which clinical decisions may be made in the common scenario of subclonal biomarkers with therapeutic relevance" [46].

Nakamura et al. conducted a review of targeted therapies for gastric cancers that include HER2-targeted therapy, FGFR2-targeted therapy, EGFR-targeted therapy, antiangiogenic therapy, MET-targeted therapy, PARP inhibitors, and Claudin 18.2 targeted therapy. Much of this information on molecular subtypes was derived from TCGA. The authors also cite molecular heterogeneity as the major reason for the failure of biomarker-based therapies in clinical trials [47].

4.10 Renal Cell Carcinoma

In the double-blind, randomized phase III study ECOG-ACRIN E2810, the VEGFR inhibitor pazopanib was evaluated in mRCC patients who underwent metastasectomy and had no evidence of disease to test whether disease-free survival would be improved. In this study, 129 patients were enrolled to receive pazopanib at a dosage of 800 mg once daily in randomization vs. placebo for 52 weeks. "The trial did not meet its primary endpoint; the 3-year DFS values were 27.4% (95% CI 17.9–41.7) and 21.9% (95% CI 13.3–36.2) for pazotinib and placebo, respectively. Three-year OS was 81.9% (95% CI 72.7–92.2) and 91.4% (95% CI 84.4–98.9) for pazopanib and placebo, respectively." The authors concluded that pazopanib did not lead to improved DFS, serving as the primary endpoint when compared with blinded placebo [48].

While mTOR inhibitors such as everolimus and temsirolimus have shown efficacy in mRCC, a multicenter, prospective phase II study evaluating sapaisertinib—a mTOR kinase kinase inhibitor that was evaluated in a patient population of treatment-refractory mRCC patients—demonstrated minimal activity. The primary and secondary endpoints of the study were ORR, CR, and PR and the best overall response was defined by RECIST and by PFS, OS, and safety profiles. Tumor mutational analysis was carried out using OncoPanel, where genomic DNA underwent targeted exon capture with massively parallel sequencing. Clinical results include a confirmed ORR of two of 38 (5.3%; 95% CI 1–15.6); 39% of patients, or 15, achieved SD, and 45% of patients, or 17, had PD as the best response. TRAEs included fatigue (39%), nausea (50%), vomiting (34%), and anemia (21%). OncoPanel analysis revealed activating mutations in genes in the mTOR pathway, one PTEN frameshift deletion (p.K183Ifs*15), one inactivating TSC1 missense mutation (p.F188S), one PTEN frameshift deletion, one MTOR missense mutation (p.N1992K), and one PTEN in-frame mutation [49].

4.10.1 Major TKI Trials for RCC

ASSURE: Sorafenib vs. sunitinib vs. placebo was evaluated; 5-year DFS benefit was "47.7% in the sunitinib and 50% in the placebo arm (HR, 0.94; 97.5% CI 0.74–1.19)."

S-TRAC: Sunitinib vs. placebo (HR, 0.76; 95% CI 0.59–0.98) was evaluated.

PROTECT: Pazopanib vs. placebo was evaluated; DFS, the primary endpoint, was not met (HR, 0.86; 95% CI 0.70–1.06).

ATLAS: Axitinib vs. placebo was evaluated; due to a failure to show DFS in a predetermined interim analysis, the study was terminated (HR, 0.87; 95% CI 0.66–1.147).

EVEREST: Everolimus vs. placebo was evaluated; DFS improvement was seen in the everolimus arm versus placebo (HR, 0.85; 95% CI 0.72–1.00), "although it fell short of [the] prespecified significance value."

4.10.2 Major Immunotherapy Trials for RCC

KEYNOTE-564: Pembrolizumab vs. placebo was evaluated; DFS was 77.3% vs. 68.1% in the placebo group (HR, 0.68; 95% CI 0.53–0.87).

IMmotion10: Atezolizumab vs. placebo was evaluated; DFS was reported as 57.2 months in the treatment arm compared with 49.5 months for placebo (HR, 0.93; 95% CI 0.75–1.15). Also, 67% versus 65% were the 2-year DFS rates.

PROSPER RCC: Nivolumab vs. observation was evaluated; with an HR of 0.97 (95% CI 0.74–1.28), between the two groups, no difference in DFS was observed, and mDFS was not reached. OS data, insignificant at the time of data presentation, are not yet mature (HR, 1.48; 95% CI 0.89–2.48).

Checkmate 914: Part A: Nivolumab + ipilimumab vs. placebo was evaluated; part B Nivolumab + ipilimumab vs. placebo + placebo vs. nivolumab + placebo was evaluated; DFS (HR, 0.92; 95% CI 0.71–1.19) was taken at a median follow-up of 37 months. DFS at 24 months was 76.4% and 74% for nivolumab + ipilimumab vs placebo.

"Rampart: durvalumab vs. durvalumab + tremelimumab vs. observation."

The review authors note that the despite evidence in clinical trials, TKIs in the adjuvant setting do not lend themselves to being studied by landmark clinical trials given that OS was unchanged, such that the use of adjuvant tyrosine kinase inhibitors in renal cell carcinoma remains controversial [50].

A gene-expression-based biomarker signature was developed and validated for recurrent ccRCC to facilitate risk stratification. Whole transcriptomic sequencing was performed to create a 15-gene (15G) signature, which was used to predict RFS/DFS,which was independently "associated with worse DFS and DSS (DFS: HR, 11.08 (95% CI 4.9–25.1); (DSS: HR, 9.67 (95% CI 3.4–27.7)) in a multivariable model adjusting for clinicopathologic parameters (including stage, size, grade, and necrosis." The study authors concluded that "our study has identified a 15G score that provides prognostic information independent of clinicopathologic variables in patients with ccRCC after nephrectomy. This signature also provides insights into the molecular mechanisms of ccRCC and may serve as a valuable tool for the identification of novel therapeutic targets. Pending further validation and clinical grade assay development, this signature has the potential to successfully stratify patients for appropriate management" [51].

4.11 Prostate Cancer

A fascinating report on NGS tissue testing evaluated the validity of tumor genomic testing for a large cohort of men with mCRPC in the phase III, randomized, prospective, open-label, global PROfound trial, which demonstrated the clinical feasibility of the PARPi olaparib. The authors defined this type of testing as definitive for the future of molecular targeted therapies when reported in 2022. The

FoundationOneCDx tissue test was used to prospectively identify patients with HRR genes to evaluate NGS tissue-testing outcomes against preanalytic testing to identify pertinent factors that influence such testing. The PROfound study led to real-time sequencing by providing a large set of prostate cancer samples available when determining eligibility for clinical studies. With 69% of patients (n = 4425) having NGS tissue-testing results in the cohort, the evaluation of sample characteristics showed that when high-quality tumor tissue samples are available for NGS and the determination of results, the relevance of adding CGP for administering PARPi therapies in this patient population is demonstrated. Positive results showed that tumor content, DNA yield, and tissue volume indicated an increase in the proportion of NGS results. Furthermore, 50–1000 ng of DNA was needed for library construction. Higher DNA yield occurred in metastatic samples when compared to primary samples, and "of the metastatic samples, those taken from lymph nodes had higher tumor content and DNA yield, and bone samples had the lowest tumor content and DNA yield."

Other Key Results

- Both DNA yield (median 357.8 vs. 88.3 ng) and the overall proportion of samples generating an NGS for the cohort of samples with a tissue volume $\geq$0.6 mm^3 was higher (58.9%; 95% CI 57.4–60.3) than for the 0.2–< 0.6 mm^3 cohort (32.1%; 95% CI 24.4–40.6).
- DNA yield served as the main variable that determined whether a result from NGS could be obtained, with other variables, such as sample age and percentage tumor content (area under the curve (AUC) 0.9061; AUC 0.6292; and AUC 0.5965), having a potential effect but to a lesser extent.

The study authors concluded that within their modeling analysis, multiple factors generate an NGS result, with some factors having greater predictive value than others. In the PROfound study, DNA yield and percentage tumor nuclei strongly affected the results generated through NGS when shown by the majority of samples that progressed through testing with an obtained NGS, as shown by their model while "meeting validated quality control criteria of the molecular test used in the trial." They also noted that liquid biopsy advances, with LB's ability to identify alterations, can provide therapy options when tumor tissue is unavailable for NGS analysis. However, they added that "plasma DNA has a tumor content below 30%," with a lack of DNA clearance for performing copy number analysis, and specificity is low, with cfDNA being negative and unable to rule out tissue positivity [52].

The open-label phase2 TRITON2 study evaluated rucaparib in mCRPC patients with DNA repair deficiency and demonstrated clinically meaningful activity, having an ORR of 44% (95% CI 31–57%) in 27/62 patients, as assessed by an independent review. In the BRCA subgroup, the confirmed ORR was 46% (95% CI 35–57%) in patients with IRR evaluable disease. In this subgroup, target lesions were reduced to 30% from the baseline. "The DOR by IRR was 15.5 mo (95% CI 6.4—not reached)." Patients with BRCA2 alterations had a confirmed ORR of 48%, and the ORR among patients with BRCA1 alterations was 30%; ORR was similar between somatic and germline mutations and between those with or without co-occurring PTEN, RB1, or

TP53 alterations. PALB2 alterations were associated with a 100% ORR, with a median DOR of 10.1 mo. TEAEs were nausea (51%), fatigue (59%), and anemia (48%). Grade 3 TEAEs were anemia (29%) and fatigue (11%). AEs led to treatment interruption in 58% of patients, or 160 patients, which led to a 38% dose reduction (or 106 patients) and treatment discontinuation in 32 patients, or 12% of them. No incidences of myelodysplastic syndrome or AML were reported. As the study authors state, in BRCA-altered mCRPC patients, the TRITON2 demonstrates the efficacy of rucaparib, which demonstrated some activity in patients with less-common alterations, such as PALB2 [53].

Combination treatments in the first-line setting for mCRPC of Androgen Receptor Signaling Inhibitors (ARSIs) and PARPis were evaluated in the MAGNITUDE, PROpel, and TALAPRO-2 trials. In the phase III PROpel study, "abiraterone plus olapraib versus abiraterone plus placebo resulted in an ITT analysis of PFS of 16.6 months in the abiraterone plus placebo arm (HR 0.66) and 24.8 months in the combination treatment arm," irrespective of HRR status. Another result favoring the combination arm was that mOS improved at 42.1 versus 34.7 months, and this trend was reflected in non-HRR-mutant, HRR-mutant, BRCA mutated, and non-BRCA mutated subgroups, with the most positive improvement seen in the BRCA mutated subgroup (HR 0.29, 95% CI 0.14–0.56), which led to the conclusion that olaparib and abiraterone yielded superior results and clinical improvements even though the incidence of grade 3 or higher AEs was greater in the combination arm (47% versus 38%), although the side effect profile was consistent with prior data. Anemia, the most common event, occurred in 46% of patients, and severe grade 3–4 anemia occurred in 15.1%. No incidences of MDS were reported. In the phase III MAGNITUDE trial, patients were stratified according to HRR biomarker status while assessing the safety and efficacy of Abiraterone Acetate + Prednisone/Prednisolone (AAP) with niraparib, and combination improved rPFS in the HRR+ cohort with BRCA1/2 mutations (HR0.53). Negative results were reported in the HRR- group. Grade 3 anemia occurred in 28.3% and hypertension in 14.6% of patients. Another biomarker-guided trial evaluating PARP1-ARSI combination treatment was TALAPRO-2, which evaluated the treatment of talazoparib plus enzalutamide in the first-line setting of mCRPC patients. HRR status stratified patients, and the combination group had an rPFS that had not been reached and was 27.5 months in the placebo plus enzalatuamide group, representing a 37% improvement in mPFS according to imaging, in which the greatest benefit was seen in BRCA1/2 positive patients. According to the analysis, there was treatment benefit in the HRR-deficient group, with an HR of 0.46, with a benefit also seen in the unselected gene alteration group, with an HR of 0.66, "exceeding the prespecified HR of 0.696 for significance," demonstrating that PARPis efficacy benefit is shown by biomarkers in the treatment of mCRPC and support the selection and stratification of patient cohorts by using HRR status as a stratification biomarker [2].

The PI3K/AKT (AKT serine/threonine kinase)/mTOR signaling pathway is associated with prostate cancer progression because PTEN loss results in aberrations in the signaling pathway, resulting in poor efficacy and treatment resistance. Due to cross-talk inherent in the PTEN pathway leading to toxicities at therapeutic doses and the destruction of normal cells, targeting PTEN is challenging. The ProCAID trial evaluated capivasertib as a selective pan-AKT inhibitor in combination with docetaxel, where it met the secondary endpoint of OS but did not lead to improved PFS or PSA reduction. However, subgroup analysis showed that this improvement was seen with progression on ARSIs. According to the authors, the "improvement in OS was intriguing and hypothesis generating," despite it being a negative result, resulting in the phase III CAPItello 280 that will examine the combination with placebo in patients progressing on ARSIs in any setting, which might lead to potential targeted therapies. Ipatasertib, also an AKT inhibitor, was investigated in IPATential 150, a double-blind phase III trial randomizing patients for treatment with ipatasertib and abiraterone/prednisolone versus abiraterone/prednisolone alone; the rationale was that the approach was characterized by "dual-activation pathway enhancing synergistic antitumor activity for a better clinical outcome." According to the review authors, "the combination of ipatasertib and abiraterone had better rPFS (HR 0.65, 95% CI 0.45–0.95), with the study being positive in patients who had PTEN loss" on IHC [2].

4.12 Other Solid Tumors

Biliary tract cancers encompass a range of tumors, including cholangiocarcinomas and gallbladder cancer, and only 10%–40% are considered resectable. IDH1-mutant (isocitrate dehydrogenase-1) mutated BTCs show improvement with ivosidenib and FGFR-2 fibroblast growth factor receptor 2 inhibitors such as infigratinib (18.8%), pemigatinib (35.5%), and futibatinib (41.7%). BRAFV600E mutated BTCs were amenable to a combination of dabrafenib and trametinib, with an ORR of 20–50%.

One review outlined "recent advances in precision medicine and immunotherapy for patients with cholangiocarcinoma (CCA)," a bile duct cancer with harsh immunosuppressive environment containing dense stroma and MDSCs. Revealing targetable mutations, the treatment landscape of cholangiocarcinoma is changing as a result precision cancer medicine. Also, 15–20% of patients with extrahepatic cholangiocarcinoma and 40–50% of patients with intrahepatic cholangiocarcinoma were found to have targetable mutations, including TMB-high tumors, MSI-high tumors, IDH1 mutations, FGFR2 fusions, HER2 amplification/overexpression, NTRK and RET fusions, and BRAF V600E mutations. Data continue to emerge for other potential targets, such as DNA repair deficiencies, KRAS G12C mutations, and MDM2 amplifications. They have a good possibility of leading to effective therapies with molecular profiling, accompanying surgical resection and triplet regimen cisplatin, gemcitabine, and nab-paclitaxel (GAP) as acceptable options for the frontline treatment of advanced BTC. FDA-approved targeted therapies include "futibatinib, an irreversible pan-FGFR inhibitor, reversible FGFR1-3 inhibitor pemigatinib, and infigratinib, another reversible FGFR1-3 inhibitor." Other investigational agents include BRAF/MEK inhibitors dabrafenib and trametinib, HER2-alterations targeted therapies, and antibody drug conjugates for targeting cell surface receptors, such as trastuzumab deruxtecan. These therapies have been shown in studies to demonstrate robust ORRs and positive clinical outcomes. National Comprehensive Cancer Network (NCCN) guidelines include treatment with "nivolumab alone (ORR, 3.3–20%) and lenvatinib combined with pembrolizumab (ORR, 10%) for refractory advanced BTCs on the basis of phase II studies." As the review authors conclude, CCA has entered the molecular therapy era in the context of the FDA approvals of pemigatinib, infigratinib, futibatinib, and ivosidenib, with the increasing likelihood of more approvals for targeted therapies [54].

The targeted therapy selpercatinib was evaluated in rearranged during transfection (RET) tumors for the durability of response in RET-activated medullary thyroid cancer and RET-fusion-positive thyroid cancer as a tumor-agnostic therapy in the phase I/II, open-label LIBRETTO-001 trial, building on initial reports. NGS, FISH, and PCR molecular testing were used to confirm mutational status. In RET-mutant medullary thyroid cancer (MTC) for treatment-naive patients, the ORR was 82.5% (95% CI 75.3–88.4), and in cabozantinib/vandetanib-naive patients, it was 84.5% (95% CI 76.6–90.5). "Median DoR was not reached." At a median follow-up of 42.4%, mPFS was not reached. RET-fusion-positive thyroid cancer (TC) was separated into two groups: those with and those without systemic radioiodine treatment. In the treatment-naive cohort, the "ORR was 95.8% (95% CI 78.9–99.9)," whereas in patients receiving treatment, it was 85.4% (95% CI 70.8–94.4)—with CRs in 20.8% and 12.2% of patients, respectively. The most common grade 3 serious AEs were increased ALT (MTC, 9.0%, TC, 6.1%) and hypertension (MTC, 21.6% TC, 15.2%). The authors concluded that selpercatinib led to "durable and robust responses in treatment-naive and previously treated patients in RET-mutant MTC and RET-fusion positive TC" [55].

Adult-onset neuroblastoma (AON) has differing clinical presentation than child-onset neuroblastoma, described as "a rare embryonal tumor of the sympathetic nervous system, [it] is most commonly diagnosed in infants and young children, and < 10% of cases are diagnosed beyond age 5 years. [Neuroblastoma] is extremely rare in adults and differs significantly in biology and clinical behavior from childhood-onset disease." One study showed the clinical efficacy of the ALK inhibitors lorlatinib in tumors with the ALK mutation. Lorlatinib AEs included "weight gain and hyperlipidemia resulting in dose reduction or discontinuation of ALKi in several patients."

Key Results

- For patients receiving lorlatinib, PFS and OS were 40.1 ± 4.7 and 47.5 ± 4 months from the initiation of lorlatinib, respectively; there was only one patient death in the lorlatinib arm, with a median follow-up of 21 months from the initiation of lorlatinib.
- For the entire arm of 15 patients, 5-year OS from of 15 patients was 89% ± 10%.

The investigators concluded that although lorlatinib exhibited clinical response, dose reductions necessitated monitoring for adverse events [56].

In HNSCC, Harvey Rat sarcoma (HRAS) is an actionable alteration evaluated in a study reported by Coleman et al., which was more prevalent in human papillomavirus (HPV)–negative patients, and which could affect "future treatment strategies" for a tumor type with poor outcomes in the recurrent and metastatic setting. Genomic profiling was conducted, and DFS was the primary endpoint. The study suggested that the FTase inhibitor tipifarnib was a targeted agent for HRAS mutations in the tumor; however, the response is not in a codon site in the HRAS mutation. One of the key results was that for HRAS-mutant HNSCC, a complex mutational profile was revealed through genomic analysis. Coexisting with the HRAS mutation, CASP8, TERT, and NOTCH1 are the most frequent mutations. The authors concluded that understanding "the mutational, genomic landscape of HNSCC has led to the development of better therapeutic approaches in this disease and our data provide additional insights into this rare genomic subset of HNSCC which may be of interest in future clinical trial design" [57].

Zhou et al. revealed in a preclinical study the discovery of periostin (POSTN) correlated with tumor-associated macrophage density, which when markedly reduced, increased survival in mouse models with tumor growth inhibition. The tumor-supportive MD type tumor associated macrophages (TAMs) in macrophages were specifically attenuated through the disruption of POSTN by recruiting TAMs through integrin alpha-beta. Blocking this signaling pathway inhibited TAM recruitment, underscoring the potential of ameliorating the treatment of GBM by "targeting POSTN-mediated TAM recruitment," which could have implications for the clinical development of an antitumor agent because macrophage recruitment by the rPOSTN protein was significantly attenuated by the integrin signaling disruption by the RGD inhibitory peptide in U937 cells. This study becomes significant in the context of recent studies that suggest that TAMs may promote the progression of GBM tumors via their recruitment through secreting IL-6 and IL-10, which play a tumor-promoting role in the progression of GBM by promoting cancer cell proliferation. The preclinical study also provided evidence that "TAMs in GBMs are mainly monocyte-derived macrophages (CCR2C/CX3CR1/from peripheral blood) but not resident microglia (CX3CR1C/CCR2/from brain)." Through the bioluminescent imaging of orthotopic tumors, the role of POSTN was derived from experiments that evaluated the tumor growth on GBM xenografts of the effect of POSTN knockdown in vivo on TAM density that led to the dramatic inhibition of tumor growth in the "xenografts derived GSCs expressing POSTN shRNA relative to those expressing non-targeting shRNA." Mice that were implanted with glioblastoma stem cells expressing POSTN shRNA versus controls demonstrated the downregulation of POSTN, as shown through immunofluorescent staining and Kaplan–Meier survival curves; other significant findings were that POSTN shRNA had extension in survival relative to the control cohort, and in addition, there were dramatic reductions in TAMs and POSTN detected in GSC tumors that expressed POSTN shRNA. Additionally, the density of TAMs was decreased by more than 65% in tumors derived from GSCs expressing POSTN. The significance of the study was shown by the different monocyte populations that existed in GBM tumors, which contained abundant CCR2C cells (monocyte-derived TAMs) but not CX3CR1C cells or microglia, whereas the opposing population were in normal brain tissues that contained CX3CR1c cells, but not CCR2C cells. POSTN-recruited

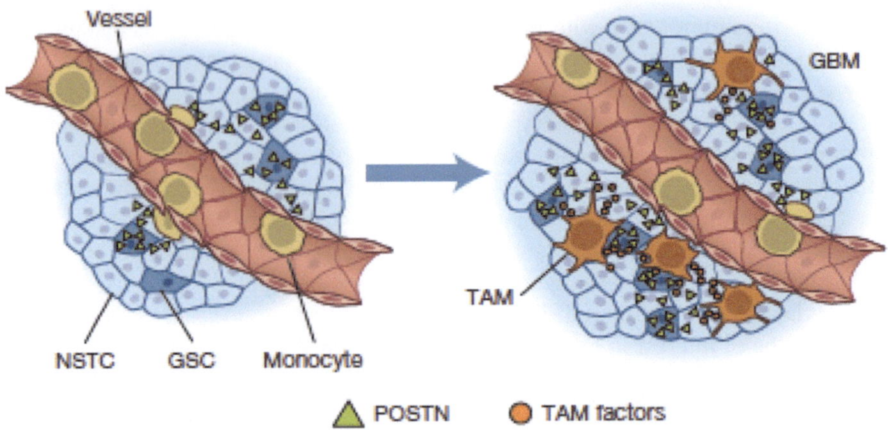

Fig. 4.6 TAMs inhibit GBM tumor growth. (Adapted from Zhou et al.)

TAMS displayed and maintained the M2 subtype in GSC-derived xenografts. An increase in M2 TAMs was seen in xenografts overexpressing POSTN relative to vector control, as shown through graphical analysis. Immunofluorescent staining also showed that when in GSCs silenced POSTN, the relative fraction of M1 TAMs increased in xenografts, and M2 macrophage markers Lyve1 and STAB1 were downregulated in the CD11bC cell population when drawn from POSTN-shRNA-expression xenografts. CCL17 and IL1b markers, however, were upregulated. The study authors concluded that disrupting POSTN may lead to the in vivo reduced recruitment of the M2 type of macrophage that supports tumor growth, with no disruption to vascularization and vessel density as a result of POSTN (Fig. 4.6) [58].

4.13 HRD Evaluation in Prostate Cancer and Ovarian Cancer

Homologous recombination deficiency (HRD) pathway mutations are identified through DNA signature methods, and the biomarker plays a central role in biomarker evaluation for the PARP therapy of solid tumors such as prostate cancer. Brown et al. conducted an analysis on HRD in prostate cancer through RNA signature methods. HRD detection was on a continuous scale. Deep deletions, pathogenic somatic and pathogenic germline mutation, and an overlapping loss of heterozygosity (LOH) defined 78% of "BRCA1/2 biallelic loss[, which] was classified as HRD-RNA+, which was associated with AR gene alterations and higher prevalence of p53; however, the most positive HRD-RNA samples were not associated with DNA-based alterations. HRD-RNA+ (13%, n = 126) and 87% (n = 859) characterized these tumors" (Table 4.2). In patients with biallelic loss of BRCA1/2, HRD-RNA+ was detected at a rate of 78% (7/9). In this retrospective study, the investigators concluded that the patients with PCa with functional HRD can be candidates for PARPi treatment through the use of then new RNA-based HRD assay that they developed, even though these patients lack conventional HRR gene alterations [59].

In the context of HRD, a widely used commercial test is the Myriad homologous recombination deficiency used in several phase III trials; however, alternatives for clinically validated HRD status have been developed, where a new biomarker for HRD was developed by using TCGA database and, "as part of the ENGOT HRD European Initiative, applied to 469 samples from the PAOLA-1/ENGOT-ov25 trial." PFS results in the olaparib + bevacizumab and placebo + bevacizumab arms as evaluated in the ovarian cancer "were compared with the Myriad myChoice Genomic Instability Score (GIS)"; this commercially available test used to predict PARPi treatment response is limited, however. The PAOLA-1/ENGOT-ov25 phase III trial aimed to answer the need for the clinical validation and evaluation of the performance of HRD tests on 469 patients.

Key Results

- "Using the Geneva test (OncoScan + nLST (large-scale state transitions)), analysis of the PAOLA-1 samples, using the Geneva test (OncoScan + nLST (large-scale state transitions))," proved superior to the Myriad myChoice (BRCAm or GIS+) test, yielding a "lower failure rate (27 of 469 vs. 59 of 469) and an HR of 0.40 (95% CI 0.28–0.57) compared with the HR" of 0.37 from Myriad myChoice (HR 0.37) for in the nLST-positive samples.
- "The Geneva test also identified a novel subpopulation of patients that had a favorable 1-year PFS of 85% but a poor 2-year PFS of 30% on treatment with olaparib + bevacizumab" [60].

Two studies evaluating olaparib in mUC and mPCa showed clinical efficacy in phase II studies (the latter was the basket TAPUR study). Metastatic urothelial cancer (mUC) was shown to harbor somatic DDR alterations (ATM, BRCA1, BRCA2, H2AX, XRCC3, RAD51, MRE11, RAD50, and NBS1), and clinical results were revealed in an open-label, single-arm, multi-institutional trial. Patients received 300 mg of olaparib after progression on platinum chemotherapy. ORR served as the primary endpoint, and safety, PFS, and OS served as the secondary endpoints.

Key Results

- Eight patients, or 42.1%, had "pathogenic BRCA2 mutations, and two patients carried alteration in other HR genes, with ten patients or 52.6% having alterations in HR genes."
- PR was not achieved in any patients, "although six patients achieved SD lasting 2.13–16.1 months (median, 7.69). The mPFS was 1.9 months (range, 0.8–16.1), and the mOS was 9.5 months (range, 1.5–22.1)," leading to conclusions that the therapy had limited antitumor activity with no patients achieving an objective response, which the authors posit implicated cross-resistance to chemotherapy and poorly characterized DDR alterations" [61].

The results from the TAPUR study showed that mCRPC patients with the BRCA1/2 alteration receiving olaparib at 600 mg daily had a DCR of 69% (95% CI 51–81) (investigator assessed) with an ORR of 58% (95% CI 37–77) among the 26 evaluable patients.

Other Key Results

- The median radiographic PFS and the mOS were 38.4 (95% CI 16.3–52.1) weeks and 76.4 (95% CI 49.3–106.0) weeks, respectively.
- Grade 3–4 AEs (serious AEs), including anemia, decreased white blood cell (WBC) count, aspiration, and fatigue, were experienced by six of 30 (20%) patients. In contrast to mUC patients, single-agent olaparib demonstrated clinical activity in heavily pretreated mCRPC patients.

Tumor heterogeneity, the vasculature of the tumor microenvironment, and the pharmacokinetic and pharmacodynamic properties of olaparib may contribute to these contrasting results, which may be the subject of future studies comparing the agent in these differing tumors [62].

The aforementioned studies demonstrate an association between PARP inhibitor survival outcomes and the presence of genomic alterations and biomarkers such as somatic and germline BRCA ½ and HRD, respectively, which has been discussed extensively in the literature. However, one retrospective real-world study showed that the identification of biallelic BRCA1/2 mutation in the presence of HRD was not confirmed in patients not receiving either PARP inhibitor or immunotherapy, finding no association between BRCA and HRR status and OS in this cohort of patients with advanced solid tumors, such as NSCLC, breast cancer, pancreatic cancer, colorectal cancer, and prostate cancer. HRs were 0.79, 0.86, and 1.18 for BRCAm vs. BRCAwt, HRRm vs. HRRwt, and HRDpos vs. HRDneg, respectively (confidence intervals omitted); the authors concluded that future studies should inform on the impact of PARPi treatment and immunotherapy in patients with advanced solid tumors [63].

HRD evaluations were also performed to validate different assays and compare with the FDA-approved Myriad myChoice assay by measuring genomic instability and by analyzing genomic scars that are inclusive of LOH and telomeric allelic imbalance. The comparisons were done for ovarian cancer for biomarker assessment to administer PARP inhibitors olaparib, niraparib, and veliparib through HRD determination. The goal was to "technically validate and harmonize different independent and decentral HRD test solutions," including the Myriad myChoice assay, to "ensure patient stratification."

Key Results

- Of the analyzed samples, 59 achieved full concordance with Myriad myChoice HRD positive/negative. A true positive and true negative result was recorded for all samples, such that "all evaluated assays had 100% concordance."
- In 25 of the remaining 58 samples, HRD positive and negative achieved concordance, with the exception of one, including seven samples that did not have a Myriad myChoice score. Between two and all tested assays, the differences for

33 samples varied when compared with testing with Myriad myChoice versus all evaluated assays.
- No concordance (SP62, SP89) was shown in comparison to Myriad myChoice (SP31, SP93, SP101), in comparison to the investigational assays, or in comparison to five samples (SP31, SP62, SP89, SP93, and SP101).

The study authors concluded that their study was one of the first to evaluate the HRD status concordance "generated by several molecular assays," of which Myriad myChoice is an example in assessing HRD-associated gastrointestinal cancer in the clinic, and by comparing it with a "multitude of assays, the data are well in range or even better than variability data for a variety of biomarker assays" [64].

4.14 Results from Adaptive Basket Clinical Trials: Targetable Alterations for Advanced Solid Tumors

The TAPUR study is a precision medicine adaptive clinical trial that evaluates commercially available drugs targeting genomic alterations, outside of their approved indications identified by genomic tests. The study reports the results of the CRC patient cohort with BRAF mutations that was treated with both vemurafenib and cobimetinib, which due to its aggressive nature and poor survival outcomes has an urgent clinical need. In BRAF-mutated mCRC, the combination of dabrafenib (a BRAF inhibitor) and trametinib (an MEK inhibitor) resulted in an ORR of 12% and an mPFS of 3.5 months. For this study, the primary endpoint is disease control with evidence of stable disease. PFS, OS, DoR, safety, and SD duration served as the secondary endpoints. DoR was "defined as the time from first documented response until disease progression." The duration of stable disease is defined as the time from study treatment initiation until disease progression.

Key Results Of 27 evaluable patients,

- "PR [was] in eight patients and SD16+ in six patients.
- The OR rate was 30% (95% CI 14–50), and the DC rate was 52% (95% CI 35–65).
- [Also,] mPFS was 15.7 weeks (95% CI 12.1–18.1 weeks); mOS was 38.9 weeks (95% CI 26.1–49.4 weeks)."
- Fatigue, diarrhea, hypercalcinemia, and upper gastrointestinal (GI) hemorrhage were reported as AEs, and "no grade 4 or 5 AEs were reported."

Other clinical studies evaluated agents for BRAFV600E mCRC tumors, such as the BEACON trial, which showed positive results for "encorafenib plus binimetinib plus cetuximab (triplet) and encorafenib plus cetuximab (doublet)," including improved median OS. Here, mPFS was "4.5, 4.3, and 1.5 months in the triplet, doublet, and control groups, respectively," demonstrating that poor outcomes were shown in control arms. The BRAFV600E mutation was identified as a targetable alteration in advanced solid tumors for the BRAF and MEK inhibitors cobimetinib plus vemurafenib in findings from the TAPUR clinical trial. DC as defined by CR, PR, and SD of at least 16 weeks' duration was the primary endpoint. In this trial, 31 BRAF mutation patients with solid tumors were enrolled, of which 28 patients were evaluable for efficacy. The mutations identified were K601E ($n = 2$), BRAF V600E ($n = 26$), and other mutations ($n = 3$). Treatment dosages were "cobimetinib (60 mg orally once daily for 21 days, followed by 7 days off) and vemurafenib (960 mg orally twice daily) until clinical and/or radiographic evidence of PD" or patient preference, unacceptable toxicity, and physician recommendation.

Key Results

- CR: Two patients with breast and ovarian cancers (V600E)
- PR: 14 (13 V600E, one N581I)
- SD16+: Three (two V600E, one T599_V600insT)
- DC rate: 68% ($p < 0.0001$; one-sided 90% CI 54–100)
- OR rate: 57% (95% CI 37–76)
- Grade 3–5 AEs or serious AEs in 19 patients, with one death as a result of treatment-related kidney injury [65]

Another study analyzing the results from basket trials for advanced solid tumors revealed the pan-cancer presence of "RET amplification as a novel putative genomic drivers" in a cohort of patients (results from the TCGA were also reported but not reiterated here).

Key Results

- 26 of 32,505 solid cancers, or 0.08%, was the frequency of wild-type rearranged during transfection (wtRET) amplification in the DFCI cohort, with 0.05% (26 of 53,152) in the MSKCC cohort.
- In terms of the genomic and clinicopathologic features of RET-amplified cases, three patients had concurrent driver mutations in MET amplification, KRAS, and EGFR exon 20 insertion; eight had no other codriver alterations; and, significantly, 11 NSCLCs harbored RET amplifications.

NSCLC, prostate cancer, breast cancer, and hepatobiliary cancer carried the RET amplification; the median RET copy number in RET-amplified cases was 7.5 (range, 6–36) in one cohort, whereas the median RET copy number was 5.7 (range, 4–27.7) in the other cohort.

The investigators concluded that wtRET amplification is representative of a novel genomic subtype with important implications for targeted treatment strategies across multiple tumor types. A study by Porcelli et al. also identified another oncogenic RET alteration (RET Δ898-901) through NGS in medullary thyroid cancer that showed secondary acquired resistance to selpercatinib, a TKI, due to an "acquired complete genetic loss of CDKN2A, CDKN2B, and MTAP genes," allowing for a customized treatment strategy," according to the study authors [66].

Another study, by Cheng et al., conducted an analysis of RET-fusion-positive Chinese patients with NSCLC treated with selpercatinib in the phase II LIBRETTO trial while also evaluating intracranial activity. "Patients received oral selpercatinib

160 mg, twice daily, until progression. Objective systemic and intracranial response was independently assessed per RECIST v1.1."

Key Results

- Of a total of the eight out of 36 patients included, 1/8, or 13%, had no previous systemic therapy but had prior brain surgery; 3/8, or 38%, had brain radiotherapy.
- The PR in 6/8 (75%) patients and SD in 2/8 (25%) served as the best overall systemic response.
- Confirmed intracranial response occurred in 4/5 (80%), with 3/5 PR and 1/5 CR among patients with measurable baseline CNS lesions.
- Only 2/8 patients among the best overall intracranial response had CNS-only disease progression, with CR being achieved in 3/8 patients, PR in 3/8 (38%) and SD in 1/8 (13%); non-PD/non-CR in 1/8 (13%); and 2/8 patients (25%) "had CNS-only disease progression," leading to the conclusion that selpercatinib had durable intracranial activity and clinical meaningful benefit in Chinese patients with BM in RET-altered NSCLC [67].

A phase II basket TAPUR study, in two results, revealed the results of the combination therapies P + T in lung cancer and endometrial cancer (EC). EC patients with ERBB2 or ERBB3 overexpression, amplification, and mutation were treated with P + T. Of the 17 tumors with ERBB2/3 and/or overexpression, eight had both ERBB2/3 mutations and ERBB2 amplification, and three had ERBB2 mutations.

"Patients were treated with an initial dose of 840 mg of IV infusion of pertuzumab over 60 minutes, then additional 420 mg of IV infusions over 30–60 minutes once every three weeks and an initial dose of 8 mg/kg of IV infusion of trastuzumab over 90 minutes and then additional 6 mg/kg of IV infusions over 30–60 minutes once every three weeks."

DC occurred in 10 patients, with two PRs and eight SD16+; 10 harbored ERBB2 amplification; and 6 of 10 with DC had more than one ERBB2/3 alteration. Furthermore, mPFS and mOS were 16 weeks (95% CI 10–28) and 61 weeks (95% CI 24–105), respectively, with DC and OR rates of 37% (95% CI 21–50) and 7% (95% CI 1–24) observed, respectively. Toxicity profiles were manageable. The authors concluded that in heavily pretreated patients, "P + T has antitumor activity in EC with ERBB2 amplification that warrants further study."

The BRAFV600E alteration is most commonly identified in melanoma; however, non-BRAFV600E mutations have also shown to be targetable, particularly by MAP-kinase therapies, as shown in a recent meta-analysis. Non-BRAFV600E mutations include in-frame deletions, fusions, and missense mutations. A literature search was conducted along with ASCO, AACR, and ESMO abstracts. Inclusion criteria were individual patient data describing class 2 or class 3 BRAF mutation. The evaluation of RR and that of PFS were gauged as primary outcomes. Patients with PR and CR were considered to have a treatment response; those with SD and PD that were categorized as nonresponders. Also, "class 2 BRAF-mutant tumors" had "higher RRs than class 3 mutants" among the varied tumor types, and among those with class 2 mutations, the RRs of mitogen activated protein kinase targeted therapies (MAPK TTs) were lowest in CRC (20%) but highest in other tumor types

(48%). RR was also observed in patients responding to EGFR and MEK inhibitors. The study authors noted that non-V600 BRAF mutations, especially class 2, can serve as driver oncogenes targeted by certain therapeutic approaches [68].

Additional studies focusing on HER2 cancers were performed, indicating association with indels and other types of alterations through genomic profiling and targeted gene sequencing. In a retrospective study, targeted gene sequencing was performed on HER2 and cancer-related genes.

- Of a "total of 25 indels in HER2 exon 18/19,
  - 17 recurrent were identified in 20 of 53,591 patients with lung cancer (0.037%)
  - two of 5888 patients with CRC (0.034%)
  - two of 3774 patients with breast cancer (0.053%)
  - one of 14 patients with UC of the renal pelvis (7.1%).
- Patients harboring HER2 exon 18/19 did not harbor any driver mutations, and in lung cancer, comparable mutation profiles existed between two established HER2 drivers, namely exon 20 insertions and S310 mutations and HER2 exon 18/19 indels."

The study significantly "revealed a class of rare but unique indels in HER2 exon 18/19, which may act as driver mutations in several cancer types" in which the indel led to differential response to TKIs [69].

Sokol et al. conducted a fascinating study on positing the mutual exclusivity of MSI-H and HRD -H status of BRCA ½ mutations in conferring PARP insensitivity to "dissect driver versus bystander status." According to the authors, the results indicated that two PC patients who had coexisting mutations in BRCAm and MSI-H showed resistance to PARPi but sensitivity to anti-PD-L1. HRR genes include "ATM, BARD1, BRCA1, BRCA2, BRIP1, CDK12, CHEK1, CHEK2, FANCL, PALB2, RAD51B, RAD51C, RAD51D, and RAD54L." The report describes two case studies of men with prostate cancer who had lower PSA levels and showed the stabilization of bone metastasis upon being identified as BRCA1/2 positive, which was refractory to Olaparib (300 mg twice daily), which was administered after androgen therapy and responded to pembrolizumab treatment. The study authors concluded that when reviewing genomic reports that show both BRCA mutation and MSI-H status, they should be interpreted as mutually exclusive phenomena because deciphering whether cancer is driven primarily by HRR deficiency or MMR is difficult, as is making a recommendation based on patients' data that they should be "preferentially" administered with PD-1 inhibitors as opposed to PARP inhibitors [70].

4.15 Resistance and Response in Solid Tumors (Fig. 4.7)

Resistance to targeted therapies is the result of a number of aspects of tumor biology, the tumor microenvironment, and the alternative signaling pathways that emerge after treatment. Combination therapies have been shown to overcome treatment, such as with immunotherapies that target multiple pathways in tumor

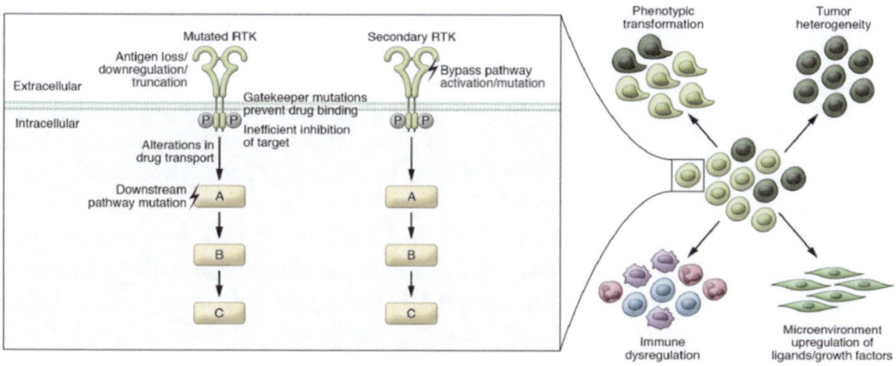

Fig. 4.7 Resistance mechanisms to targeted therapies against kinases in cancer. (Adapted from Waarts) [5]

progression. Tailoring therapy is another modality through which resistance can be overcome because clinicians are able to target specific signaling pathways, identify molecular alterations, and "bypass" mechanisms of resistance [71].

Kinase domain mutations prevent drug binding to targets and are the most frequent resistance mechanisms. Monoclonal antibody resistance results from tumor heterogeneity and the upregulation of ligands and growth factors in the tumor microenvironment (TME) (Fig. 4.7).

Resistance to targeted agents has also been identified through targeted next-generation sequencing. Zurita et al. conducted a fascinating study titled "Genomic Biomarkers and Genome-Wide Loss-of-Heterozygosity Scores in Metastatic Prostate Cancer Following Progression on Androgen-Targeting Therapies." The investigators used the Foundation One and Foundation One CDx assays to curate longitudinal clinical data via the technology-enabled abstraction of EHR conduct correlative analysis. They showed that in mCRPC, diagnostic biopsies should guide PARPi therapy because the number of HRR gene aberrations remains stable along the progression of mPC disease. Furthermore, gLOH served as a marker in the ADT-naive group of poor prognosis with incrementally greater increases in gLOH of up to 10%, leading to an increased risk of CRPC progression or death, with "progression to androgen- targeted therapies being linked to enrichment in AR, MYC, TP53, PTEN, RB1, and PI3K/PTEN pathway aberrations, as well as in genomic instability as per increasing gLOH scores, independent of BRCA1/2 status. "A significant enrichment in more-advanced disease states (from ADT-naive to CRPC and to NHT-CRPC) was observed for aberrations in AR (0.1% vs. 28% vs. 40%), MYC (5.5% vs. 18.2% vs. 20%), TP53 (35.4% vs. 47.7% vs. 51.5%), PTEN (27.6% vs. 38.6% vs. 36.4%), and RB1 (3.8% vs. 5.3% vs. 7.9%; all adjusted p values < 0.05" [72].

Right-sided CRC is found to be resistant to the anti-EGFR monoclonal antibody cetuximab; however, the underlying resistance mechanisms have not been investigated. One study showed that when CRC was divided into consensus molecular subtypes, CMS2 patients ($n = 52$; BRAF mutation enriched in CMS1) had the highest ORR, at 90.4% (47/52), and no patients experienced PD. CMS1 patients ($n = 26$) had the lowest ORRm at 42.3% (11/26) including four patients with PD, suggesting that comparing right-sided CMS2 tumors and left-sided CMS2 tumors yielded very little significant difference in response rates (93% left vs. 80% right), leading to the implication that anti-EGFR treatment should be an option for CMS2 tumors, irrespective of primary tumor location [73].

Treatment selection pressure occurs in the context of G1 cell-cycle arrest in that RB1 mutations in breast cancer can serve as a molecular escape mutation by tumors, as seen in a longitudinal study focused on ctDNA reports that described the emergence of RB1 mutation when a palbociclib combination encountered drug resistance. Of the patients, 3% (9/348) reported RB1 loss on CDK4/6i treatment, with a significantly shorter mPFS of 3.6 months (95% CI 2.2 to no response) when compared with their RB1 wild-type tumors.

According to Sato et al., who identified novel driver oncogenic mutations and the mechanisms of acquired resistance for the further development of personalized cancer medicine, the nine members of the SRK family of kinases—SRC, YES1, FYN, FGR, LCK, HCK, BLK, LYN, and FRK—can cooperate with RTKs while performing crucial regulatory functions in mediating cell invasion due to migration and adhesion, leading to the activation of downstream signaling pathways that are implicated in tumor progression. The SRK/ABL kinase inhibitors include bosutinib and dasatinib for approved usage in Ph+ chromosome-positive leukemias driven by BCR/ABL fusion. In their article "SRC Family Kinase Inhibition Targets YES1 and YAP1 as Primary Drivers of Lung Cancer and as Mediators of Acquired Resistance to ALK and Epidermal Growth Factor Receptor Inhibitors," the investigators explore how YES1 amplification can serve as an oncogenic driver for promoting tumorigenesis and how YES1/YAP1 amplifications act as mediators of acquired resistance to ALK and of EGFRs and TKIs [13].

The NOXA mRNA destabilization was identified by Montero et al. as a common mechanism conferring resistance to targeted therapies. Targeted therapies, BRAF and EGFR inhibitors among them, deplete the proapoptotic factor NOXA, thus creating a dependence on antiapoptotic proteins MCL-1, an adaptation of pathway signaling destabilizing mRNA transcripts and leading to increases in cytotoxic responses in cell lines and murine melanoma models by interrupting antiapoptotic adaptive resistance. The authors demonstrated that targeted therapies induce rapid dependence on MCL-1, and MAPK inhibition suppresses the proapoptotic factor NOXA while also destabilizing the NOXA mRNA. Targeted therapies create a vulnerability to MCL-1 inhibitors, which when evaluated in vivo in sequence with BRAF inhibition demonstrated a cytotoxic response. Small molecule inhibitors, including BRAF inhibitors, gefitinib for EGFR mutant cell lines, imatinib for KIT mutant cell lines, and crizotinib for ALK mutant cell lines, were dosed at a high potency and were strongly sensitized, leading to enhanced targeted activity in the presence of MCL-1 suppression. MCL-1 expression inhibited the BRAF inhibitor-led cytotoxicity, showing that MCL-1 is "necessary and sufficient for resistance to multiple targeted therapies." The mechanisms of this adaptive dependence were then evaluated by determining the effect of targeted therapies on the BCL-2 family of proteins, and a loss of NOXA expression was found. NOXA is a protein that binds to and inactivates MCL-1, especially seen in cell lines treated with MEK and BRAF inhibitors but also in imatinib-treated KIT mutated GIST cell lines, crizotinib-treated ALK mutant cell lines, lapatinib-treated HER2-amplified breast cancer lines, and geftinib-treated EGFR lung cancer cell lines. MAPK-mediated suppression on NOXA were mRNA related with downregulated levels, and the MCL1 and BCL-2 family members were not changed. Additionally, siRNA-targeted ERK1/2 experiments showed that decreased NOXA protein was associated with the suppression of the MAPK pathway. The constitutive expression of NOXA strongly sensitized cells to BRAF inhibitors, the data suggesting that the MAPK pathway is the necessary expression of NOXA, considered a functionally important MCL-1 antagonist. Because NOXA binds to MCL-1, a hypothesis surrounding the loss of NOXA to free MCL-1 from its bound form to associate with the proapoptotic BCL-2 family members was generated. Immunoprecipitation experiments showed that the pro-apoptotic BAX/BAK activating factor BIM associates with MCL-1 and inhibits it, which strongly increased upon treatment with targeted agents, suggesting that the targeted inhibition of the MAPK pathway induces MCL-1 dependence This suggests that cancer cell priortreatment with MAPK pathway inhibitors promotes sensitivity to MCL-1 inhibitors, which is less effective when administered in the opposite sequence, as shown by tumor-bearing mice being treated with vemurafenib and dabrafenib; "dependence on MCL-1 was induced with the suppression of the NOXA protein and association of BIM to MCL-1 promoted." The in vivo sequential targeting of BRAF and MCL-1 was then conducted. No overt toxicity was observed, and the growth inhibition of tumors was demonstrated but reversed upon treatment discontinuation, showing that BRAF and MCL-1 inhibition "led to profound tumor regression" and prolonged survival when compared to dabrafenib alone. The study authors showed through data that CR can be achieved with MAPK inhibition, leading to in vivo MCL-1 independence with therapeutic targeting through BRAF and MCL-1 inhibitors. They gained insights into the mechanisms behind how cancer cells can evade apoptosis despite the targeted suppression of oncoproteins, through adaptation rather than genetic mechanisms; and they showed that that overcomes targeted therapy resistance in vivo through targeting apoptotic cells [74].

4.16 Targeted Therapies in Preclinical and Early Stages

SAFFRON-104 is a multicohort phase Ib/II study that evaluated sitravatinib as a spectrum-selective TKI that can target with/without tislelizumab, an anti-(PD-1) antibody, in patients with advanced HCC. Sitravatinib is an oral TKI that targets TAM and VEGFR-2 and that reduces immunosuppressing by promoting macrophage activity and reducing T-reg cells.

Phase I determined the RP2D of sitravatinib in combination and as monotherapy and phase II evaluated sitravatinib monotherapy in pretreated HCC as well as the combination therapy in anti-PD-L1–naive and –treated patients. ORR and safety were the primary endpoints. The study presented the safety and preliminary clinical activity of sitravatinib with or without tislelizumab in patients with advanced HCC.

Key Results

- Sitravatinib RP2D: 120 mg orally once daily while both as monotherapy and in combination with tislelizumab, grade ≥ 3 treatment-related adverse events were reported in 14 (51.9%) and 42 (50.0%) patients, respectively. The ORR = 25% (95% CI: 8.7–49.1) in HCC-pretreated patients receiving sitravatinib monotherapy.
- In dual combination therapy, the ORRs were as follows.
  - Anti-PD-(L)1–naive HCC—11.5% (95% CI 2.4–30.2)
  - Anti-PD-(L)1–treated HCC—9.5% (95% CI 1.2–30.4)
  - Anti-PD-(L)1–naive GC/GEJC—16.1% (95% CI 5.5–33.7)
- Sitravatinib monotherapy was administered to all patients at either the 80 mg of QD dose ($n = 3$) or the 120 mg of QD dose ($n = 24$) in phases I and II combined or the safety analysis set that had reported a TRAE. Furthermore, 81/84 patients were treated with sitravatinib plus tislelizumab and received the sitravatinib 120 mg of QD dose, of whom 90.1% ($n = 73/81$) experienced a TRAE; 90.1% of patients had events that were considered treatment related (sitravatinib), whereas 82.7% had events tislelizumab related. Most common TRAEs (occurring in > 30.0% of patients) were proteinuria, increased alpha-1 antitrypsin (AAT), palmar/plantar erythrodysesthesia syndrome, hypertension, and diarrhea.
- TEAEs leading to death occurred in 12 patients in the sitravatinib dose of 120 mg of QD and tislelizumab arm. Moreover, 8.6% of deaths ($n = 7$) were unexplained, and fatal TEAEs were reported in ≥ two patients, including death and respiratory failure.
- The ORR in the combination treatment was as follows.
  - 11.5% (95% CI 2.4–30.2) in patients with anti-PD-(L)1–naive, pretreated HCC
  - 9.5% (95% CI 1.2–30.4) in patients with anti-PD-(L)1–treated HCC
  - Median PFS was 6.8 months (95% CI 2.8–8.3) and 4.2 months (95% CI 2.7–6.8) in patients with anti-PD-(L)1–naive and anti-PD-(L)1–treated HCC, respectively.
  - Median OS was 20.5 months (95% CI 7.4–NE) and 12.4 months (95% CI 7.0–14.1), respectively, in the phase II safety analysis set.
- 120 mg of QD was the phase I determined RP2D of sitravatinib, both as monotherapy and in combination with tislelizumab.
- All patients experienced TRAEs in the sitravatinib monotherapy group and 90.5% in patients receiving sitravatinib with tislelizumab, most of whom were manageable through dose reduction or interruption or supportive therapy. Half of all patients, or 51.9% treated with monotherapy experienced grade ≥ three TRAEs and 50.0% treated with combination, of whom 3.7% and 10.7% led to treatment discontinuation, respectively.

The study authors concluded that "[s]itravatinib with/without tislelizumab was generally well tolerated and showed preliminary antitumor activity in patients with advanced HCC" [75].

The RET fusion was identified as a tissue-agnostic target by Subbiah et al. in the phase 1/2 ARROW trial, illustrating the precision oncology paradigm that identifies oncogenic alterations through NGS and genomically targeted therapies for multiple tumor types. The pan-cancer efficacy of pralsetinib, which targets the RET fusion, was evaluated in thyroid cancer, NSCLC, and other RET-altered tumors. The RET oncogene encodes a transmembrane RTK that when mutated induces oncogenic transformation through the aberrant activation of the RET RTK. Pralsetinb is a selective RET inhibitor, for which preclinical and clinical evidence suggests that targeting RET fusions prevents oncogene addiction across tumor types. The ARROW trial revealed the safety and efficacy of RET-altered NSCLC and thyroid cancer. In that trial, 587 patients were enrolled, 29 of whom had RET-fusion-positive NSCLC or thyroid cancer, with 28 patients receiving a starting dose of 400 mg of QD. Four patients remained on treatment at data cutoff, and 25 patients discontinued treatment due to disease progression or adverse events (neutropenia and thrombocytopenia). Moreover, ctDNA identified CCDC6 (six patients (26%)), KIF5B (six patients (26%)), and NCOA4 (three patients (13%)) as RET-fusion "partners." ORR was the primary endpoint of phase 2, which was 57% (CI 35–77), or 23 eligible patients, with three having CR and ten having confirmed PR. Tumor shrinkage was seen in 91% of patients after baseline.

Key Results

- Four tumor responses were found, with one CR confirmed, 2/3 cholangiocarcinoma and 2/3 sarcoma patients with one CR, 2/3 neuroendocrine cancer patients, one HNC patient, and one unknown primary tumor with CR.
- Another cholangiocarcinoma patient "had a single timepoint response before discontinuing treatment due to an AE. DOR rates were 69% (95% CI 44–94) at 6 months and 39% (95% CI 8–69) at 12 months."
- TEAEs occurred in all patients, of whom 21 were grade 3 or greater events. TRAEs occurred in 25 patients (86%), of whom 20, or 69%, experienced a grade ≥ 3 TRAE. Increased AST was seen in 11 patients, increased alanine aminotransferase (ALT) was seen 10 patients, and neutropenia was seen in 10 (38%, 34%, and 34%, respectively).
- Two patients experienced grade 4 events, with one patient having thrombocytopenia, pancytopenia, and acute kidney injury.
- The study investigators concluded that "pralsetinib achieved robust and durable anti-tumor activity regardless of tumor type in advanced and metastatic RET-fusion-positive tumors, with an ORR of 57%. No new safety signals were observed, with the data suggesting that broad RET testing via NGS may be conducted to identify candidates who may benefit from treatment with pralsetinib" [76].

Yarchoan et al. conducted a first-in-human trial of TPST-1120, a first-in-class oral inhibitor of a fatty acid ligand-activated transcriptional factor that leads to the upregulation of genes involved in fatty acid oxidation and peroxisome proliferator-activated receptor alpha (PPAR-alpha). The investigators hypothesized that the PPAR-alpha would be a novel target for an antitumor agent because TPST-1120 in preclinical models led to tumor reduction when combined with immune checkpoint inhibitors. TPST-1120 was evaluated in a phase I, open-label, dose-escalation study with and without nivolumab in several cancers, including RCC, cholangiocarcinoma, and HCC. The endpoints were safety and antitumor activity. The metabolic aspects of tumorigenesis are the increase in glycolysis known as the Warburg effect and other pathways, including fatty acid oxidation, which leads to increased stemness, drug resistance, and metastasis (5–7). PPAR-alpha is a unique ligand-activated transcription factor that regulates genes in fatty acid oxidation (FAO), angiogenesis, and inflammation and dampens Th-1 promoting inflammation during metabolic disturbances that involve antagonizing proinflammation transcription factors NFκB and AP-1. TPST-1120 was shown to be a competitive antagonist of human PPAR-alpha in nanomolar quantities, achieving high specificity, as shown in xenograft and syngeneic tumor models. Safety was assessed on the basis of the incidence of AEs, a physical exam, and laboratory results. In this trial, 39 patients were enrolled, with 21 in the monotherapy cohort (pancreatic cancer, $n = 8$; CCA, $n = 5$; CCR, $n = 4$) and 18 in the nivolumab+TPST-1120 cohort (CCA, $n = 9$; RCC, $n = 5$). Prior systemic therapies were a median of three for the monotherapy (2–9) and three for combination patients (1–6). No dose limiting toxicities (DLTs) were observed during dose escalation; however, an maximum tolerated dose (MTD) was not established as a compound as monotherapy or in combination with nivolumab. TRAEs included nausea (20%), fatigue (15%), and diarrhea (10%) in the monotherapy cohort and fatigue (33.3%), nausea (17%), and a grade 3 TRAE of arthralgia ($n = 1$) at 400 mg twice daily. Hepatic enzymes increased along with the muscle spasms at a dosing of 600 mg twice daily. SD was achieved in 10 patients, or 53% of them, and PD was reported in six patients, or 32% of them, which constituted best overall response (BOR). Tumor shrinkage was observed in four patients, or 21% of them, with no target lesion growth showing a change from the baseline. The RCC responder had prior lines of anti-PD-1 treatment (ipi + nivo, followed by cabozantinib and everolimus). Biomarker exploration revealed modulated genes that included FCGRIIA, ITGAX, TAP1, and TNFRSF1A. The OBD for monotherapy and combination therapy was 600 mg twice daily. The study authors concluded in this FIH study that TPST-1120 as a novel investigational agent inhibited PPAR-alpha and can therapeutically target cancer cells, being both well tolerated as a monotherapy and in combination with nivolumab. Clinical activity was also shown in pancreatic cancer, CCA, and late-stage CRC given that an ORR of 20% was shown across all doses. The authors also characterized the antitumor activity of the agent as dual: transrepression associated with immunomodulatory activity that is linked to the PPAR response element–mediated transcription-controlling lipid metabolism [77].

In *Nature Medicine*, a phase I trial evaluating the KRASG12C investigational agent D3S-001 in advanced solid tumors was published by Cho et al. D3S-001 is a next-generation KRAS-G12C inhibitor that enhances efficacy by overcoming growth-factor-induced nucleotide exchange. The primary endpoints were safety and determining MTD. The secondary endpoints included ORR, DCR, and biomarker exploration. Codon 12 of the RAS protein impairs GTPase activating protein–facilitated hydrolysis, leading to KRAS overactivation and driving cancer progression. G12C mutation retains the intrinsic hydrolytic function, and the targeting GDP-bound form can impact cancer outcomes. First-generation KRASG12C inhibitors include adagrasib and sotorasib for the treatment of NSCLC; however, ORRs remain modest (31.9% and 28.1%, respectively). One of the objectives for this study was to achieve optimal target inhibition at therapeutic doses and pharmakinetic exposures. EGF-stimulated nucleotide also complicates the issue because it shifts from the GDP-bound inactive form to the GTP-bound active form, which is particularly relevant for CRC. The investigators aimed to achieve target effectivity at clinically relevant doses and to trap KRAS-G12C proteins in their inactive form in the presence of growth factors that lead to nucleotide exchange. In preclinical models, D3S-001 was shown to enhance target engagement and overcome nucleotide exchange, displaying improved potency while depleting active KRAS in the cell. Antitumor activity was demonstrated in mouse NSCLC, CRC, and PDAC models, and CNS penetration was observed, leading to intracranial tumor regression. This phase1/2 trial was designed to investigate these effects in human populations. In the phase 1a dose-escalation phase, MTD was not determined; however, no DLTs were seen in the dosages given. TRAEs, including hyperkalemia, hypertriglyceridemia, and nausea (all $n = 1$), occurred in two of 40 patients, and abnormal hepatic function occurred as well (increased gamma-glutamyl transferase (GGT), AST, ALT, 1,1,2). Serious treatment-related AEs were not reported. Nausea occurred in 19 patients, or 45.2% of them; diarrhea in 13, or 31.0%; and increased amylase in eight, or 19%. NSCLC patients ($n = 25$) who had prior PD-L1 treatment experienced hepatotoxicity in the form of increased ALT, AST, and GGT that were mostly grade 1 in severity. The confirmed ORR among "34 response-evaluable patients was 73.5% (95% CI 55.6–87.1) and DCR was 97.1% (95% CI 84.7–99.9)." "Among G12Ci-naive responders, the estimated 6-month DOR rate was 78.4% (95% CI 55.6–90.4). Among all 36 G12Ci-naive patients, the estimated 6-month PFS rate was 68.6% (95% CI 50.5–81.3)." In biomarker analysis, all 34 patients had KRASG12C ctDNA positivity at baseline, with 25 patients having a rapid reduction in mutant allele frequency. In phase Ib dose expansion, 20 patients with KRASG12Ci-pretreated NSCLC were enrolled and received D3S-001 at a dose of 600 mg once daily. The best response in a pretreated population (sotorasib, gleirasib, garsorasib, adagrasib, and olmorasib) was PR in eight patients (40%), SD in seven (35%), and unknown in five (25%). Prior treatment was discontinued due to PD and toxicity in one patient. Tumor shrinkage was seen in 12 of 20 patients in the dose-expansion cohort. Eight patients had a 100% reduction in KRAS G12C MAF, and that reduction was > 90% for 11 patients. All six radiographic responders were G12C positive at baseline, and five exhibited the complete clearance of MAF. The study authors concluded that D3S-001 demonstrated a favorable safety profile in the dose-escalation part with complete target inhibition, with promising antitumor activity across all tumor types in KRAS-G12Ci-naive patients (ORR 73.5%; DCR 97.1%.) "Confirmed ORRs in NSCLC, CRC, and PDAC were 66.7%, 88.9% and 75.0%, respectively."

Furthermore, 20 NSCLC patients in an expansion cohort had disease progression on first-generation KRAS-G12C, with D3S-001 demonstrating a DCR of 80% and an ORR of 30%. The study reported clinical data on single-agent activity for the GDP-bound KRAS inhibitor, as shown in a cohort of NSCLC patients with disease progression on G12Ci, eliciting a diversity of resistance mechanisms and further providing clinical validation for the D3S-001 mechanism of action for its further translation over first-generation G12Ci-enhanced activity. This finding highlights its promise to overcome the limitations of an earlier G12Ci and represents "a next-generation high-potency inhibitor for the backbone of treatment for KRASG12C mutated solid tumors" [78].

References

1. Rai V, Yash G, Srivastava SP, Shukla A, Bano N, et al. Targeted therapies in cancer treatment: unveiling the latest breakthroughs and promising approaches. J Res Appl Sci Biotechnol. 2023;2(6):175–83.
2. Kulasegaran T, Oliveira N. Metastatic castration-resistant prostate cancer: advances in treatment and symptom management. Curr Treat Options in Oncol. 2024;25:914–31.
3. Trédan O, Pouessel D, Penel N, Chabaud S, Gomez-Roca C, et al. Broad versus limited gene panels to guide treatment in patients with advanced solid tumors: a randomized controlled trial. Nat Med. 2024;31:1502.
4. Forrest SJ, Gupta H, Ward A, Li YY, Doan D, et al. Molecular profiling of 888 pediatric tumors informs future precision trials and data sharing initiatives in pediatric cancer. Nat Commun. 2024;15:5837.
5. Waarts MR, Stonestrom AJ, Park YC, Levine RL. Targeting mutations in cancer. J Clin Invest. 2022;132:e154943.
6. Punekar SR, Velcheti V, Neel BG, Wong W. The current state of the art and future trends in RAS- targeted cancer therapies. Nat Rev Clin Oncol. 2022;19:637.
7. Bettaieb A, Paul C, Stéphanie P, Shan J, Lotfi C, et al. Precision medicine in breast cancer: reality or utopia? J Transl Med. 2017;15:139.
8. Mayer EL, Ren Y, Mahtani R, Ma C, DeMichele A, et al. PACE: a randomized phase II study of Fulvestrant, Palbociclib, and Avelumab after progression on cyclin-dependent Kinase 4/6 inhibitor and Aromatase inhibitor for hormone receptor–positive/human epidermal growth factor receptor–negative metastatic breast cancer. J Clin Oncol. 2024;42(17):2050.
9. Rastogi P, Goetz MP, Cicin I, O'Shaughnessy J, Martin M, et al. Adjuvant Abemaciclib Plus Endocrine therapy for hormone receptor–positive, human epidermal growth factor receptor 2–negative, high-risk early breast cancer: results from a preplanned monarchE overall survival interim analysis, including 5-year efficacy outcomes. J Clin Oncol. 2024;42:987–93.
10. Heiss JL, Chang E, Gao X, Troung T, Brave MH, et al. US Food and Drug Administration approval summary: Talazoparib in combination with enzalutamide for treatment of patients with homologous recombination repair gene-mutated metastatic castration-resistant prostate cancer. J Clin Oncol. 2024;42(15):1851.
11. ASCO Educational Guidelines. J Clin Oncol, 2024.
12. Chavez-MacGregor M, Maio J, Pusztai L, Goetz MP, Rastogi P, et al. Phase III randomized, placebo-controlled trial of endocrine therapy ±1 year of Everolimus in patients with high-risk, hormone receptor–positive, early-stage breast cancer. J Clin Oncol. 2024;42:3012.
13. Sato H, Kubato D, Qiao H, Jungbluth A, Rehtkman N, et al. SRC family Kinase inhibition targets YES1 and YAP1 as primary drivers of lung cancer and as mediators of acquired resistance to ALK and epidermal growth factor receptor inhibitors. JCO Precis Oncol. 2022;6:e2200088.

14. Cortes J, Hurvitz SA, O'Shaunessey J, Delaloge S, Iwata H, et al. Randomized phase III study of Amcenestrant Plus Palbociclib versus Letrozole Plus Palbociclib in Estrogen receptor-positive, human epidermal growth factor receptor 2-negative advanced breast cancer: primary results from AMEERA-5. J Clin Oncol. 2024;42:2680.
15. Lu Y-S, Mahadin EIB, Azim H, Eraip Y, Sim Y, et al. Final results of RIGHT choice: Ribociclib Plus Endocrine therapy versus combination chemotherapy in premenopausal women with clinically aggressive hormone receptor–positive/human epidermal growth factor receptor 2–negative advanced breast cancer. J Clin Oncol. 2024;42:2812.
16. Batalini F, Madison RW, Sokol ES, Jin DX, Chen K-T, et al. Homologous recombination deficiency landscape of breast cancers and real-world effectiveness of poly ADP-ribose polymerase inhibitors in patients with Somatic BRCA1/2, Germline PALB2, or homologous recombination deficiency signature. JCO Precis Oncol. 2023;7:e2300091.
17. Gerratana L, Davis AA, Velimirovic M, Reduzzi C, Clifton K, et al. Cyclin-dependent Kinase 4/6 inhibitors beyond progression in metastatic breast cancer: a retrospective real-world biomarker analysis. JCO Precis Oncol. 2023;7:e2200531.
18. Brett JO, Dubash TD, Johnson GN, Niermieko A, Mariotti V, et al. A gene panel associated with Abemaciclib utility in ESR1-mutated breast cancer after prior cyclin-dependent Kinase 4/6-inhibitor progression. JCO Precis Oncol. 2023;7:e2200532.
19. Janne PA, Planchard D, Kobayashi K, Cheng Y, Lee CK, et al. CNS efficacy of Osimertinib with or without chemotherapy in epidermal growth factor receptor–mutated advanced non–small-cell lung cancer. JCO Precis Oncol. 2023;42:808.
20. Remon J, Besse B, Aix SP, Callejo A, Al-Rabi K, et al. Overall survival from the EORTC LCG-1613 APPLE trial of Osimertinib versus Gefitinib followed by Osimertinib in advanced EGFR-mutant non–small-cell lung cancer. J Clin Oncol. 2024;42:1350.
21. Thummalapalli R, Bernstein E, Herzberg B, Li BT, Iqbal A, et al. Clinical and genomic features of response and toxicity to Sotorasib in a real-world cohort of patients with advanced KRAS G12C-mutant non–small cell lung cancer. JCO Precis Oncol. 2023;7:e2300030.
22. Perol M, Solomao BJ, Goto K, Park K, Nadal E. CNS protective effect of Selpercatinib in first-line RET fusion-positive advanced non–small cell lung cancer. J Clin Oncol. 2024;42:2500.
23. Li W, Xiong A, Yang N, Fan H, Yu Q, et al. Efficacy and safety of Taletrectinib in Chinese patients with ROS1+ non-small cell lung cancer: the phase II TRUST-I study. J Clin Oncol. 2024;42:2660.
24. Blakely CM, Urisman A, Gubens MA, Mulvey CK, Allen GM, et al. Neoadjuvant Osimertinib for the treatment of stage I-IIIA epidermal growth factor receptor–mutated non–small cell lung cancer: a phase II Multicenter Study. J Clin Oncol. 2024;42:3105.
25. Solomon BJ, Liu G, Felip E, Mok TSK, Soo RA, et al. Lorlatinib versus Crizotinib in patients with advanced ALK-positive non–small cell lung cancer: 5-year outcomes from the phase III CROWN study. J Clin Oncol. 2024;42:3400.
26. Pike LRG, Maio E, Boe LA, Patil T, Imber BS, et al. Tyrosine Kinase inhibitors with and without up-front stereotactic radiosurgery for brain metastases from EGFR and ALK oncogene–driven non–small cell lung cancer (TURBO-NSCLC). J Clin Oncol. 2024;42:3606.
27. Giustini N, Patel SP, Myall NJ, Moura JFP, Kulkarni A, et al. Resistance to EGFR Tyrosine Kinase inhibitor therapy in non–small-cell lung cancer via newly acquired targetable oncogenic driver alterations with an emphasis on BRAF: case series and literature review of treatment. JCO Precis Oncol. 2022;6:e2100551.
28. Urbanska EM, Sorensen JB, Melchior LC, Costa J, Santoni-Rugui E. Durable response to combined Osimertinib and Pralsetinib treatment for Osimertinib resistance due to novel intergenic ANK3-RET fusion in EGFR-mutated non–small-cell lung cancer. JCO Precis Oncol. 2022;6:e2200040.
29. Ambrosini M, Del Re M, Manca P, Hendfar A, Drilon A, et al. ALK inhibitors in patients with ALK fusion–positive GI cancers: an International Data Set and a Molecular Case Series. JCO Precis Oncol. 2022;6:e2200015.

30. Drilon A, Tan DSW, Lassen UN, Leyvraz S, Liu Y, et al. Efficacy and safety of Larotrectinib in patients with Tropomyosin receptor Kinase fusion–positive lung cancers. JCO Precis Oncol. 2022;6:e2100418.
31. Ahn ER, Rothe M, Mangat PK, Garret-Mayer E, et al. Pertuzumab Plus Trastuzumab in patients with endometrial cancer with ERBB2/3 amplification, overexpression, or mutation: results from the TAPUR study. JCO Precis Oncol. 2023;7:e2200609.
32. Ganti AK, Rothe M, Mangat PK, Garret-Mayer E, Dib EG, et al. Pertuzumab Plus Trastuzumab in patients with lung cancer with ERBB2 mutation or amplification: results from the targeted agent and profiling utilization registry study. JCO Precis Oncol. 2023;7:e2300041.
33. Lin NU, Murthy RK, Abramson V, Anders C, Bachelot T, et al. Tucatinib vs placebo, both in combination with Trastuzumab and Capecitabine, for previously treated ERBB2 (HER2)-positive metastatic breast cancer in patients with brain metastases updated exploratory analysis of the HER2CLIMB randomized clinical trial. JAMA Oncol. 2023;9(2):197–205.
34. Gluz O, Nitz UA, Christgen M, Kuemmel S, Holtschmidt J, Schumacher J. Efficacy of Endocrine Therapy Plus Trastuzumab and Pertuzumab vs De-escalated chemotherapy in patients with hormone receptor–positive/ERBB2-positive early breast cancer the Neoadjuvant WSG-TP-II randomized clinical trial. JAMA Oncol. 2023;9(7):946–54.
35. Mouabbi JA, Raghavendra AS, Bassett RL, Hassan A, Tripathy D. Survival outcomes in patients with hormone receptor–positive metastatic breast cancer with Lowor no ERBB2 expression treated with targeted therapies plus endocrine therapy. JAMA Netw Open. 2023;6:e2313017.
36. Girod M, Dalle S, Mortier L, Dalac S, Leccia M-T, et al. Non-V600E/K BRAF mutations in metastatic melanoma: molecular description, frequency, and effectiveness of targeted therapy in a large National Cohort. JCO Precis Oncol. 2022;6:e2200075.
37. Lee C-k, Kim HS, Jung M, Kim H, Bae WK, et al. Open-label, multicenter, randomized, biomarker-integrated Umbrella trial for second-line treatment of advanced gastric cancer: K-Umbrella gastric cancer study. J Clin Oncol. 2024;42:348.
38. Battaglin F, Ou F-S, Qu X, Hochster HS, Niedzwiecki D, et al. HER2 gene expression levels are predictive and prognostic in patients with metastatic colorectal cancer enrolled in CALGB/SWOG 80405. J Clin Oncol. 2024;42:1890.
39. Domingo E, Kelly C, Hay J, Sansom O, Maka N, et al. Prognostic and predictive value of immunoscore in stage III colorectal cancer: pooled analysis of cases from the SCOT and IDEA-HORG studies. J Clin Oncol. 2024;42:2207.
40. Nowak JA, Twombly T, Shi O, Haruki K, Fujiyoshi K, et al. Improved survival with adjuvant cyclooxygenase 2 inhibition in PIK3CA-activated stage III colon cancer: CALGB/SWOG 80702 (Alliance). J Clin Oncol. 2024;42:2853.
41. Ranganathan M, Sacca RE, Trottier M, Maio A, Kemel Y, et al. Prevalence and clinical implications of mismatch repair-proficient colorectal cancer in patients with lynch syndrome. JCO Precis Oncol. 2023;7:e2200675.
42. Benusiglio PR, Elder F, Touat M, Perrier A, Sanson M, et al. Mismatch repair deficiency and lynch syndrome among adult patients with Glioma. JCO Precis Oncol. 2023;7:e2200525.
43. Hino K, Nishina T, Kajiwara T, Bando H, Nakamura N, et al. Association of ERBB2 copy number and gene Coalterations with Trastuzumab efficacy and resistance in human epidermal growth factor receptor 2–positive Esophagogastric and gastric cancer. JCO Precis Oncol. 2022;6:e2200135.
44. Gupta R, Meric-Bernstam F, Rothe M, Garret-Meyer E, Mangat PK, et al. Pertuzumab Plus Trastuzumab in patients with colorectal cancer with ERBB2 amplification or ERBB2/3 mutations: results from the TAPUR study. JCO Precis Oncol. 2022;6:e2200306.
45. Hegewisch-Becker S, Mendez G, Chao J, Nemecek R, Feeney K, et al. First-line Nivolumab and Relatlimab Plus chemotherapy for gastric or gastroesophageal junction adenocarcinoma: the phase II RELATIVITY-060 study. J Clin Oncol. 2024;42:2080.

46. Nakamura Y, Ozaki H, Ueno M, Komatsu Y, Se Y, et al. Targeted therapy guided by circulating tumor DNA analysis in advanced gastrointestinal tumors. Nat Med. 2025;31:165.
47. Nakamura Y, Kawazoe A, Lordick F, Janjigian YY, Shitara K. Biomarker- targeted therapies for advanced- stage gastric and gastro- oesophageal junction cancers: an emerging paradigm. Nat Rev Clin Oncol. 2021;18:473.
48. Appleman LJ, Kim SE, Harris WB, Pal SK, Pins MR, et al. Randomized, double-blind phase III study of Pazopanib versus placebo in patients with metastatic renal cell carcinoma who have no evidence of disease after Metastasectomy: ECOG-ACRIN E2810. J Clin Oncol. 2024;8:2061.
49. McGregor BA, Xie W, Adib E, Stadler WM, Zakharia Y. Biomarker-based phase II study of Sapanisertib (TAK-228): an mTORC1/2 inhibitor in patients with refractory metastatic renal cell carcinoma. JCO Precis Oncol. 2022;6:e2100448.
50. Boyle JJ, Pfail JL, Lichtbroun BJ, Singer EA. Adjuvant therapy for renal cell carcinoma: endpoints, outcomes, and risk assessments. JCO Precis Oncol. 2023;7:e2200407.
51. Mehra R, Nallandhighal S, Cotta B, Knuth Z, Su F, et al. Discovery and validation of a 15-gene prognostic signature for clear cell renal cell carcinoma. JCO Precis Oncol. 2024;7:e2300565.
52. Hussain M, Corcoran C, Sibilla C, Fizazi K, Saad F, et al. Tumor genomic testing for >4,000 men with metastatic castration-resistant prostate cancer. Clin Cancer Res. 2022;28:1518–30.
53. Abida W, Campbell D, Patnaik A, Bryce AH, Shapiro J, et al. Rucaparib for the treatment of metastatic castration-resistant prostate cancer associated with a DNA damage repair gene alteration: final results from the phase 2 TRITON2 study. Eur Urol. 2023;84(3):321–30.
54. Karasic TB, Eads JR, Goyal L. Precision medicine and immunotherapy have arrived for Cholangiocarcinoma: an overview of recent approvals and ongoing clinical trials. JCO Precis Oncol. 2023;7:e2200573.
55. Wirth LJ, Brose MS, Subbiah V, Worden F, Solomon B, et al. Durability of response with Selpercatinib in patients with RET-activated thyroid cancer: long-term safety and efficacy from LIBRETTO-001. JCO Precis Oncol. 2024;8:3187.
56. Stiefel J, Kushner BH, Roberts SS, Iglesias-Cardenas F, Kramer K, Modak S. Anaplastic Lymphoma Kinase inhibitors for therapy of neuroblastoma in adults. JCO Precis Oncol. 2023;7:e2300138.
57. Coleman N, Marcelo KL, Hopkins JF, Khan NI, Du R, et al. HRAS mutations define a distinct subgroup in head and neck squamous cell carcinoma. JCO Precis Oncol. 2023;7:e2200211.
58. Zhou W, Ke SQ, Huang Z, Flavahan W, Fang X, et al. Periostin secreted by glioblastoma stem cells recruit M2 tumour-associated macrophages and promote malignant growth. Nat Cell Biol. 2015;17:170.
59. Brown LC, Zhu J, Mauer E, Thiede SM, Macera L, et al. RNA-based homologous recombination deficiency signature detects homologous recombination deficiency-RNA+ patients with and without homologous recombination repair gene pathogenic alterations in men with prostate cancer. JCO Precis Oncol. 2023;7:e2300378.
60. Doroshow DB, O'Donnell PH, Hoffman-Censits JH, Gupta SV, Vaishampayan U, Heath EI, Garcia P, Zhao Q, Yu M, Milowsky MI, Galsky MD. Phase II trial of Olaparib in patients with metastatic urothelial cancer Harboring DNA damage response gene alterations. JCO Precis Oncol. 2023;7:e2300095.
61. Christanat J, Ho L, Clement S, Genestie C, Sehouli J. Normalized LST is an efficient biomarker for homologous recombination deficiency and Olaparib response in ovarian carcinoma. JCO Precis Oncol. 2023;7:e2200555.
62. Yang ES, Halabi S, Rothe M, Garret-Meyer E, Mangat PK, et al. Olaparib in patients with metastatic prostate cancer with BRCA1/2 mutation: results from the TAPUR study. JCO Precis Oncol. 2023;7:e2200505.
63. Shao C, Ren Y, Zhou H, Chen C, Dettman EJ, et al. Association between homologous recombination repair biomarkers and survival in patients with solid tumors. JCO Precis Oncol. 2023;7:e2300195.

64. Pfarr N, Schwarzenberg von K, Zocholl D, Merkelbach-Bruse S, Siemenowski J, et al. High concordance of different assays in the determination of homologous recombination deficiency–associated genomic instability in ovarian cancer. JCO Precis Oncol. 2024;8:e2300348.
65. Meric-Bernstam M, Rothe M, Mangat PK, Garrett-Meyer E, Gutierrez R, et al. Cobimetinib plus Vemurafenib in patients with solid tumors with BRAF mutations: results from the targeted agent and profiling utilization registry study. JCO Precis Oncol. 2023;7:e2300385.
66. Porcelli T, Moccia M, De Stefano M, Ambrosio R, Capaluongo E, et al. D898_E901 RET deletion is oncogenic, responds to Selpercatinib, and treatment resistance can Arise via RET-independent mechanisms. JCO Precis Oncol. 2023;7:e2300052.
67. Cheng Y, Huang D, Zhou J, Zhou C, Sun Y, et al. Intracranial activity of Selpercatinib in Chinese patients with advanced RET fusion-positive non-small-cell lung cancer in the phase II LIBRETTO-321 trial. JCO Precis Oncol. 2023;7:e2200708.
68. Danker M, Wang Y, Fazelzad R, Johnson B, Nebhan CA, et al. Clinical activity of mitogen-activated protein kinase–targeted therapies in patients with non–V600 BRAF-mutant tumors. JCO Precis Oncol. 2022;6:e2200107.
69. Yin Y, Song L, Shi D, Li X, Yang M, et al. Identification of recurrent insertions and deletions in Exon 18 and 19 of human epidermal growth factor receptor 2 as potential drivers in non-small-cell lung cancer and other cancer types. JCO Precis Oncol. 2022;6:e2100325.
70. Sokol ES, Jin DX, Fine A, Trabucco SE, Maund S, et al. PARP inhibitor insensitivity to BRCA1/2 Monoallelic mutations in microsatellite instability-high cancers. JCO Precis Oncol. 2022;6:e2100531.
71. Gadade DD, Jha H, Kumar C, Khan F. Unlocking the power of precision medicine: exploring the role of biomarkers in cancer management. Future J Pharm Sci. 2024;10:5.
72. Zurita AJ, Graf RP, Villacampa G, Raskina K, Sokol E, Jin D, Antonarakis ES, Li G, Huang RSP, Casanova-Salas I, Vivancos A, Carles J, Ross JS, Schrock AB, Oxnard GR, Mateo J. Genomic biomarkers and genome-wide loss-of-heterozygosity scores in metastatic prostate cancer following progression on androgen-targeting therapies. JCO Precis Oncol. 2022;6:e2200195.
73. Chowdhury S, Gupta R, Millstein J, Lin K, Haridas V, Zeineddine MA, Parseghian C, Lenz HJ, Kopetz S, Shen JP. Transcriptional profiling and consensus molecular subtype assignment to understand response and resistance to anti-epidermal growth factor receptor therapy in colorectal cancer. JCO Precis Oncol. 2023;7:e2200422.
74. Montero J, Gstalder C, Kim DJ, Sadowicz D, Miles W, et al. Destabilization of NOXA mRNA as a common resistance mechanism to targeted therapies. Nat Commun. 2019;10:5157.
75. Li J, Bai Y, Chen Z, Guo YY, et al. SAFFRON-104: a phase Ib/II study of Sitravatinib alone or with Tislelizumab in advanced hepatocellular carcinoma and gastric cancer/gastroesophageal junction cancer. Cancer Immunol Immunother. 2024;73:219.
76. Subbiah V, Cassier PA, Siena S, Garralda E, Paz-Ares L. Pan-cancer efficacy of pralsetinib in patients with RET fusion–positive solid tumors from the phase 1/2 ARROW trial. Nat Med. 2022;28:1640.
77. Yarchoan M, Powderly JD, Bastos BR, Karasic TB, Crysler OV. First-in-human phase I trial of TPST-1120, an inhibitor of PPARα, as monotherapy or in combination with Nivolumab, in patients with advanced solid tumors. Cancer Res Commun. 2024;4:1100.
78. Cho BC, Lu S, Lee MA, Song Z, Park JJ. D3S-001 in advanced solid tumors with KRASG12C mutations: a phase 1 trial. Nat Med. 2025;31:2768.
79. Oh DY, Bang YJ. HER2-targeted therapies — a role beyond breast cancer. Nat Rev Clin Oncol. 2020;17:33–48.

Chapter 5
Targeted Therapies for Hematologic Malignancies

Targeted therapies for hematologic malignancies or blood cancers (Table 5.1) are developed in tandem with those for solid tumors: Molecular profiling as a result of sequencing identified targetable signaling pathways. Schmidt et al. conducted a comprehensive review of targeted therapies for hematologic malignancies, or non-solid tumors, including a discussion on the pathophysiology and mechanisms of action and their categorization into small molecule inhibitors and monoclonal antibodies.

The mechanism of action of nonreceptor and receptor tyrosine kinases is dependent on their cellular localization. An FLT3 inhibitor is a tyrosine kinase inhibitor (TKI) whose activation is conducted by binding to its ligand cytokine FLT3LG, and it has roles in the MAPK, PI3K, and STAT5 pathways. A common mutation in acute myeloid leukemia (present in almost a third of patients), the FLT3 mutation is present as internal tandem duplications or affects the tyrosine kinase (TK) domain, both of which lead to constitutive proliferation and cellular survival. FLT3 inhibitors gilteritinib and midostaurin inhibit FLT and are type I inhibitors in their active conformation. FLT3 internal tandem duplication (ITD) inhibitors can adapt to both their inactive conformation and their active conformation, whereas FLT3-TKD mutations favor the active conformation. Sorafenib falls under the category of type II inhibitors that inhibit FLT3-ITD and bind to the active conformation. JAK inhibitors are of the non-RTK type and mediate immunological cytokine triggered signaling and hematopoietic signaling. JAK activation results from the binding of cytokines to their receptor, which leads to the phosphorylation of this receptor and creates a scaffolding of the STAT, PI3K, and MAPK pathway. A constitutive activation of the JAK2 mutation (JAK2 V617 for exon 12) is a common JAK-STAT dysregulation in BCR::ABL1 negative myeloproliferative neoplasms (MPNs). Common mutations in genes CALR and MPL are associated with BCR::ABL1 negative MPNs. The thrombopoietin receptor is encoded by MPL, and with the mutated

P. Hays, *Personalized Medicine in Oncology*,
https://doi.org/10.1007/978-3-032-14437-9_5

Table 5.1 FDA-approved kinase inhibitors

Drug name	Medically relevant targets	Indications in hematooncology
Tyrosine kinase inhibitors		
BCR::ABL1 inhibitors		
Asciminib	BCR::ABL1	CML
Bosutinib	BCR::ABL1	CML
Dasatinib	BCR::ABL1	CML, Ph + ALL
Imatinib	BCR::ABL1, PDGFR	CML, Ph + ALL, HES and/or CEL, MDS/MPN, off label: Ph + AML, Ph + MPAL
Nilotinib	BCR::ABL1	CML
Ponatinib	BCR::ABL1 (including T315I)	CML, Ph + ALL
BTK inhibitors		
Acalabrutinib	BTK	MCL, CLL
Ibrutinib	BTK	MCL, CLL, WM
Zanubrutinib	BTK	MCL, WM, MZL
FLT3 inhibitors		
Gilteritinib	FLT3	AML
Midostaurin	FLT3, KIT (see below)	AML
Sorafenib	FLT3	Off-label: AML (post ASCT maintenance therapy in *FLT3* mutated AML)
KIT inhibitors		
Avapritinib	KIT D816V	ASM
Midostaurin	KIT (including D816V)	ASM, SM-AHN, mast cell leukemia
JAK inhibitors		
Fedratinib	JAK2	MF
Pacritinib	JAK2	MF
Ruxolitinib	JAK1/2	MF, PV
BRAF inhibitors		
Dabrafenib	BRAF	Off-label: HCL
Vemurafenib	BRAF	Off-label: HCL
PI3K inhibitors		
Copanlisib	Pan-PI3K, predominant activity: PI3Kα and PI3Kδ	FL
Duvelisib	PI3Kδ and PI3Kγ	CLL, FL
Idelalisib	PI3Kδ	CLL, FL

Adapted from Schmidts et al. [1]

CALR associated with MPL, it activates JAK2 signaling, a feature of MPN neoplasms regardless of the individual driver mutation. Ruxolitinib, fedratinib, and pacritinib are US Food and Drug Administration (FDA)–approved JAK inhibitors at the ATP binding site that bind to JAK2 in its active conformation. Ruxolitinib is an inhibitor of both JAK1 and JAK2, and pacritinib and fedratinib and specifically bind JAK2; however, none of the inhibitors are specific to JAK2V617F, nor is any of them effective in myeloprofilitive neoplasms (MPN), regardless of the driver mutations present (JAK2 V617F, JAK2 exon 12, MPL, or CALR) [1].

Targeted therapies transitioned from being administered at a dose below the maximum-tolerated dose on the basis of toxicities after chemotherapy to being administered on the basis of an optimal biologic dose for maintaining efficacy and mitigating adverse events, beginning with the development of imatinib. This was shown through patients experiencing longer-than-normal expected lifetimes, where the TKIs given several years earlier had toxicities not observed within that therapeutic window. Currently, targeted therapies are prescribed according to the concept of the optimal biologic dose [2]. A fundamental element of the cell cycle and organism health, apoptosis has long been recognized as relevant in tumorigenesis in forming a barrier against it in many hematologic malignancies. Because of this, the intrinsic apoptotic pathway is frequently exploited as a much-sought-after therapeutic target in hematologic malignancies. Of the most commonly occurring hematologic malignancies (HMs) in adult populations, chronic lymphocytic leukemia is the most common chronic leukemia, and overall, acute myeloid leukemia is the most common acute leukemia; both are sensitive to cell death induced via apoptosis [3].

BCR::ABL1Inhibitors are based on breakpoint cluster region (BCR) genetic fusion and Abelson protein kinase 1 (ABL), leading to the constitutive activation of the ABL1 kinase that promotes cellular proliferation and increased cellular survival. Chronic myeloid leukemia (CML) was the first hematologic malignancy that showed activity against BCR::ABL1 inhibitors such as first-generation imatinib; second-generation bosutinib, dasatinib, and nilotinib; and third-generation ponatinib. Asciminib binds to the ABL1 myristoyl pocket and is one of the first allosteric TKIs [1].

Other targeted therapies that have been developed are the hedgehog inhibitor glasdegib, which targets the hedgehog pathway, whose central effector is the zinc finger proteins in the GLI category that acts as a transcriptional activator. Glasdegib binds to the smoothened protein, thereby inhibiting this pathway and thus preventing downstream activation through translocation. Selinexor is an exportin 1 inhibitor and targets the XPO1 binding pocket that plays a critical role in nuclear export and proto-oncogenesis. XPO1 has been shown to be overexpressed in many blood cancers, including multiple myeloma (MM).

Selinexor, through covalent binding to cysteine, inhibits XPO1-mediated export and targets the cargo binding pocket of the protein, leading to the nuclear retention of tumor suppressor proteins and mRNA. This nuclear accumulation leads to apoptosis. Isocitrate dehydrogenase (IDH) inhibitors (IDH1 and IDH2) play parts in the Krebs cycle that catalyzes the oxidation of the isocitrate-2-oxoglutarte enzyme. Mutations in IDH1 and IDH2 display a gain-of-function phenotype leading to hypermethylation and are associated with myeloid neoplasms. Ivosidenib and enasidenib fall under this class of targeted therapies, have been approved for the treatment of acute myeloid leukemia (AML), and serve as allosteric inhibitors. Due to their association with IDH1/2 mutations, both lead to 2-hydroxyglutarate production inhibition and differential block suppression. Ivosidenib competes with magnesium, a IDH1 cofactor, bringing to a halt the formation of the catalytically active site. Enasidenib, on the other hand, prevents IDH2 transition into the catalytically active, closed conformation [1].

5.1 BTK Inhibitors and Degraders

Ibrutinib is regarded as a highly potent BTK inhibitor and covalently binds to cysteine 481 residue in the BTK active site. BTKs are part of the BCR pathway, which is instrumental for proliferation and B-cell survival, and drugs that inhibit this pathway via inhibited BTK are effective in the management of chronic lymphocytic leukemia (CLL) and have dramatically improved clinical outcomes with a progression-free survival (PFS) and an overall survival (OS) of 75% and 83% reported, respectively, with consistently impressive objective response rates (ORRs) in both, with an estimated 7-year PFS of 83% for frontline patients and 34% for R/R patients. The RESONATE-1 and RESONATE-2 trials compared ibrutinib to ofatumumab and chlorambucil in R/R and frontline therapy, respectively, and showed superior PFS and OS [4]. Due to the off-targeted effects of second-generation cBTKi drugs on 19 other kinases as a result of a nonselective mechanism, these drugs have been developed with lower off-target activity with improved tolerability and similar efficacy. Third-generation BTKi drugs, on the other hand, have a unique binding mechanism that is reversible or noncovalent agnostic to C481 residue and may be a further option for cases of resistance and intolerance. Second-generation BTK inhibitors include acalabrutinib and zanubrutinib for CLL. Two phase 3 trials, namely ASCEND and ELEVATE-TN, evaluated acalabrutinib. The ELEVATE-TN trial led to longer median progression-free survival (mPFS) in older patients with comorbidities in the acalabrutinib arm as monotherapy when compared to the agent in combination with obinutuzumab and the chlorambucil-obinutuzumab chemo-immunotherapy combination, leading to its approval in the front line as monotherapy and in combination. A similar ORR was reported in the ASCEND trial, which compared the agent as monotherapy with either bendamustine–rituximab (BR) or idelalisib–rituximab in patients who had at least one prior treatment (81% vs. 75%), with a prolonged PFS due to acalabrutinib's tolerability versus the investigator's choice regimen. Acalabrutinib was evaluated in the ELEVATE-RR trial in R/R CLL/SLC patients in a cohort with high-risk cytogenetics composed of the del (17p) (45.2%) of patients) and/or del (11a) (64.2% of patients) and compared with ibrutinib with the primary endpoint being noninferiority (HR 1.00 and 38.4-month PFS). According to one report, acalabrutinib was associated with lower rates of atrial fibrillation and flutter, cardiac adverse events with flutter being a key secondary endpoint (9.4% with acalabrutinib vs. 16% with ibrutinib) and hypertension (9.4% vs. 23.2%) [4].

Zanubrutinib is a second-generation BTK inhibitor that is also selective and irreversible, designed to minimize adverse effects as a result of off-target kinase inhibition and maximize BTK inhibition. The phase 3 ALPINE trial showed improved PFS (94.9% vs. 84%) and improved ORR (78.3% vs. 62.6%), and in R/R CLL patients, it had lower rates of atrial fibrillation in all cytogenetic subgroups when compared to ibrutinib. Zanubrutinib was also evaluated in the phase 3 multicenter SEQUOIA trial that spanned 14 countries, as frontline monotherapy for chronic lymphocytic leukemia/small cell lymphocytic leukemia (CLL/SLL) in treatment-naive patient, resulting in a PFS of 86% vs. 70%, respectively. Another irreversible covalent BTKi, orelabrutinib, has been approved in China for R/R CLL patients as evaluated in a phase 2 study of 80 patients, and it has been shown to have robust clinical outcomes with an ORR of 91% (complete response (CR) in 10%), with no cases of atrial fibrillation reported.

5.2 Mechanisms of Resistance to Covalent BTK Inhibitors

The most commonly acquired mutation associated with resistance to covalent BTK inhibitors that resulted in impaired drug binding is in the C481 residue detected in over 50% of patients through sequencing. Autonomous BCR signaling also results from the PLC γ2 gain-of-function mutations observed upon progression. The L528W residue mutation is associated with resistance to zanubrutinib, as shown by studies that demonstrated that ATP binding interference results from the mutation when the agent is bound to BTK, leading to a protein without kinase activity and to progression (54%, or seven of 13 patients, compared to 4%, or one of 24 patients) when compared to ibrutinib. Further analysis showed that increased measurable disease and eventual disease progression resulted when the BTK L528W mutation was initially detected, as one report stated [4].

The development of third-generation, noncovalent BTK inhibitors (ncBTKi) that had a novel binding mechanism at the ATP binding pocket resulted from the situation where cBTKi led to intolerance and disease progression with long-term adherence as a result of the acquired mutation in C481. Consequently, ncBTK inhibitors, subsequent to either progression that developed or intolerance to cBTK1, were developed as a therapeutic option. Third-generation BTK inhibitors, including luxeptinib, showed antitumor efficacy and favorable safety profiles in a phase 1a/b dose-escalation study. Nemtabrutinib is a covalent reversible BTC inhibitor existing in both WT and C481S mutated BTK (ibrutinib resistant) with a selective inhibition of the TEC, Trk, and SRC family of kinases, resulting in, the transcription of NF- κB genes, the reversible inhibition of BTK and MEK1 BTK-dependent functions such as BCR signaling. The suppression of activated C481S BTK and PLC γ2 mutants also occurs, rendering it a viable therapeutic option in ibrutinib-resistant cases. In the phase ½ dose-escalation BELLWAVE-001 study, in R/R CLL/SLL patients, antitumor activity and a favorable safety profile were shown. Pirtobrutinib (previously LOXO-305) was shown to be a significantly selective ncBTKi that demonstrates a 300-fold selectivity for BTK over other kinases, with equal potency and decreased potential for off-target toxicities resulting from the inhibition of wild-type and C481 mutant BTK. Pirtobrutinib was evaluated for relapsed B-cell malignancies in the BRUIN open-label, multicenter phase 1/2 study, enrolling a cohort with efficacy observed at all dose levels; however, no MTD was established. Updated results were presented at ASH 2022: A PFS of 19.6 months and an ORR of 82% were reported with 13.9 months of median follow-up in 247 evaluable BTKi-pretreated CLL patients who had a median of three lines of previous therapies. A subgroup composed of 100 patients who failed both BTKi and BCL2 inhibitors showed a median PFS of 16.8 months and an ORR of 79%, with consistent response rates across all subgroups (previous therapies, mutation, and age). The study authors concluded that pirtobrutinib appears to be very well tolerated. PD associated with newly acquired non-C481 BTK mutations demonstrated in vivo resistance to ncBTK1 and served as a mechanism of resistance. Longitudinal sequencing "demonstrated the gatekeeper T474I mutation as a driver of resistance for one patient with another patient whose progression correlated with the expansion of an L528W mutation." The BRUIN trial provided a dataset that included a cohort of 49 patients with PD, and it reiterated these findings in that newly acquired BTK mutations occurred in 45% of patients, with 22% at the T474 gatekeeper residue and 11% at the L528 residue. Cotreatment with zanubrutinib and pirtobrutinib demonstrated cross-resistance in two patients progressing on both therapies; however, variation exists in the clinical responses. One patient treated with onset pirtobrutinib (cancer cell fraction 2.2%) progressed after 23 months of therapy, whereas another patient had nodal progression with fully clonal L528W following 6 months of pirtobrutinib treatment. These studies are relevant in impacting the sequencing of treatment for future studies to understand the mechanisms of resistance for pirtobrutinib and other noncovalent BTKi, an example of which is evaluating earlier settings and comparing them to ibrutinib and chemoimmunotherapy. Cross-resistance with covalent inhibitors raises concerns. The use of BTK degraders as treatment for CLL is being implemented. The mechanism of action is through its design of a linker and degradation machinery that links an E3 ubiquitin ligase and a target protein binding arm that breaks down BTK. Examples are as follows:

- NX-2127, through its immunomodulatory properties and properties as a first-in-class BTK degrader, modulates cereblon, an E3 ligase in hematopoietic cells, resulting in the degradation of both WT and mutant BTK proteins.
- NX-2127 was evaluated in a phase 1a/1b clinical trial in patients with R/R CLL and other B-cell malignancies, with a median age of enrolled patients at 75 years. Preliminary results reported at ASH 2022 showed that with 14 of 23 CLL patients actively maintaining treatment, an ORR of 33% (95% confident interval (CI) 12–62%) was demonstrated at a median follow-up of 5.6 months. Reported adverse events were grade 3 neutropenia (36%), thrombocytopenia (8.3%), atrial fibrillation (16.6%), and anemia (11.1%).
- NX-5948 is also a BTK degrader but has no effect on IZKF3; however, no results are reportable in an ongoing phase1a dose-escalation trial.
- BGB-16673, an investigational compound, is being evaluated in preclinical studies and has demonstrated effects against both wild-type and mutant BTK in targeted BTK degradation activity. Additionally, it is being evaluated in two trials with patients with B-cell malignancies being enrolled.
- In an ongoing phase 1a trial, HSK29116 is being evaluated and is also considered a BTK degrader. No results for either BGB-16673 or HSK29116 have been reported [4].

Alsouqi and Woyach reported on the three cBTK inhibitors that have been FDA approved and administered in the clinic for CLL: ibrutinib, acalabrutinib, and zanubrutinib. All three agents have shown efficacy and safety and demonstrated superiority over standard chemoimmunotherapy (CIT) in both frontline and R/R settings. A treatment paradigm resulted, in which CLL had significantly improved response rates, survival, and toxicity profiles. Ibrutinib is considered an effective first-generation inhibitor but is associated with off-target toxicity due to its nonselective inhibition. Acalabrutinib and zanubrutinib are second-generation BTKis that have higher selectivity. These inhibitors are particularly effective for patients with high-risk disease, TP53 mutation del (17p), and immunoglobulin heavy chain (IGH) status. Ibrutinib irreversibly inhibits BTK activity, leading to CLL cell apoptosis, the abrogation of downstream survival pathways, and blocked stimulatory survival signals by binding covalently to a cysteine residue. PCYC-1102 was the pivotal phase Ib/II open-label trial that evaluated ibrutinib at a dosage of 420 mg daily in frontline settings that included a high-risk population, with safety, ORR, and PFS being the primary endpoints. The key result was that at a median follow-up of 87 months and 82 months, respectively, in the R/R setting, ORR was 87% and 89%, respectively. Furthermore, mPFS was 52 months overall and 26 months in del (17p) patients; 28% of patients experienced hypertension and 24% of patients developed pneumonia. Progression occurred in 41 patients. Four further trials were conducted to establish ibrutinib's approval and implementation in the clinic for the treatment of CLL. The RESONATE trial enrolled 391 patients and evaluated the agent versus the CD20 antibody ofatumumab, with a third of the patients having del (17p). Also, mPFS was 44.1 months for ibrutinib versus 8.1 months for ofatumumab. Extensive crossover to the ibrutinib arm occurred, leading to similar OS rates. Grade 3 atrial fibrillation occurred in 12% of patients, and hypertension occurred in 9% of patients. The RESONATE-3 phase 3, randomized open-label trial evaluated ibrutinib versus chlorambucil in untreated patients older than 65 years ($n = 269$). Median PFS was not reached in the ibrutinib arm and not reached in the comparator arm after a median follow-up of 7.4 years. PFS was estimated at 59% versus 9% for each arm, respectively. OS at 7 years was 78%; ORR was 92%, with a CR rate of 34%. Grade 3 hypertension occurred in 12% of patients with atrial fibrillation occurring in 6% of patients. The Alliance A041202 trial enrolled 547 treatment-naive CLL patients and compared ibrutinib with ibrutinib and rituximab (IR) or chemoimmunotherapy (CIT) with bendamustine and rituximab (BR). A 48-month PFS was 76% in each of the arms containing ibrutinib and 47% in the BR arm. The trial authors concluded that the "benefit of ibrutinib regimens over CIT remained consistent among subgroups of TP53 mutated disease, del (11q), or IGHV unmutated CLL with no additional PFS benefit with the addition of rituximab." The ILLUiminate study was also an open-label, randomized phase III study ($n = 229$) that was composed of high-risk features (65% del (17p), TP53) and evaluated previously untreated patients and comorbidities with CLL/SLL aged ≥ 65 years or < 65 years, featuring agent combinations of ibrutinib and obinutuzumab versus CIT with chlorambucil and obinutuzumab (ChO). Median PFS was not reached in the in the I-O arm versus 22 months in the ChO arm. The estimated 42-month PFS was 74% and 39% in the I-O arm and ChO arm, respectively, with greater benefit observed in the high-risk population. In CLL patients in high-risk categories (TP53 mutation del (17p)), at an approved dose of 420 mg of ibrutinib orally resulted in a paradigm shift in the treatment of CLL, especially for patients with TP53 and del (17p), at an approved dose of 420 mg orally; however, caveats remain for patients with a history of cardiovascular disease such as hypertension, cardiac arrhythmia, and atrial fibrillation, although diarrhea, fatigue, and nausea, which are common and mild side effects, and asymptomatic lymphocytosis are also associated with the administration of ibrutinib. Acalabrutinib is a second-generation BTKi with greater specificity, leading to fewer side effects, and has been evaluated as monotherapy in the phase I/II ACL-CL-001 and ELEVATE-TN, in comparison with investigator's choice in the ASCEND trial, and in a head-to-head comparison with ibrutinib in the phase III ELEVATE R/R study. Key results from these trials include the following: For ACL-CL-001, an R/R cohort of 134 patients had a dosing of 100 mg twice daily, with 73% of patients having IGHV mutated disease, and at a median follow-up of 41 months, mPFS was not reached; ORR was 94%; grade 3 or higher AEs, including neutropenia, pneumonia (11%), hypertension (14%), and anemia (7%), occurred in 5% of patients. The treatment-naive cohort had an ORR of 97% at a median follow-up of 53 months in a patient population with 2% unmutated IGHV disease and 18% TP53 aberration. ELEVATE-TN had a treatment-naive cohort ($n = 535$) randomized to receive acalabrutinib–obinutuzumab, acalabrutinb monotherapy, or ChO. Median PFS in the AO and A arms was not reached at a median follow-up of 74.5 months compared to 27.8 months in the ChO arm (HR 0.14 and 0.23), respectively. The results revealed an "estimated 72-month PFS of 78%, 62%, and 17% in the acalabrutinib-obinutuzumab arm, acalabrutinib arm, and ChO arm, respectively." The most common adverse events reported in each of the arms were in the acalabrutinib–obinutuzumab and acalabrutinib groups, including diarrhea (6% and 2%), neutropenia (31% and 12%), and thrombocytopenia (8% and 3%). Other events included hypertension occurring in 4% and 5%, respectively, with grade 3 or higher atrial fibrillation occurring in 2% in both groups. In the ASCEND trial, 42-month OS was 78% versus 65%, and 42-month PFS was 62% in the acalabrutinib arm versus 19% at a 4-year follow-up, and atrial fibrillation (8%) and hypertension (8%) were common AEs. Second primary malignancies occurred in 7% of patients, excluding nonmelanoma skin cancer. In the ELEVATE R/R study ($n = 533$ with confirmed del (17p) or del (11q)), the primary endpoint was PFS, with safety serving as the secondary endpoint. Median PFS in both arms was 38.4 months with a significantly lower incidence of atrial fibrillation in the acalabrutinib arm and fewer bleeding events occurring (38% vs. 51.3%). Second primary malignancies occurred in 24 (9%) versus 20 (7.6%) patients. Acalabrutinib has approval for a dose of 100 mg twice daily in both newly diagnosed and previously treated CLL and is monotherapy when compared to ibrutinib given its lower risk of hypertension and atrial fibrillation. The other second-generation BTKi approved for CLL is zanubrutinib, which, like acalabrutinb, has higher selectivity and was evaluated in two trials: SEQUOIA as a monotherapy versus BR in frontline settings and in ALPINE in a head-to-head comparison with ibrutinib. Key results from both trials include cohorts with and without del (17p); mPFS for the BR group was 42.2 months and not reached in the zanubrutinib group (HR 0.03 (95% CI 0.21 to 0.43)). At 42 months, PFS was 82.4% in the zanubrutinib group. For the ALPINE trial ($n = 652$) at 36 months, PFS was 65.8%

versus 54.3, respectively. High-risk categories of del (17p)/TP53 mutations also showed clinical benefit, where PFS rates were 60.1% versus 43.3%. The 36-month OS rate was 82.6% versus 79.7%, with significantly higher ORR/CR rates: 85% versus 79.7%. Decreased atrial fibrillation risk is also associated with zanubrutinib and is approved for CLL in frontline and R/R patients, though the choice of BTKs should be individualized. The combination of BTKi with BCL-1 inhibitor venetoclax with or without CD20 monoclonal antibodies has led to great excitement and has been evaluated in four comparator trials: CLARITY (phase II, intravenous (IV) combination with R/R CLL), CAPTIVATE (international phase II study, IV in frontline setting); GLOW (phase III trial comparing ChO with IV in frontline setting in patients between 65-75 years old. populations and pediatric populations with comorbidities); FLAIR (phase III trial comparing CIT with IV).

5.2.1 *Key Results*

- CLARITY: $n = 53$; the uMRD rate after 12 months was 53%; ORR was 89%.
- CAPTIVATE: Primary endpoint 1-year DFS with placebo versus IV ($n = 164$). Here, 75% achieved uMRD, and DFS was 100% versus 95%. Fixed duration treatment, with three cycles of ibrutinib followed by 12 cycles of ibrutinib + venetoclax. There was a CR rate of 55% in all cohorts, and in patients with del (17p), the CR rate was 56%. CR rate was observed as 55% in the total population and 56% of patients with del (17p).
- GLOW: $n = 211$; the primary endpoint was PFS, IGHV unmutated disease appeared in 66.9% of patients; 4.3% had TP53 mutations, 18% had del (11q); and 42-month PFS was 74.6% versus 24.8% in the ChO group. IV combination had a clinical benefit in the mutated IGHV arm with a 42-month PFS of 90% versus 69.8%.
- FLAIR: $n = 523$; the 3-year PFS was 97.2% in I+V arm and 76.8% in CIT arm with patient population subgroups, including 1.3% having del (17p) and 49.9% having unmutated IGHV at a median follow-up of 43.7 months. IV achieved a undetectable minimal residual disease (uMRD) of 92.7% in peripheral blood and 65.9% in the bone marrow after 5 years. Second-generation venetoclax combinations are also undergoing evaluation, including one phase II trial of acalabrutinib administered for the first cycle; venetoclax was added starting at cycle 4; and obinutuzumab was added starting at cycle 2 (a total of six cycles). CR evaluated via uMRD in the bone marrow at cycle 16 served as the primary endpoint (38% after 16 cycles in previously untreated CLL). A combination trial of zanubrutinib, obinutuzmab, and venetoclax was conducted; however, treatment was discontinued when uMRD was met in both blood and bone marrow. With the clinical benefits of uMRD and remissions achieved, this combination is undergoing extensive evaluation. As the authors conclude, BTK inhibitors are targeted therapies that have improved patient care for CLL over the past decades, leading to durable responses and higher remission rates and fewer toxic adverse events

when compared with the standard of care. In frontline settings and R/R disease, cBTK inhibitors acalabrutinib, ibrunitinb, and zanubritinib are FDA-approved agents and "provide several advantages over conventional CIT, such as CD20 monoclonal antibodies, purine analogues, or alkylating agents. Overall, the three covalent BTK inhibitors provide excellent disease control with tolerable safety profiles in patients with CLL" [5].

5.3 BCL-2 Inhibitor: Venetoclax (Fig. 5.1)

Antiapoptotic BCL-2 normally binds BAX and BIM proteins, preventing the mitochondrial release of cytochrome c and apoptosis. Venetoclax (VEN) binds BCL-2, freeing BAX and BIM and inducing apoptosis. The upregulation of non-VEN binding proteins BCL-XL and MCL-1 prevent apoptosis induction. Mutations in BCL-2's binding pocket and the BAX protein inhibit VEN-induced apoptosis. Mutations in other pathways can also lead to MCL-1 upregulation and BAX downregulation. Finally, metabolic changes in mitochondria, including elevations in oxidative phosphorylation (OXPHOS), can prevent apoptosis.

A fascinating study was conducted by Aoki et al. and reported in *JCO* that applied spatial biology to tumor microenvironment (TME), which predicted outcomes in R/R Hodgkin lymphoma. About one-third of patients with classical Hodgkin lymphoma succumb after CT and allogeneic stem cell transplantation (ASCT) . The authors spatially resolved the TME to reveal novel biomarkers associated with therapy failure in this disease. They found that in early r/r chronic Hodgkin's lymphoma (CHL) samples, imaging mass cytometry (IMC) data revealed

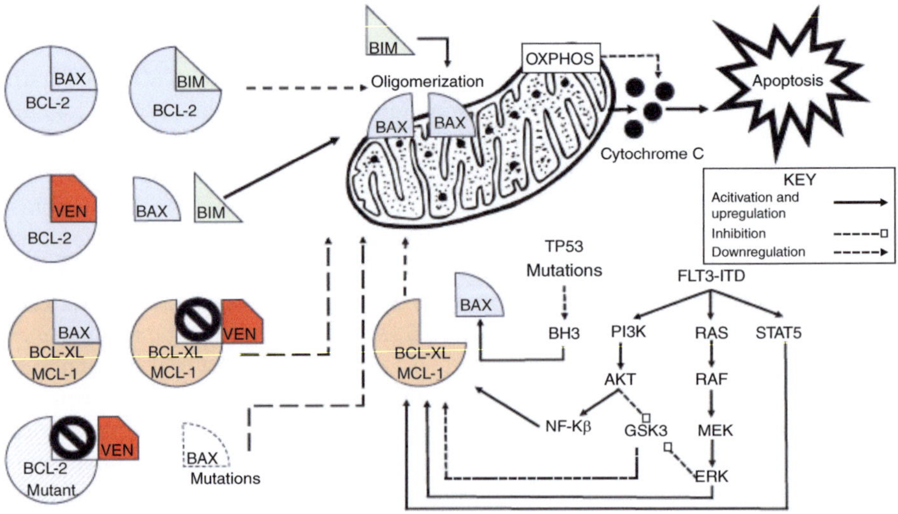

Fig. 5.1 Antiapoptotic BCL-2. (Adapted from Forsberg and Klonopeva)

shared patterns in the TME, and late relapse samples revealed more-divergent patterns. The interaction of CXCR5+ Hodgkin Reed Sternberg cells with ligand-expressing CXCL13+ macrophages displayed "prominent crosstalk axis in relapsed CHL." They developed a novel prognostic model by using the TME biology that can be applied to relapsed CHL biopsies [6].

Acute myeloid leukemia has a common mutation associated with it, namely FLT3 internal tandem duplication (ITD) mutations, which confer an increased risk of relapse. AHCT is considered the standard of care after first remission. Before or after hematopoietic cell transplant (HCT), the presence of MRD is a predictor of clinical outcomes. Although not usually considered a marker of MRD, PCR and NGS are now considered methods to detect low levels of the FLT3-ITD mutation in patients in remission, and retrospective studies have shown that it correlates with relapse. Gilteritinib is clinically efficacious for R/R FLT3 mutated AML and is a well-tolerated, potent oral FLT3 inhibitor. A study published in the *Journal of Clinical Oncology* in 2024 demonstrated in a randomized study of post-HCR maintenance that RFS was higher in the gilteritinib arm; however, the result was not considered statistically significant (HR, 0.679 (95% CI 0.459 to 1.005)). According to the study investigators, before or after HCT, 50.5% of participants had detectable MRD, even in subgroup analysis, and gilteritinib was shown to be beneficial in this population (HR, 0.515 (95% CI 0.316 to 0.838)). Patients who showed no detectable MRD had no benefit (HR, 1.213 (95% CI 0.616 to 2.387)), whereas MRD at a level of 1×10^{-6} or greater was associated with decreased OS and RFS, regardless of treatment arm [7, 8].

A recent review on oral therapy for AML elaborated on molecularly targeted agents for the malignancy that showed appreciable benefit for older, less-fit patients in remission or undergoing maintenance therapy in the form of reduced hospital visits. Common mutations include FLT3 with internal tandem duplications and in the RAS oncogene that activate KRAS, NRAS, KRAS, NF1, and PTPN11. Venetoclax showed superior clinical responses (CRs) in patients between the 65 to 75 years old with AML unfit for chemotherapy (71%), especially when combined with targeted therapies. A phase I study of venetoclax in combination with decitabine and cedazuridine and venetoclax combined with gilteritinib was conducted with an FLT3 inhibitor in another arm. Venetoclax was given in three cycles: day 1, 100 mg; day 2, 200 mg; day 3, 400 mg; and then indefinite single-agent gilteritinib. Primary endpoints were the MTD of gilteritinib and CR/CR with incomplete blood recovery. A CR rate of 87% and a 6-month OS of 70% were achieved. Enasidenib and ivosidinib were evaluated as oral agents against IDH1 and IDH2 mutations and were shown to be effective and well tolerated. A phase Ib/II study had patients on venetoclax and cedazuridine and decitabine and either ivosidenib (against IDH1) or enasidinib (against iDH2) for the treatment of R/R AML given in 28-day cycles (27 evaluable patients). On day 14, a bone marrow biopsy was carried out. The composite CR was 72% (100% for the newly diagnosed group and 53% for the R//R group). In 42% of the R/R group and 83% of the newly diagnosed group , MRD negative-composite CR was achieved according to flow cytometry. Four nonhematologic AEs were reported (hyperbilirubinemia, $n = 2$; 7%) in the newly diagnosed group [8].

A recently developed targetable mutation, NPM1-mutant (nucleophosmin) or KMT2A-rearranged, has been discovered in AML, leading to the development of menin inhibitors. Menin serves as a crucial cofactor for binding the important HOX gene promoters. Preserved throughout all the fusion proteins, it binds the first 10 amino acids of KMT2A protein. The genetic ablation of menin reverses aberrant HOX gene expression and halts oncogenesis in mouse models of KMT2A leukemia. Because this gene expression is specific for leukemic cells and not hematopoietic cells, the organism can tolerate loss of gene expression. Small molecule inhibitors of the menin–KMT2A interaction were developed as a result of the identification of the KMT2a binding pocket, disrupting the binding of KMT2A to menin and disrupting the binding of the complex to target gene promoters. In one phase I trial, the ORR of R/R KMT2Ar leukemia patients was 54% in 13 of 24 evaluable patients with an undetectable MRD of 67%. Combining this agent with venetoclax appears promising, according to these recent reports [8].

Venetoclax was administered to patients with low-dose cytarabine (LDAC) in a phase II prospective study to target MRD and low-blast relapse in AML. In this study, 48 patients with either oligoblastic relapse ($n = 33$) or MRD ($n = 26$) were enrolled. According to the study, markers of "molecular MRD relapse included NPM1, CBFB::MYH11, and RUNX1::RUNX1T1." Moreover, 21 patients, or 44% of them, underwent hematopoietic cell transplantation. Grade 3 or greater anemia (32% vs. 4%) and infections (36 vs. 8%) were observed in patients with oligoblastic relapse. The authors concluded that for "AML in first remission and either MRD or oligoblastic relapse, venetoclax plus LDAC is well tolerated and highly effective" [9].

A targeted therapy combination composed of venetoclax and the MEK 1/2 (mitogen activated protein kinase) inhibitor cobimetinib showed less-than-spectacular results for the treatment of R/R AML in a phase 1b dose-expansion trial in that adverse events occurred at a greater frequency than each agent as monotherapy. Limited responses also occurred, and although R2PD was achieved, no expansion was pursued. Two-dimensional dose escalation was conducted with VEN dosed daily and cobimentinib dosed on days 1–21 in a 28-day cycle. VEN has shown activity in this population, with a CR rate of 19%, as have Cob and other MEK1/2 inhibitors, namely trametinib, selumetinib, and binimetinib, in RAS mutated AML. The synergistic induction of apoptosis in the combination was observed when studying in vitro AML models, and a reduction in leukemic burden was observed when studying in vivo models, significantly enhancing cell death and suppressing cell growth, leading to "MCL-1 downregulation" and the "upregulation of proapoptotic BIM." The rationale for administering the combination is that the overexpression of MCL-1 is associated with VEN resistance (acquired) and that targeting MCL-1 indirectly through MAPK may led to beneficial outcomes. Diarrhea was the most frequent event (80%) in the 32-patient cohort and led to the mandatory antidiarrheal prophylaxis. Vomiting at a rate of 40%, febrile neutropenia at a rate of 40%, and fatigue at a rate of 40% were also shown. Because the overall benefit–risk profile was low in that serious AEs were reported in 80% of patients, including pneumonia (20%) and sepsis (20%), the combination was discontinued. Fatal AEs also occurred in six patients due to lung infection ($n = 2$), sepsis ($n = 2$), respiratory failure ($n = 1$), and lung disorder ($n = 1$). Treatment withdrawal due to AEs occurred in 23.3% of patients. Efficacy CRc and antileukemic response were 15.6% (5/32) and 18.8% (6/32), respectively, with blast count reduction observed. Median OS was 3.6 months (2.0–8.6). MRD was not achieved. In terms of biomarker response, p53 expression was associated with nonresponse, whereas IDH1/2 and NRAS/KRAS signaling pathways were associated with antileukemic response. Although the authors admitted that the safety profile was expected, the response rate suggested no added benefit with the combination that may have been due to the patient characteristics of the cohort (ages 65–75, frail), and no downregulation of MCL-1 was reported. The study investigators also suggest that effect strategies may need to "target MCL-1 directly rather than indirectly through complex signaling pathways," with too much or too little RAS signaling implicated, and they suggest that the safety and dosage learning from this study may optimize patient selection and the design of VEN combination with MAPK pathway inhibitors [10].

Immunoscore (IS) was found to have prognostic and predictive value in stage III CRC, as found in a pooled analysis of cases from IDEA-HORG and SCOT studies enrolling patients receiving FOLFOX chemotherapy. Patients with myelodysplastic syndromes were evaluated for "the optimal timing of allogeneic hematopoietic stem cell transplantation, with clinical and genomic-based decision support systems" as the only potential curative treatment. In a retrospective study analyzing 7118 patients, a decision strategy was built over an 8-year time horizon to estimate the average survival. The molecular international prognostic scoring system (IPSS-M) insightfully determined that those with either low or moderate-to-low risk benefited from delayed transplantation over immediate transplantation and that those in the low or moderate risk and moderately high, high, and very high categories had a prolonged life expectancy. The decision changed the "transplantation policy," resulting in a significant increase in life expectancy in a significant proportion of patients under the IPSS-M-based policy, providing clinical evidence for incorporating genomic features such as 5q and p53 [11].

One review focused on targeted and immune approaches for myelodysplastic syndromes, noting that hypomethylating agents, or the standard of care, have a CR rate of 10–15%, with a real-life median OS of 15–17 months, partly because the affected population was between 65 to 75 years old. The problem, as cited by the review authors, is that the IDH-FLT3 mutation is rare in myelodysplastic syndrome (MDS). Genetically agnostic small molecule inhibitors pevonedistat and venetoclax, anti-CTLA4 and anti-PD-1/PD-L1 antibodies, and anti-TIM-3 and anti-CD47 antibodies are being clinically evaluated. The VIALE-A trial showed median improvement from the combination of azacytidine and venetoclax compared to the control group (14.7 months vs. 9.6 months; HR, 0.66 (95% CI: 0.52–0.85)). A single-arm, open-label, dose-escalation phase Ib study was conducted to evaluate venetoclax and azacitadine in treatment-naive HR-MDS. Results were presented at ASH meetings, showing that across "all mutations, including TP53 (83%), ASXL1 (82%), and RUNX1 (71%), clinical responses (CRs and mCRs) were observed." Other key results included "[g]rade 3 or 4 adverse events observed in 96% of the patients with neutropenia (84%), including 42% thrombocytopenia and 45% febrile neutropenia." Median OS was 28.2 (95% CI 17.7, NR). Median OS for 31 patients achieving CR was 28.6 months. Other agents being tested are pevonedistat, a first-in-class inhibitor of the NEDD8 activating enzyme that "blocks the ubiquitination of select proteins upstream of the proteasome" and IDH mutation target ivosidenib, and ipilimumab and nivolumab, and two first-in-class inhibitors of the NEDD8-activating enzyme. Two MDS patients received ipilimumab in one study, with one patient developing AML. Although these therapies show promise, the risk profile of MDS patients may prevent durable outcomes and manageable safety profiles [12].

In acute myeloid leukemia, a 2019 study showed data on outcomes for a number of genetic abnormalities identified, particularly for patients undergoing allogeneic hematopoietic stem cell transplantation (allo-HSCT). EV11 was prognostic for "poorer overall survival (HR 2.06, 95% CI 1.28–3.31), relapse-free survival (HR 2.28, 95% CI 1.35–3.86), and event-free survival (HR 1.79, 95% CI 1.15–2.77) within all t(11q23) AMLs." Midostaurin and quizartinib are TKIs that show clinical activity in FLT3 mutated AML patients. Midostaurin shows clinical activity against PDGFR, VEGFR2, KIT, PRKC, and FLT3, and is one of a broad spectrum of kinases in combination with cytotoxic chemotherapy that result in improved median OS (74.7 months vs. 25.6 months, HR 0.78, $p = 0.009$). Quizartinib was shown to be highly potent as an oral agent and selective FLT3-mutated AML, with a reported CRR of 46% (62/136) among 136 patients. IDH1 inhibitor ivosidenib has been given FDA approval for relapsed and refractory AML patients. The relevant points of this study were shown to be the use of gene mutational profiling for patients between the ages 65 to 75 unfit for intensive chemotherapy and the identification of specific gene mutations that influence prognosis and treatment decisions, particularly regarding allo-HSCT [13].

Forsberg and Klonopleva reported on overcoming venetoclax resistance in hematologic malignancies with discovery of the therapeutic landscape for acute myeloid leukemia. The response, though heterogenous, ranged between 10% and 50%, with a 40% relapse. Venetoclax activates antiapoptotic proteins such as the BCL-2 family of proteins and is subject to intrinsic and acquired resistance that occurs through the upregulation of compensatory cell signaling pathways such as the mutant FLT3-ITD, the PI3K/AKT/mTOR, and the MAPK/ERK. Combination therapies designed through the incorporation of non-BCL-2 inhibitors, FLT-3 inhibitors, and next-generation BCL-2 agents, in addition to VEN, are becoming increasingly attractive alternatives for resolving VEN resistance. VEN is one of many agents in the BCL-2 inhibitors category that plays a crucial role in mitochondria-mediated intrinsic resistance, which can be broken down into the BCL-XL, antiapoptotic BCL-2, MCL-1, BCL-W, and A1/BFL-1 proteins and the proapoptotic BAX and BAK proteins. VEN's mechanism relies on the activation of executors and the oligomerization and binding of proapoptotic proteins BAK and BAX that lead to the activation of caspases and cell death by disrupting the outer membrane permeability of the mitochondria, releasing cytochrome c and other apoptogenic factors. VEN, a BH3 mimetic, binds with high affinity for and selectively to the BH3 binding groove of BCL-2 proteins, releasing regulating proteins that result in leukemic cell death. When compared to its predecessor, navitoclax, it a has significantly milder thrombocytopenia because it does not inhibit BCL-XL. The interaction of BCL-2 pathways with other signaling pathways that are involved in cellular life and regulation have been transformed into another mechanism for VEN resistance, one being the PI3K/AKT/mTOR pathway that regulates apoptosis, autophagy, and cell proliferation. Downstream proteins such as GSK3, FOXO, and NF-kappaB promote the transcription of the BCL-2 family of proteins, resulting in the upregulation of BCL-XL and the phosphorylation of BAD, shifting binding from BCL-XL to 14-3-3 proteins, which leads to VEN resistance. The activation of the NF-kappaB pathway promotes the expression of MCL-1 and BCL-XL that promote protumorigenic cytokines such as IL-10 and CD40L, resulting in the increased expression of BCL-XL and MCL-1. The upregulation of the MAPK/ERK pathway leads to VEN resistance, as in vitro models have shown. Further, relapsed AML patients have an increased rate of FLT3-ITD mutations, which confers poor prognosis. NF-kappa B inhibitors as well as PI3K inhibitors have inducted VEN sensitivity in cell lines. In murine xenograft models, midostaurin and gilteritinib, first-generation and second-generation FLT3 inhibitors, are active and demonstrated increased efficacy, which has also been reiterated in early clinical trials in humans, such as a phase 1 open-label study that treated 61 patients between 65 to 75 years with R/R AML with FLT3 mutation. This cohort received a combination of VEN and gilteritinb that achieved a CR rate of 75%, with a median OS of 6.7 months. However, AEs included myelosuppression and 80% experiencing grade 3 or 4 cytopenia. AZA +VEN + giliternib also showed efficacy in a similar population, with a “very respectable” 95% CR rate and a day 14 finding of aplastic marrow in a bone marrow collection. Mutations in BCL-2 such as Gly101Val and D013Y have also been associated with VEN resistance. As the authors conclude, “Venetoclax has had major impacts on the treatment of AML and CLL [1–11]. However, resistance continues to be a concern recognizing the mechanisms of venetoclax resistance and investigating means of overcoming them is deeply important to the landscape of hematologic malignancies” [3].

5.4 Chronic Lymphocytic Leukemia

In CLL patients, Richter transformation refers to the occurrence of aggressive lymphoma, most commonly large B-cell lymphoma. Prognosis remains poor, although treatments are available for large B-cell lymphoma (LBCL), with median OS ranging from 3 to 12 months. RT has unmet needs requiring new treatment modalities. Of 69 patients, 44 received axi cel, 17 received tisa cel, seven received liso cel, and one received brex leu. Moreover, 11 patients experienced greater than grade 3 CRS, and 25 patients had Immune Effector Cell–Associated Neurotoxicity Syndrome (ICANS). ORR was 63%, with 46% achieving CR. With a “median follow-up of 24 months, median PFS was 4.7 months (95% CI 2.0 to 6.9), the 2-year PFS was 29% (95% CI 18 to 41). Median OS was 8.5 months (95% CI 5.1 to 25.4). Median DOR was 27.6 months (95% CI 14.5 to not reached) for patients achieving CR.” The study authors concluded that CAR-T demonstrates clinical efficacy for patients with Richter transformation (RT) [14].

A study identifying clonal hematopoiesis showed that ctDNA detection may reveal occult HM in patients with solid tumors, whose significance in the progress of the study was shown. Adults with solid cancers underwent liquid biopsy analysis, and molecular reports revealed pathogenic alterations and potential CH alterations in these adults, who were referred for hematology consult. JAK2, MPL, or MYD88 underwent hematology consult irrespective of VAF, and DNMT3A, TET2, ASXL1, IDH1, IDH2, SF3B1, or U2AF1 with VAF $\geq$ 10% were also referred.

- Specifically 110 patients, or 7.7% of them, carried at least one high-risk CH mutation: JAK2 ($n = 28$), ASXL1 ($n = 18$), DNMT3A ($n = 32$), TET2 ($n = 19$), SF3B1 ($n = 5$), IDH1 ($n = 4$), IDH2 ($n = 3$), MPL ($n = 3$), or U2AF1 ($n = 2$).
- In 45 patients, MTB was advised for hematologic consultation.
- Overall, nine of 18 patients were actually addressed, and confirmed hematologic malignancies occurred in six patients: two essential thrombocytopenia, two patients with MDS, one with a Waldenström macroglobulinemia, and one with a marginal lymphoma [15].

5.4.1 A TME Model Enabling Targeted Therapy Drug Sensitivity

Li et al. constructed a TME model of CLL that potentially enables targeted therapy drug sensitivity to guide precision medicine. They reported on the development of an affordable and reasonably constructed cell model that has compatibility with drug sensitivity screens and ex vivo functional assays. For 24 hours, CLL cells are cultured in fibroblasts coexpressing the ligands BAFF, CD40L, and APRIL. For at least 13 days, the survival of primary CLL cells is sustained by the transient co-culture and mimics in vivo drug resistance signals. Resistance to the Bcl-2 antagonist venetoclax correlates with in vivo responses. This assay is significant for identifying treatment vulnerabilities and guiding precision medicine for relapsed CLL patients, and taken together, "the presented CLL microenvironment model enables the clinical implementation of functional precision medicine in CLL." Molecular alterations leading to disease progression enabled functional precision medicine to test the sensitivity of different drugs directly on tumor cells; that was, however, made challenging by the rapid, spontaneous apoptosis of tumor cells outside of the TME and needed to be overcome by the signals being present during drug testing so that measured ex vivo sensitivity reflected in vivo sensitivity to treatment. Key ME factors included APRIL, BAFF, and CD40L that would support ex vivo survival.

Key Results

- CLL signaling in several pathways related to cell proliferation, including mTOR (pS2448), p38 MAPK (pT180/Y182), NF-κB p65 (pS529), and AKT (pS473), was induced, as revealed by co-culture with GFP-APRIL + CD40L fibroblasts, as shown through high-throughput protein profiling.

- At a time point at which the viability of unstimulated CLL cells was less affected by spontaneous apoptosis Bcl-2 antagonists, CLL sensitivity to venetoclax after CD40L/APRIL/BAFF stimulation was tested; unstimulated or stimulated CLL cells with physiologically relevant concentrations (1–10,000 nM) were treated with BGB- 11417 or venetoclax for 24 hour. This was corroborated by previous findings that CD40L induces Bcl-2 antagonist venetoclax resistance, leading to the activation of PI3K/AKT, p44/42 MAPK, JAK/STAT, and NF-κB through the activation of PI3K/AKT, p44/42 MAPK, JAK/STAT, and NF-κB.
- After CD40L/APRIL/BAFF CLL cells were treated with 10 nM BGB-11417 and with 60% cell viability treatment with 10 nM venetoclax, 50% viability was found; however, high sensitivity was reported in unstimulated CLL cells.
- When CLL cells co-cultured with CD40L/APRIL/BAFF fibroblasts were compared to CLL cells co-cultured with control fibroblasts, this further supported the notion that microenvironmental factors lead to CLL drug resistance, and it showed significantly higher cell viability for each concentration (except 10,000 nM) of venetoclax and BGB-11417.

A case study of a patient revealed that ex vivo sensitivity correlated with in vitro sensitivity, which guides precision medicine. A 64-year-old patient presented with refractory disease, and peripheral blood mononuclear cells. (PBMCs) were isolated to study the sensitivity of ibrutinib, venetoclax, and idelasib, with idelasib resulting in the inhibition of BTK and venetoclax inducing the cleavage of caspase-3. The patient received idelasib, but treatment stopped due to adverse events. After relapse with venetoclax, samples were isolated to guide the next line of therapy, being under clinical investigation, and were found to be Bcl-2 antagonist BGB-11417 and proteasome inhibitors (bortezomib and ixazomib citrate). Sensitivity remained high at T1 to other Bcl-2 antagonist combinations, as observed for cobimetinib (MEK inhibitor) + venetoclax combinations and for copanlisib (PI3K inhibitor) + BGB-11417, and the case illustrated that the model and ex vivo testing can indicate drug sensitivity, but not tolerability. The study authors concluded that in vivo responses to respective treatments were associated with ex vivo sensitivity to targeted therapy when measured either at cell viability or at protein level [16].

5.4.2 A New Druggable Molecular Pathway in CLL

Ikhiel et al. evaluated the potential of the protein complex neurotensin receptor 2/ tropomyosin related kinase B (NTSR2/TrkB) oncogenic pathway in CLL cells, which is relevant because existing targeted therapies have low long-term efficacy and lead to therapeutic resistance. The binding domain of NTRSR2 and a peptide complex targeting TRKB were identified, in which the latter decreases the interaction of the two proteins, affects the SRC family kinase pathway, and leads to apoptosis, demonstrating a cytotoxic effect in vivo and ex vivo in a cohort of 30 CLL patients. A new druggable molecular pathway may have been found given that both targets are constitutively active or highly expressed in B cells. The study provided evidence that the interaction between TRKB and NTRS2 was primarily associated with the C-terminal domain of NTSR2.

Key Results

- A competitor for the 0 Trans-Activator of Transcription ("TAT") cell-penetration peptide sequence and the NTSR2–TRKB interaction was added for enhancing cell penetration, leading to the inhibition of this interaction through a generated Pep that corresponds to the C-terminal sequence of the NTSR2 protein.
- The TAT-Pep peptide induced the cell death of CLL-B cells through a cohort of 30 patients at an IC50 of 10 μm by using an MEC-1 cell line. A 1.6-fold increase in cell death occurred when compared to controls at 5 um that progressively increased two-fold at 10 μm, and a 2.8 fold increase occurred at 30 μm, together demonstrating that the TAT-Pep-V5 peptide effectively enters CLL-B cells and binds to the intracellular domain of the TRKB protein.
- A significant implication for disrupting leukemic cell growth and survival pathways was shown through the successful binding of TRKB to TAT-Pep-V5 peptide, demonstrating its potential as an effective inhibitor of the NTSR2–TRKB interaction, which has also been shown to be a therapeutic peptide inhibiting the expression of antiapoptotic proteins and affecting the activation of SRC family kinase.
- After the TAT-Pep treatment of CLL-B cells, a decrease in the antiapoptotic proteins BCL-2, BCL-XL, and MCL-1 occurred regarding antiapoptotic expression, possibly due to the inactivation of SRC kinase. Also, mRNA levels were evaluated for all three antiapoptotic proteins after peptide treatment to determine whether the mechanism of regulation after observed modifications was transcriptional and post-transcriptional, with results implying that regulation might occur transcriptionally with significantly lowered expression for all three demonstrated.

As the authors discuss, an unexplored pathway in CLL demonstrates its therapeutic potential, showing that the development of new therapies for achieving more-durable and better responses in patients is necessitated by targeting exploring pathways in CLL, with the purpose of demonstrating its therapeutic potential. Peptide-based solutions show a potential solution to overcoming drug resistance through disruptions to protein–protein interactions by instead interacting with binding partners of the target protein, which overcomes induced resistance in alternative signaling pathways and target genes and plays a pivotal role is the induction of leukemic B-cell death by targeting the NTSR2–TRKB interaction [17].

5.4.3 *The Discovery of Pathogenic Genes in CLL Cells*

The discovery of pathogenic genes, including BCL2, BCL3, and CCND1, was advanced through the identification in CLL cells of infrequent balanced translocations with the immunoglobulin heavy chain locus (14q32). The investigators hypothesized that this finding may have unrecognized significance because it followed the identification in a CLL patient of a "t(X;14)(q28;q32) translocation that placed the mature T cell proliferation 1 gene (MTCP1) adjacent to the immunoglobulin locus." Walker et al. reported on human MTCP1 overexpression in the B-cell compartment only in mouse models that led to the production of CD5+/CD19+ leukemia, recapitulating many of the features of human CLL. A therapeutic response to ibrutinib was shown as further evidence when the translocation of BCL2 created a similar situation to a CLL patient with the t(X;14)(q28;q32) translocation in that the prior translocation led to the colocation of "the mature T cell proliferation 1 (MTCP1) coding region with the IGH locus."

According to the authors, increased MTCP1 expression in CLL was prognostic of poor outcomes and elevated mRNA expression of MCTP1 in CLL cells when compared to normal B cells was an associated factor. This further led to the demonstration of the potential of the role of using MTCP1 as a target for mitigating pathogenic mechanisms driving CLL and the ability of MTCP1 to result in aggressive CLL-like leukemia, and it demonstrated the need for further interrogating this phenomenon thanks to the discovery of the in vivo model for optimal translatability to the clinical setting. Additionally, t(X;14)(q28;q32) translocation was identified in CLL for investigating "unexplored mechanisms" and evaluating "therapeutic strategies."

Key Results

- A 2-fold increase in the expression of MTCP1 as a single continuous variable was observed to be associated with shorter PFS when adjusting for each study arm and also led to spontaneous and lethal leukemia through B-cell-specific MTCP-1 overexpression.
- The percentages of transgenic mouse models under the control of a promoter-enhancer expressing MTCP1 developing a CLL-like leukemia were 70% and 28% for founder lines. When MTCP1 is expressed in CLL patients, it is associated with poor outcomes, and aggressive human CLL is recapitulated by MTCP1-driven leukemia, the "accumulation of abnormal B lymphocytes in Eμ-MTCP1 mice showing a CD19+CD5+CD93−B220dim phenotype, with dim surface expression of IgM, IgD, and CD23 confirming a B1a cell phenotype."
- Kaplan–Meier curves demonstrated survival in Eμ-MTCP1 mice, and the median survival time was 10.8 months (95% CI 9.5–12) for Eμ-MTCP1 founder line Z36, and 14.5 months (95% CI: 13.1–16) for founder line Z20 ($p < 0.001$), respectively. Eμ-MTCP1 leukemia development was also impaired by ibrutinib treatment.
- Mice treated with ibrutinib at 30 mg/kg/day with monthly assessments of circulating CD5+/CD19+ and CD19+/B220dim leukemia cells led to a considerable survival prolongation in mice receiving ibrutinib at 12 months and a lower leukemic burden at 6 and 12 months in all treated mice.
- Similarly, ibrutinib administration led to a reduction in the rate of disease development between 6 weeks and 12 weeks after enrollment and prolonged survival compared to those receiving vehicle.

The study authors conclude that a pathogenic role of MTCP 1 in CLL is highly suggested by the discovery of a translocation that juxtaposes IGH locus and the observed MTCP1 gene with its overexpression in CLL, and the study remains significant because it demonstrates how whole-genome sequencing (WGS) assessment and classic cytogenetics blend the discovery of rare recurrent balanced translocations for finding previously unrecognized oncogenes. Additionally, the evidence from the transgenic mouse model and human cells presents a previously undiscovered causal relationship between CLL and MTCP1 [18].

5.5 Lymphoma

5.5.1 Clinical Studies for Mantle Cell Lymphoma

Novel approaches for classical mantle cell lymphoma, a subset of non-Hodgkin's lymphoma (NHL), were evaluated in SHINE, NCTN-E1211, ENRICH, and GELTAMO studies in efforts to elicit deeper and more-durable responses to bendamustine and rituximab combination treatments. In SHINE, BTKis were incorporated into the frontline settings in a randomized phase 3 study. Ibrutinib alone was shown to have an mPFS of 52.9 months, whereas it was 80.6 months in the ibrutinib and BR combination treatment at a median follow-up of 84.7 months, with a 25% reduction in the risk of death or progression and with a similar OS of 7 years. These limitations were due to TRAEs and more disease progression in the monotherapy group. In the NCTN-E211 trial, the proteosome inhibitor bortezomib and lenalidomide were evaluated to determine whether the regimen had additive and synergistic benefits to BR in the frontline setting. Median PFS, ORR, and CR did not differ between the bortezomib group and the lenalidomide group (64.1 vs. 64 months; 88.9% with CR 65.5% vs. 89.5% with CR 60.5%, respectively). Grade 3 or higher adverse events were higher in the bortezomib group (88.1% vs. 77.5%). The ENRICH study showed whether durable PFS could be achieved with a combination of BTKi and anti-CD20 therapies without chemotherapy in the form of alkylating agents. In a single-arm cohort of 50 patients, an ORR of 96% with a CR of 71% was achieved; however, most patients had disease progression due to toxicities. The phase 2 GELTAMO study featured patients with low-burden disease where ibrutinib with eight total doses of rituximab was administered for at least 2 years, showing an ORR of 82%, a CR of 75%, and 87% MRD negativity in 23 patients eligible for peripheral blood testing [19].

Mantle cell lymphoma (MCL) with the advent of targeted and cellular therapies has been shown to have more-favorable outcomes with more cases of indolent disease presenting for a watchful approach, as opposed to aggressive disease requiring intensive therapy. As patients experience longer remissions, surveillance becomes necessary, typically carried out through imaging. One study evaluated the CloneSEQ assay, the only FDA-approved assay for assessing MRD through immunoglobulin high-throughput sequencing that could serve as a less costly, more sensitive alterative that eliminates the risk of radiation exposure that utilizes ctDNA. In this study, 34 patients with low risk, an mPFS of 13.76 years, and an OS of 86% that underwent a median of 5.5 MRD tests were enrolled. Patients with radiographic relapse had peripheral blood MRD+, with the first MRD+ test between 0 and 24 months (median 34 days). Only one patient with PD had an MRD- result. Among 22 patients in continuous clinical remission from MCL, 21 remained MRD-, where one patient who developed myelodysplastic syndrome underwent allogeneic transplant and died from AML. According to the study investigators, several patients were able without surveillance imaging to enjoy 2- to 4-year intervals while still getting reassurance every few months from the negative cloneSEQ testing, suggesting that the assay following first-line therapy for MCL patients is an effective form of surveillance [20].

5.6 Acute Lymphoblastic Leukemia

In a retrospective study on relapsed Ph+ ALL in a pediatric patient population, olverembatinib, a third-generation TKI, was shown to deliver complete remission and less than 0.01% MRD (negative) in four out of five patients. A good safety profile with grade 2 myopathy was also shown in two patients and grade 3 fever in one patient. The median cumulative dose was 600 mg. Olverembatinib is a potent third-generation TKI that was shown to be effective in resistant CML patients harboring the T315I mutation, with 50–83% achieving a complete cytogenetic response and 40–59% achieving a molecular response. In a US-based population of CML patients resistant to BCR::ABL1 inhibitors, the drug achieved a complete cytogenetic response in 42.9% of patients. The drug was also found to be well tolerated, with common grade 3 events of thrombocytopenia and neutropenia observed. In a retrospective study of 12 patients with Ph+ ALL and T315I mutation who had hematological relapse (n = 4), molecular positive disease (n = 4), or molecular relapse (n = 2) after prior TKI, olverembatinib treatment alone or with chemotherapy induced complete remission in seven patients. These studies led to the hypothesis that the drug could induce remission in this pediatric population (n = 7). Six patients received olverembatinib after relapse on dasatinib and chemotherapy treatment. One of each was at their second or third relapse, with four patients at their first relapse. Single-agent olverembatinib at days 6, 2, and 16 after relapse were administered for three patients—numbers 1, 4, and 6, respectively—with the other four patients receiving the drug in combination with cytotoxic chemotherapy between days 4 and 85 after relapse. Monotherapy achieved CR with negative MRD on days 28 and 29. Two patients on combination treatment attained remission with negative MRD tested on days 20 and 39. In addition to excellent hematologic effects, olverembatinib led to leukemia control in central nervous system (CNS). One patient with CNS leukemia (with a white blood cell (WBC) count of 4865 cells/μL and 86.13% blasts) at the time of relapse had their WBC count reduced to 1200 cells/μL after receiving a single dose of the drug. Safety profiles were also favorable and evaluable in six patients. The most frequent effect was grade 2 myopathy in a lower extremity and grade 2 extremity pain in two patients between 59 and 136 days of treatment. One patient had a grade 3 fever and pneumonia. Hematologic toxicity was not observed in three patients receiving only olverembatinib. The study authors concluded that olverembatinib induced remission in patients with relapse Ph+ ALL in prior treatment in dasatinib [21].

Patel et al. reported in *CLML* on a potential tumor-agnostic therapy for advanced hematologic malignancies in their study on the investigational agent INCB053914, a pan-PIM kinase inhibitor (proviral integration site of Moloney murine leukemia virus) alone or in combination with standard-of-care agents (cytarabine, azacitidine, or ruxolitinib) in a dose-escalation/dose-expansion phase 1/2 study. The compound showed efficacy in preclinical models and was evaluated for safety and efficacy in AML, MDS/MF, MM, and lymphoproliferative neoplasms in parts 1/2 monotherapy ($n = 58$) and parts 3/4 combination therapy ($n = 39$). The most common toxicities were AST and ALT elevations (each $n = 4$) and fatigue. PIM kinases were found to be overexpressed in a number of hematologic neoplasms (including diffuse large B-cell lymphoma (DLBCL)) and are implicated in several oncogenic signaling pathways, being downstream effectors in PI3K and JAK/STAT mediated activation. They regulate cell-cycle and cellular proliferation and apoptosis by phosphorylating key substrates, including the BCL-2-associated promoter proteins that are downstream of PI3K isozymes and PIM kinases, resulting in crosstalk between PIM kinases and PI3K/AKT/mTORC1 signaling pathways, leading to additive or synergistic therapeutic effects with other anticancer agents. In this study, safety, tolerability, and ORR served as the primary endpoints. In the monotherapy group, 57 of 58 patients, or 98.3% of them, had TEAEs of ALT elevation and fatigue, with 48, or 82.8%, having grade 3 or higher TEAEs, which were most commonly anemia ($n = 18$). Treatment-related events include ALT elevation that occurred in 43 patients that led to dose interruption in 29, dose reduction in three, and dose discontinuation in 12. Serious TEAEs were in the form of febrile neutropenia and pneumonia. Similar types of adverse events were reported in the combination groups (cytarabine, azacytidine, and ruxolitinib), with patients experiencing grade 4 hypophosphatemia and grade 3 ALT elevation. On the basis of dose-limiting toxicities (DLTs), the investigational agent with cytarabine was not tolerated. Treatment-related AEs occurred in five patients, mostly ALT, diarrhea, stomatitis, and AST elevation. In the azacytidine group, three patients had fatal TEAEs due to disease progression; however, none were related to the treatment. No DLTs were reported in the ruxolitinib combination therapy group. The RP2Ds for each group were identified: 80 mg of twice a day (BID) and 80 mg of BID, respectively. No confirmed responses were found in the monotherapy group, and in the combination groups, one patient achieved partial remission (with cytarabine), two CRs (50 mg with azacytidine and 80 mg with azacytidine) were found, and eight patients had a reduction in spleen volume in the ruxolitinib combination group. These data allowed the study authors to conclude that INCB053914 had promising efficacy was generally well tolerated, with AST and ALT elevations being the most common adverse events [22].

A review conducted by Haddad et al. revealed that complete molecular remission through NGS (NGS-CMR) and undetectable BCR::ABL1 transcripts via RT-PCR is the most important factor predicting relapse, with NGS-CMR being more sensitive for Ph+-ALL. The development of T315I mutation in patients is also an important factor. To increase complete molecular remission (CMR) and prevent the emergence of this mutation, a third-generation TKI, namely ponatinib, was administered in combination in the frontline setting of a Hyperfractionated Cyclophosphamide, Vincristine, Doxorubicin/Adriamycin, Dexamethasone (hyper-CVAD). In one study, the regimen increased CMR to a rate of 84% and had a 6-year OS rate of 75% with confirmed superiority over imatinib, and it was again associated with a higher rate of MRD- (34% versus 17%). In a study, 85 newly diagnosed Ph+ ALL patients were enrolled and were treated with TKIs and hyper-CVAD (ponatinib, $n = 23$, imatinib, $n = 23$; dasatinib, $n = 39$); those who achieved CMR within 6 months had improved survival. The 4-year OS rate was 66%, and the median OS was 217 months. TKIs also conferred CNS prophylaxis. Dasatinib was evaluated in a randomized phase 3 trial in 189 pediatric patients with Ph-ALL and was shown to be associated with decreased CNS relapse. A recent report highlighted the emergence of "CML-like biology" in Ph+ALL, emphasizing NGS's role in the monitoring of MRD. Because 20–30% of patients relapse despite achieving CMR with the correlation of RT-PCR for transcripts and MRD, such as RT-PCR for immunoglobulin or T-cell receptor, being poor, the emergence of blasts of myeloid lineage, and a non-leukemic compartment, investigators sought to evaluate this correlation to determine the prognostic impact of NGS-MRD in Ph+-ALL patients. They found in their analysis that 15–30% of patients in this population who achieved NGS-MRD negative at a sensitive of 1×10^{-6} still had BCR::ABL1 transcripts detectable via RT-PCR. None of these patients experienced relapsed, and none were prognostic for OS or RFS, with similar rates between RT-PCR+/NGS+ and RT-PCR+/NGS-, where patients achieved NGS-MRD and had a low risk of relapse. Other targeted therapies under clinical evaluation include the STAMP inhibitor asciminib, an allosteric ABL myristoyl pocket with activity against ABL1 kinase domain mutations, which achieved hematologic remission in seven evaluable patients in one study with a recommended phase 2 dosing achieved thanks to olverembatinib, a novel third-generation BCR::ABL TKI. Olverembatinib showed efficacy in Ph+ALL in a multicenter randomized trial dosed at 30 mg and 50 mg every day for 30 enrolled patients having failed more than two prior TKIs and a 75% complete cytogenic c response. In a recent update, of 13 R/R Ph+ALL patients, three, or 23%, of them, achieved a major molecular response, one with T315I mutation and one with resistance to prior ponatinib. The agent was well tolerated as a monotherapy and in combination with blinatumomab, with 70% of patients responding and five achieving MRD through flow cytometry and CMR as a single agent. In combination, all 13 patients achieved CR, with 77% having grade 1 CRS. As the authors conclude, the prognosis of Ph+ALL patients has improved with the implementation of TKIs and has led to reduced rates of chemotherapy-induced side effects, reduced reliance on allogeneic transplantation, and improved survival [23].

A fascinating study was conducted by Larkin et al. on polygenic pharmacodynamic markers as toxicity phenotype predictors in the treatment of ALL in a single-center study. Common antileukemic agents were evaluated that underwent comprehensive pharmacogenomic evaluation to develop during the treatment of ALL a polygenic toxicity risk score that would be utilized to be predictive of the most common toxicities.

- Increased risk of GI (p = 2.07E-05, 3 SNPs: TYMS-rs151264360/FPGS-rs1544105/GSTM1-GSTM5-rs3754446)
- Neurologic (p = 0.0005, 3 SNPs:DCTD-rs6829021/SLC28A3-rs17343066/CTPS1-rs12067645)
- Endocrine (p = 4.77E-08, 3 SNPs: AKR1C3-rs1937840/TYMS-rs2853539/CTH-rs648743)
- Heme toxicities (p = 0.053, 3 SNPs: CYP3A5-rs776746/ABCB1-rs4148737/CTPS1-rs12067645)—SNP-SNP combination pathway analysis leads to predictions in toxicity

The authors concluded that "each described high multigene/SNP-based toxicity risk score is significantly associated with a higher incidence of toxicity" [24].

5.6.1 *Rearrangements in B-cell ALL with Response to TKIs*

Another study was conducted on B-cell ALL adults who had refractoriness to chemotherapy and possessed Philadelphia-like genetics that had response to TKIs. Many of these patients have rearrangements in PDGFRβ, JAK2, EPOR, ABL1, and ABL2 genes, which show potential response to TKIs.

Key Results

- Nine had JAK2 class fusions (five JAK2 and four EPOR), and 14 had ABL class fusions (eight ABL1, one ABL2, and five PDGFRβ). Additionally, 16 of 23 received TKIs, and the remainder received chemotherapy. The study's aim was to evaluate B-cell ALL outcomes for patients harboring ABL and the non–cytokine receptor like factor 2 JAK class fusions/rearrangements, with a focus on their responses to TKIs. According to the study authors, improved long-term survival and deeper responses were achieved through the frontline use of BCR::ABL1 TKI in patients with ABL class fusions and rearrangements. Using genomic analysis through fluorescence in situ hybridization (FISH) and fusion assays in contrast to conventional cytogenetics helps to identify genetic aberrations in Ph+B-cell ALL patients [25].

5.7 Chronic Myeloid Leukemia

5.7.1 *Bosutinib*

Bosutinib is approved for the treatment of Ph+ CML, and as a second-generation TKI, its efficacy has been evaluated as a frontline therapy and in second- and later-line settings. Comparative efficacy has been shown for later-line treatment options in combination with asciminib that have also demonstrated favorable safety profiles in the context of comorbidities and associated adverse events. It is administered in the chronic or accelerated phase and has transformed a disease once with poor prognosis to a manageable, indolent one, particularly in resistant cases to prior lines of chemotherapy or first-generation TKIs as well as newly diagnosed cases. Other second-generation TKIs, such as dasatinib and nilotinib, produce higher rates of cytogenic and deep molecular response; however, they have shown no improvement in OS. The phase 3 BFORE trial in patients with newly diagnosed CML established the efficacy and long-term safety of bosutinib (400 mg/d) when compared to imatinib. Higher rates of major molecular response (MMR) were achieved (47.2% vs. 64.6%), with rates of 73.9% vs. 64.6% in a 5-year cumulative follow-up. Early response as indicated by BCR::ABL transcripts of less than 10% was higher (80.6% versus 60.5%), and 5-year progression/death at 5-years was 6.7% versus 9.3% with similar OS rates (94.5% vs. 94.6%). These results from the BFORE trial led to the approval of bosutinib in the frontline treatment of CML. Resistance to bosutinib, measured by BCR::ABL1 transcript greater than 1 after 1 year, is not clearly understood but may be related to genomic instability or DNA damage; however, it is uncommon, occurring in 10–15% of patients. The phase 1/2 Study 200 trial established an acceptable safety profile and durable efficacy for second-line bosutinib at a dose of 500 mg/d in resistant CP-CML or intolerant to imatinib, with a major cytogenetic response rate of 24 weeks being 31%. In a final analysis at a 10-year follow-up, the cumulative cytogenetic response was 50%, and the MMR was reported as being 42%. In this cohort, bosutinib was reduced from 400 mg to 300 mg in 50% of patients to manage AEs and escalated to 600 mg in 18% of patients to improve efficacy. Overall, bosutinib has efficacy and safety in later-line settings and serves as a treatment option in CML resistant or intolerant to multiple prior TKIs, which was further confirmed by the phase 4 BYOND trial, in which the cumulative confirmed major cytogenetic response (MCyR) rate by 1 year was reported at 75.8% and 62.3% in patients previously treated with one or two TKIs and those treated with three TKIs, respectively. In the same patient population, complete cytogenetic response (CCyr) rates were 83.7% (one prior line of therapy), 83.9% (two prior lines of therapy) and 73.3% (three prior lines of therapy). Also, 25.8% of patients discontinued therapy due to AEs. Bosutinib was also evaluated in comparison with asciminib and was shown to be more effective in later lines of treatment in the ASCEMBL trial, where the 6-month MMR rate did not translate into a survival benefit, and this trial had a treatment discontinuation rate of 21.1%. When evaluated in the BEST dose-optimization study, AEs in patients receiving bosutinib were observed at a 50% higher rate when compared to asciminib. Post hoc analysis of the BYOND trial showed that greater flexibility in dosing may be required for lower discontinuation rates and higher response rates. Several trials, including the BODO trial, the BEST trial and an interim analysis of DESTINY, led to dose-optimization strategies for bosutinb aiming to reduce toxicities and maximize efficacy. The BODO trial started bosutinib on 100 mg/d every 2 weeks to a maximum dose of 500 mg/d and led to 100% of patients having an any-grade TEAE, with frequently reported gastrointestinal toxicities. In the BEST trial, the agent was administered at 200 mg/d for 2 weeks with increases to 300 or 400 mg/d with cardiac ischemia, resulting in AEs of nephrotoxicity, diarrhea, skin rash, and fatigue [26].

5.7.2 *Dasatinib*

Dasatinib is also a second-generation TKI approved for the treatment of CML and was shown in a 5-year follow-up study to serve as a frontline therapy for CP-CML at a low dose (50 mg). In the chronic phase, 93 newly diagnosed CML patients received a 50 mg daily dose of dasatinib and demonstrated an MMR of 95% and a DMR of 82%; the 5-year OS was 96%. These results were significant given that dasatinib has been approved for a larger dose (100 mg) and given that the lower dose still led to better outcomes and tolerability. "At 3 months, 78 (96%) patients achieved BCR::ABL1 transcripts (IS) ≤ 10%, and at 12 months, 65 (81%) patients achieved BCR::ABL1 transcript (IS) ≤ 0.1%" Second-generation TKIs are the preferred treatment in younger patients because treatment discontinuation after DMR may lead to treatment-free remission in higher risk cases. In a head-to-head comparison with imatinib, dasatinib was shown to be superior to imatinib according to rates of CCyR (77% vs. 66%) and major molecular response (46% vs. 28%) at 12 months. Associated AEs are pleural effusions and myelosuppression (28% and 20%). Reduced dosage could potentially lead to fewer side effects and a lower dose schedule. An early molecular response (BCR::ABL1 transcripts [IS] ≤ 10% at 3 months) was associated with dasatinib at > 90%, with a 6-month MMR rate of 66% and a 12-month MR4 molecular response and with a 4-log reduction rate of 71% and an MR4.5 rate of 46%. In the study of 81 evaluable patients, a high percentage achieved BCR::ABL1 transcripts at less than or equal to 10% at 3 months. At 1 year, 80 patients were on dasatinib therapy, with 77 achieving CCyR, and only three patients remained with BCR::ABL1 transcripts greater than 1%. At 2 years, 78 patients were on dasitinib therapy, and 76 achieved CCyR, with two not having achieved CCyR.

Key Results

- The cumulative incidence of MMR at 44% and 79% was reported at 6 and 12 months, and the cumulative incidence of CCyR at 62% and 94% was observed at 6 and 12 months, respectively. MR4 at 52%, MR4.5 at 43%, and CMR at 22% were reported for the 12-month cumulative rates. The cumulative 5-year CCyR and MMR rates were 98% and 95%, respectively. MR4 83%, MR4.5 82%, and CMR at 70% were observed as high cumulative DMR rates.
- Nine patients had their dose increased to 100 mg daily, four of whom did not achieve CCyR. One patient showed persistent disease from bone marrow assessment (no molecular or cytogenetic response) and was switched to 15 mg of ponitinib daily. Nine patients were discontinued on dasatinib to achieve treatment-free remission after achieving DMR.
- Outcomes include an estimated 5-year OS rate of 96%, an EFS rate of 90%, and an FFS rate of 86%. Eight patients failed therapy on dasatinib, four being due to resistance and four others being due to toxicity.
- Grade 3 or 4 myelosuppression and thrombocytopenia, neutropenia, and anemia were low (7%; 6%, and 5%, respectively). Furthermore, 11 patients, or 13% of them, developed pleural effusion with a time to first event of 28 months; 2% had grade 3 to 4 pleural effusion. For five patients who had dasatinib reductions,

recurrent pleural effusion was reported after resuming dasatinib. Eight of the 11 patients who developed effusion were older than 65 years. Also, 23 patients, or 28% of them, had their dasatinib dose reduced due to side effects (2/22 to 40 mg daily and 20/22 to 20 mg daily) and one due to their physician's advice. "Most of the patients had grade 1 to 2 AEs, which included mainly pleural effusion, fatigue, skin abnormalities, and arthromyalgia."

As the study authors concluded, the optimization of TKI dose schedules will improve patient compliance, lead to a reduction in the rate of failure due to intolerance, and improvements in efficacy by maintaining uninterrupted TKI therapy and reducing the cost of TKI care [2].

In an observational, retrospective study, the real-world effectiveness of dasatinib versus imatinib was evaluated in newly diagnosed CML patients. Real-world outcomes in the treatment of CML-CP with first dasatinib versus imatinib was assessed, and the study found that 1 L of dasatinib had higher rates and shorter times to major molecular and DMR, and outcomes were maintained across body mass index (BMI) and age subgroups. In the first-line setting are four TKIs that have been approved by the FDA for CML: imatinib, nilotinib, bosutinib, and dasatinib. These results are consistent with the DASISION trial, which also compared the effectiveness of imatinib with dasatinib for newly diagnosed CML-CP: At the 5-year follow-up, the MMR was 76% versus 64%, and the DMR was 42% versus 33%. CcyR determined primary treatment response, which was defined as < 1% BCR::ABL-positive nuclei through fluorescence in situ hybridization (FISH), 0% Ph + metaphases measured through bone marrow cytogenetics or assessed by a physician, clinical MMR "(defined as BCR::ABL ≤ 0.1%, or 3-log reduction or physician-assessed) rate, time to MMR, and DMR (defined as BCR::ABL ≤ 0.0032% or 4.5-log reduction, or physician-assessed) rate." The dasatinib cohort ($n = 306$) had a low discontinuation of index therapy when compared to imatinib (($n = 84$ (28%) vs. $n = 47$ (15%), $p < 0.001$)), with reasons more due to pleural effusion than a lack of efficacy, adverse events, or disease progression. In terms of MMR (79% vs. 65%) and DMR (44% vs. 25%), nearly all patients achieved significantly higher rates and a shorter time to DMR (11.9 months vs. 14.7 months; 30.3 months vs. 66.1 months) with dasitinib.

- When comparing clinical response according to the risk for patients from dasatinib and imatinib, the rate of DMR was significantly greater among patients on dasatinib, and the time to DMR was significantly shorter as well (18.5 vs. 53.4 months; 60% vs. 32%). However, the time to and rate of MMR did not significantly differ. When comparing dasatinib with imatinib again for the intermediate/high-risk subgroup, DMR and MMR rates were significantly higher in patients receiving dasatinib (DMR: 36% vs. 18%; MMR: 78% vs. 57%). Median times to DMR and MMR were also significantly shorter in the dasatinib cohort versus the imatinib cohort (DMR: 43.0 months vs. not reached, MMR: 13.2 vs. 18.3 months).

As the study authors conclude, in the current real-world study, improved outcomes were consistent with the DASISION trial, with results demonstrating a shorter time to MMR and DMR, with significantly higher rates of MMR and DMR in dasatinib versus imatinib and with robust improvements across each risk subgroup, age, and BMI [27].

5.7.3 Ponatinib

Ponatinib, a third-generation, highly potent pan-BCR-ABL TKI, also underwent evaluation in a real-world setting for CML-CP patients ($n = 72$); the agent is also indicated in accelerated phase (AP) and blast phase (BP). Molecular response as estimated by < 1% BCR::ABL1 at 12 months was achieved in 51.6% of patients, and the 2-year PFS was 84%, leading to the conclusion that controlling cardiovascular risk factors and reducing doses at optimal time points may help to optimize the dosing of ponatinib. Ponatinib is indicated in patients who are resistant to first-generation and second-generation TKIs, who have received prior TKI treatment, and who have the T315I mutation, which is higher in relapsed CML patients. Other results include 43% and 25% achieving major and deep molecular response, with an estimated (2-year) PFS of 84%. However, severe arterial occlusive events were reported in 10.9% of patients after 5 months of median treatment. Additionally, 12 patients, or 16.6% of them, were ponatinib resistant and harbored the T315I mutation, and they were rescued with allogeneic transplantation on follow-up. Dosing was reduced from 45 mg to 30 mg in 10 patients due to AEs, including cytopenia and elevated lipase; "none of these patients achieved MMR nor MR < 1% BCR::ABL1 (IS)"; 12 patients had a dose reduction of 45 mg to 15 mg for MMR achievement; 50% of patients who maintained MMR who required dose reduction maintained MMR, with none of the patients losing response. Hypertension (grade 2 or grade 3) was the most common AE ($n = 11$, 15%), which was treated with 50 mg of losartan and was controlled in 81%. Severe arterial occlusive events (AOEs) were reported in eight patients after a median treatment time of 5 months (range 2–48 months), including coronary (60%), cerebrovascular (30%), and peripheral arterial (10%) events, which were mainly resolved, with two deaths reported. These events were more common in patients with a history of ischemia. AOEs related to ponatinib were reported as severe thrombocytopenia (8.3%) at dosages of 45 mg and 30 mg, with isolated elevated lipase occurring at dosages of 45 mg of ponatinib. These AEs resolved, with one patient experiencing acute pancreatitis. The study authors concluded that cardiovascular (CV) safety outcomes were consistent across other clinical trials and observational registries in this first real-world analysis of CML patients receiving ponatinib, with hypercholesterolemia and older age significantly associated with a higher risk of AOEs, mitigated by optimally controlling CV risk factors, potentially contributing to lower discontinuation rates and having a direct impact on responses and survival by optimizing ponatinib doses with reductions at precise time points [28].

5.7.4 Asciminib

Asciminib is an ABL/BCR::ABL1 TKI that was approved for the treatment of CML for patients who received previous lines of TKIs, such as first-generation TKI imatinib and second-generation TKIs bosutinib, dasatinib, and nilotinib. It inhibits the ABL1 kinase activity of the BCR::ABL1 fusion protein by binding to the ABL myristoyl pocket, allowing for specificity in targeting BCR::ABL1 and hundreds of other kinases, and was shown to have superior efficacy in the phase III ASCEMBL trial over bosutinib, with a major molecular response (MMR): BCR::ABL1 $\leq$ 0.1% of 24.9% versus 11.9% at 24 weeks and 33.0% versus 18.6% at 48 weeks. A real-world study was conducted to evaluate asciminib in clinical practice to determine potential benefits for patients with CML-CP following TKI failures in order to elucidate treatment patterns and clinical outcomes. The average age of patients was 63 years, and comorbidities included other malignancies, chronic pulmonary disease, renal disease, and congestive heart failure.

Key Results

- Asciminib was administered to 46 patients (47.4%) after two prior TKIs and 51 patients (52.6%) after three or more prior TKIs (three prior TKIs: 24.7%; four or more prior TKIs: 27.8%), and most patients were prescribed a dosage of 80 mg at the time of initiation or as either 80 mg once daily or 40 mg twice daily. Prior TKIs used at any time prior to asciminib initiation included imatinib (63.9%), bosutinib (61.9%), dasatinib (85.6%), nilotinib (53.6%), and senaib (15.5%).
- The best overall response (BCR::ABL1 $\leq$ 0.1% (MR3 or better)) was within 24 weeks post-asciminib initiation: BCR::ABL1 between $\leq$ 1% and > 0.1% (MR2) in 14.5% of patients.
- Among patients with $\geq$ 1 MR test postindex ($n = 70$), BCR::ABL1 $\leq$ 0.1% (MR3 or better) was achieved or maintained by 31.3% (95% CI).
  - Two prior TKIs at 12 weeks: 43.3% (95% CI 27.8%, 62.8%)
  - Three or more prior TKIs at 12 weeks: 21.6% (95% CI 27.8%, 62.8%)
  - Two prior TKIs at 24 weeks: 71.5% (95% CI 53.5%, 87.1%)
  - Three or more prior TKIs at 24 weeks: 33.4% (95% CI 20.4%, 51.4%)

The study featured a real-world analysis of the ASCEMBL trial and provided treatment options for a malignancy with poor prognosis and CP-CML patients who have failed prior TKI treatment with the further development of mutations, limiting therapies. In this trial, 24.9% of patients achieved a BCR::ABL1 $\leq$ 0.1%, and 41.5% achieved BCR::ABL1 in ASCEMBL and asciminib. This real study showed that deep molecular response that was achieved after previous treatment, filling an unmet need for tolerability and effectivity for a disease with no clear standard of care. However, follow-up studies are needed because results were assessed 6 months after asciminib initiation. As the study authors conclude, this real-world analysis of reported clinical outcomes post-asciminib treatment in the United States showed the treatment efficacy of the current analysis when compared to the phase III ASCEMBL trial on asciminib in patients with CML-CP that had been previously treated with two or more TKIs [29].

The EURO-SKI trial evaluated TKI CML treatments to determine prognostic factors and to carry out a final analysis for treatment-free remission with stable deep molecular remission. Of 728 patients, 434 were in major molecular response at 6 months, and 309 of 678 patients were in major molecular response at 36 months. The duration of TKI was predictive of response; BCR::ABL1 transcript served as a prognostic factor; and the presence of blasts in peripheral blood predicted treatment-free remission [30].

Targeted therapies considerably evolved from their first discovery and development as imatinib in CML in the context of new mutations and the evaluation of response through MRD. FLT3-IDH inhibitors for AML as well as ibrutinib and venetoclax for CLL mark their transition as the standard of care for hematologic malignancies. Overall, this chapter supports their continued clinical use and development and supports communicating to patients their robust efficacy and favorable safety profiles, which have been evaluated through studies.

References

1. Schmidts I, Haferlach T, Hoermann G. Precision medicine in the therapy of non-solid tumors. In: Precision medicine. Cham: Springer Nature; 2023.
2. Gener-Ricos G, Haddad FG, Sasaki K, Issa GC, Skinner J, Masarova L, et al. Low-dose Dasatinib (50 mg daily) frontline therapy in newly diagnosed chronic phase chronic myeloid leukemia: 5-year follow-up results. Clin Lymphoma Myeloma Leuk. 2023;23(10):742–8.
3. Forsberg M, Konopleva M. SOHO state of the art updates and next questions: understanding and overcoming Venetoclax resistance in hematologic malignancies. Clin Lymphoma Myeloma Leuk. 2024;24(1):1–14.
4. Easaw S, Ezzati S, Coombs CC. SOHO state of the art updates and next questions: updates on BTK inhibitors for the treatment of chronic lymphocytic leukemia. Clin Lymphoma Myeloma Leuk. 2023;23(10):697–704.
5. Alsouqi A, Woyach JA. SOHO state of the art updates and next questions | covalent Bruton's tyrosine kinase inhibitors in chronic lymphocytic leukemia. Clin Lymphoma Myeloma Leuk. 2025;25(2):89–95.
6. Aoki T, Jiang A, Xu A, Yin Y, Gamboa A, Milne K, et al. Spatially resolved tumor microenvironment predicts treatment outcomes in relapsed/refractory Hodgkin lymphoma. J Clin Oncol. 2024;42(9):1077–87.
7. Levis MJ, Hamadani M, Logan B, Jones RJ, Singh AK, Litzow M, et al. Gilteritinib as post-transplant maintenance for AML with internal tandem duplication mutation of FLT3. J Clin Oncol. 2024;42(15):1766–75.
8. Nasnas P, Ravandi F. SOHO state of the art updates and next questions: oral therapy in acute myeloid leukemia. Clin Lymphoma Myeloma Leuk. 2024;24(4):205–13.
9. Tiong IS, Hiwase DK, Abro E, Bajel A, Palfreyman E, Beligaswatte A, et al. Targeting molecular measurable residual disease and low-blast relapse in AML with Venetoclax and low-dose cytarabine: a prospective phase II study (VALDAC). J Clin Oncol. 2024;42(18):2161–73.
10. Konopleva MY, Dail M, Daver NG, Garcia JS, Jonas BA, Yee KWL, et al. Venetoclax and Cobimetinib in relapsed/refractory AML: a phase 1b trial. Clin Lymphoma Myeloma Leuk. 2024;24(6):364–74.
11. Tentori CA, Gregorio C, Robin M, Gagelmann N, Gurnari C, Ball S, et al. Clinical and genomic-based decision support system to define the optimal timing of allogeneic hematopoietic stem-cell transplantation in patients with myelodysplastic syndromes. J Clin Oncol. 2024;42(24):2873–86.
12. Mohty R, Al Hamed R, Bazarbachi A, Brissot E, Nagler A, Zeidan A, Mohty M. Treatment of myelodysplastic syndromes in the era of precision medicine and immunomodulatory drugs: a focus on higher-risk disease. J Hematol Oncol. 2022;15(1):124.
13. Miyamoto K, Minami Y. Precision Medicine and novel molecular target therapies in acute myeloid leukemia: the background of hematologic malignancies (HM)-SCREEN-Japan 01. Int J Clin Oncol. 2019;24:893.

14. Kittai AS, Bond D, Huang Y, Bhat SA, Blyth E, Byrd JC, et al. Anti-CD19 chimeric antigen receptor T-cell therapy for Richter transformation: an international, multicenter, retrospective study. J Clin Oncol. 2024;42(17):2071–9.
15. Aldea M, Tagliamento M, Bayle A, Vasseur D, Verge V, Marinello A, et al. Liquid biopsies for circulating tumor DNA detection may reveal occult hematologic malignancies in patients with solid tumors. JCO Precis Oncol. 2023;7:e2200583.
16. Hermansen JU, Yin Y, Urban A, Myklebust CV, Karlsen L, Melvold K, et al. A tumor microenvironment model of chronic lymphocytic leukemia enables drug sensitivity testing to guide precision medicine. Cell Death Discov. 2023;9(1):125.
17. Ikhlef L, Yassine M, Chandouri B, Riviere L, Naves T, Dmytruk N, et al. Targeting the NTSR2/TrkB oncogenic pathway in chronic lymphocytic leukemia. Sci Rep. 2024;14(1):6084.
18. Walker JS, Hing ZA, Sher S, Cronin J, Williams K, Harrington B, et al. Rare t(X;14)(q28;q32) translocation reveals link between MTCP1 and chronic lymphocytic leukemia. Nat Commun. 2021;12(1):6338.
19. Patel D, Kahl B. SOHO state of the art updates and next questions: tailoring upfront therapy in mantle cell lymphoma. Clin Lymphoma Myeloma Leuk. 2023;23(9):633–41.
20. Rezazadeh A, Pruett J, Detzner A, Edwin N, Hamadani M, Shah NN, et al. Immunoglobulin high throughput sequencing (Ig-HTS) minimal residual disease (MRD) analysis is an effective surveillance tool in patients with mantle cell lymphoma. Clin Lymphoma Myeloma Leuk. 2024;24(4):254–9.
21. Li X, Zhang J, Liu F, Liu T, Zhang R, Chen Y, et al. Olverembatinib treatment in pediatric patients with relapsed Philadelphia-chromosome-positive acute lymphoblastic leukemia. Clin Lymphoma Myeloma Leuk. 2023;23(9):660–6.
22. Patel MR, Donnellan W, Byrne M, Asch AS, Zeidan AM, Baer MR, et al. Phase 1/2 study of the pan-PIM kinase inhibitor INCB053914 alone or in combination with standard-of-care agents in patients with advanced hematologic malignancies. Clin Lymphoma Myeloma Leuk. 2023;23(9):674–86.
23. Haddad FG, Jabbour E, Short NJ, Jain N, Kantarjian H. SOHO state of the art updates and next questions: update on the approach to Philadelphia chromosome-positive acute lymphoblastic leukemia. Clin Lymphoma Myeloma Leuk. 2024;24(5):271–6.
24. Larkin T, Kashif R, Elsayed AH, Greer B, Mangrola K, Rafiee R, et al. Polygenic pharmacogenomic markers as predictors of toxicity phenotypes in the treatment of acute lymphoblastic leukemia: a single-center study. JCO Precis Oncol. 2023;7:e2200580.
25. Senapati J, Kantarjian H, Haddad FG, Short NJ, Welch MA, Jain N, et al. SOHO state of the art updates and next questions | next questions: acute lymphoblastic leukemia. Clin Lymphoma Myeloma Leuk. 2024;24(6):333.
26. Kantarjian HM, Jabbour EJ, Lipton JH, Castagnetti F, Brummendorf TH. A review of the therapeutic role of bosutinib in chronic myeloid leukemia. Clin Lymphoma Myeloma Leuk. 2024;24(5):285–97.
27. Klink AJ, Keating SJ, Brokars J, Feinberg B, Jabbour E. Real-world effectiveness of Dasatinib versus Imatinib in newly diagnosed patients with chronic myeloid leukemia. Clin Lymphoma Myeloma Leuk. 2024;24(3):149–57.
28. Mela Osorio MJ, Moiraghi B, Osycka MV, Pavlovsky MA, Varela AI, Bendek Del Prete GE, et al. Long-term follow-up in patients with chronic myeloid leukemia treated with Ponatinib in a real-world cohort: safety and efficacy analysis. Clin Lymphoma Myeloma Leuk. 2024;24(3):158–64.
29. Atallah EL, Wei D, Latremouille-Viau D, Rossi C. Real-world evaluation of treatment patterns and clinical outcomes among patients with chronic myeloid leukemia in chronic phase treated with asciminib in clinical practice in the United States. Clin Lymphoma Myeloma Leuk. 2025;25(3):178–187.e2.
30. Mahon FX, Pfirrmann M, Dulucq S, Hochhaus A, Panayiotidis P, Almeida A, et al. European stop tyrosine kinase inhibitor trial (EURO-SKI) in chronic myeloid leukemia: final analysis and novel prognostic factors for treatment-free remission. J Clin Oncol. 2024;42(16):1875–80.

Chapter 6
Immune Checkpoint Inhibitors

6.1 The Evolution of Immune Checkpoint Inhibitors for Solid Tumors

Immune checkpoint inhibitors (ICIs) were among the first innovative treatments in the field of cancer immunotherapies and had successes that are continuing in melanoma and non–small cell lung cancer (NSCLC) due to the immunogenic characteristics of these malignancies. NSCLC, one of the cancers that were found to have a response rate early in the development of therapy, had initial rates of around 20%. Research efforts are focusing on breast cancer and colorectal cancer (CRC) to investigate their treatment through immune checkpoint inhibitors, such as ipilimumab, nivolumab, and pembrolizumab. However, tumor heterogeneity and a hostile tumor microenvironment led to drug resistance, and incidences of nonresponders grew in the clinical setting. Drug development efforts led to next-generation agents such as atezolizumab, durvalumab, and relatlimab, a novel LAG-3 inhibitor, and TIGIT antibodies. The clinical concern of nonresponders necessitated research into the discovery of prognostic and predictive biomarkers and disease response measured to determine minimal residual disease (MRD). Combination strategies also came under development [1].

6.2 The Mechanism of Action of Anti-PD-L1 Antibodies and Anti-CTLA-4 Antibodies: First-Generation Immune Checkpoint Blockade (ICB) Targeting

CTLA-4, a molecule on Tregulatory cells, has the molecular mechanism of binding to CD80 and CD86 while competing with CD28 in this function. The binding of CD80/86 to CD28 leads to immune stimulation, whereas the binding of CTLA-4 to

P. Hays, *Personalized Medicine in Oncology*,
https://doi.org/10.1007/978-3-032-14437-9_6

CD28 leads to inhibition, the downregulation of the immune response, and thus self-tolerance. The inhibition of T-cell activation results in a decreased ability to recognize tumor cells and antigen-presenting cells. This is adaptive in a normal immune response given that the CTLA-4 pathway prevents an overactive T-cell response and halts this when no longer necessary during an immune-mediated response. However, during a malignancy, it poses a threat because activated T cells can no longer assist in recognizing cancer antigens, and in a tumor microenvironment (TME), immunosuppressive regulatory T cells, as opposed to cytotoxic T cells, are activated. Immune recognition results from the administration of an anti-CTLA-4 ICI. On a more detailed level, the balance between its trafficking to the cell membrane and subsequent internalization leads to T-cell activation through the T-cell receptor-interacting molecule (TRIM). T-cell dysfunction results from TRIM binding to CTLA-4 and transport to the cell membrane, activating both PI3 kinase and protein kinase B and thereby PKB/AKT signaling pathways. Antigen-presenting cells (APCs) are also downregulated by CTLA-4 through CD80/CD86 molecules on their surface and CTLA-4 expression on Treg cells [2].

PD-1, on the other hand, is expressed on NK cells, activated T cells, B cells, macrophages, and dendritic cells in comparison to CTLA-4, which has high tumor-specific T-cell expression. Ruli et al. describe in an elegant account how PD-1 interacts with its ligand PD-L1, both found expressed on tumor cells to avoid immune-mediated antitumor response. PD-L1 binds to PD-1, and downstream, apoptosis is reduced in regulatory T cells while being induced in T cells with specific antigens, which maintains immune regulation and reduces proinflammatory immune responsiveness. However, the T-cell dysfunction that results leads to neutralization, the dampening of the immune response, cancer growth progression, and the spread of cancer by inhibiting "what would be a protective, proper antitumor immune response." Anti-PD-1 antibodies inhibit this evasive immune mechanism and allow for the T cells to be active or in an active state and exert "an inherent anti-tumor/anti-cancer response." Anti-PD-L1 antibodies exert their effect through similar pathways, but the target of the antibody is the PD-L1 ligand. PD-L1 is expressed in gastric cancer, renal cell carcinoma (RCC), ovarian cancer, and hepatocellular carcinoma (HCC). Its overexpression on tumor cells prevents host immune response and leads to neutralization and immune inactivation, which can be stymied by anti-PD-1/anti-PD-L1 ICIs.

Sun et al. describe PD-1 inhibition on a more granular level through the expression of its two ligands, PD-L1 and PD-L2, on nonhematopoietic cells and macrophages, respectively. PD-1 binds to its ligands, leading to the SHP-2 recruiting of (Immunoreceptor Tyrosine-based Inhibitory Motifs (ITIMs) and Immunoreceptor Tyrosine-based Switch Motifs (ITSMs), the dephosphorylation of TCR signaling, and T-cell inhibition. Inhibitors targeting PD-1 and its ligand PD-L1 were clinically effective in that PD-1 is inducibly expressed on immune cells via TCR signaling and type IFN signaling. In both CD4+ and CD8+ T cells, the H3K4me3 binds to the Pdcd1 gene promoter through a loss of the DNA methylation of Pdcd1, whereas CD8+ T-cell in the promoter region of the Pdcd1 gene activation upregulates PD-1 after chronic viral infection. PD-1 transcription is activated through the binding of the STAT and NFAT2 regulatory regions in the promoter region of the Pdcd1 gene.

In turn, IL-6 and IL-12 proinflammatory cytokines increase PD-1 expression through the STAT3/STAT4 pathway. TLR/NF-kappaB signaling in macrophages also induces PD-1 expression. PD-L1 regulation and expression are more complicated and may occur at both genomic and epigenetic levels given that histone methylation and acetylation are involved. In melanoma, HDAC6 was identified to activate STAT3 and leads to PD-L1 upregulation. In pancreatic cancer and melanoma, H3K4me3 can also catalyze PD-L1 transcription. In terms of regulation at the RNA level, EGFR signaling, MAPK signaling, the PTEN/P13K/AKT signaling pathway, and HIF-1alpha pathways are key aberrant oncogenic pathways implicated in drug resistance. The mechanism of action of anti-PD-1/PD-L1 is similarly described as binding on tumor cells and antigen presenting cell (APC) membrane surfaces, and the T cell is activated, expands, and releases perforin and granzyme, leading to enhanced tumor killing, with the attenuation of Tregulatory cells [2].

Liu describe the PD-1/PD-L1 structure, function, regulation, and signaling as follows: PD-1, being a suppressive receptor, is found on T cells, B cells, and NK cells and is a member of the immunoglobulin superfamily (Fig. 6.1). PD-1 features

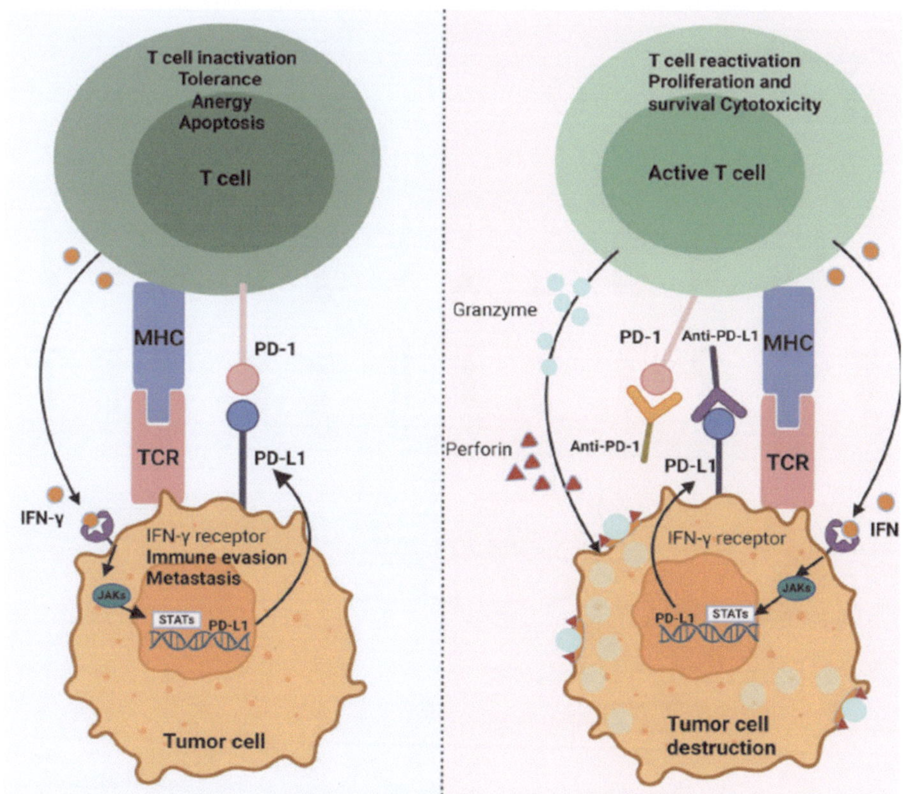

Fig. 6.1 A model of PD-L1 and PD-1 interactions. (Adapted from Liu et al. [3]. Permission to reuse under Creative Commons CC BY 4.0)

an intracellular region, an extracellular immunoglobulin variable (IgV) domain, and a transmembrane segment, of which the intracellular part includes an ITIM and an ITSM, which are needed for PD-1 signaling. PD-L1 has a cytoplasmic tail, an extracellular domain with IgV-like and immunoglobulin C (IgC)–like structures, and a transmembrane component. It is expressed on APCs and tumor cells. The pathway ensures "immune system equilibrium" by dampening T-cell activation and effector functions while PD-1 and PD-L1 interactions trigger SHP-2 signaling pathways that inhibit TCS and CD28 costimulatory signals. T-cell apoptosis, cytotoxic activity, cytokine production, and suppressed T-cell proliferation prevent autoimmune disease but in the case of cancer, tumor cells exploit it in the TME to escape immune detection. Transcription factors NF-kappaB, AP-1, and IRF enhance PD-1 gene transcription. IFN-gamma and TGF-beta also enhance PD-L1 by activating IRF-1. HIF-1alpha leads to increased PD-L1 gene expression under hypoxic conditions. Cytokines such as IFN-gamma, TNF-alpha and IL-1- also markedly boost PD-L1 expression levels that are secreted by tumor cells that are infiltrating immune cells, such as dendritic and T cells. PD-L1 and PD-1 model interaction is displayed in Fig. 6.2. The PD-1/PD-L1 pathway enhances the Treg suppressive function that

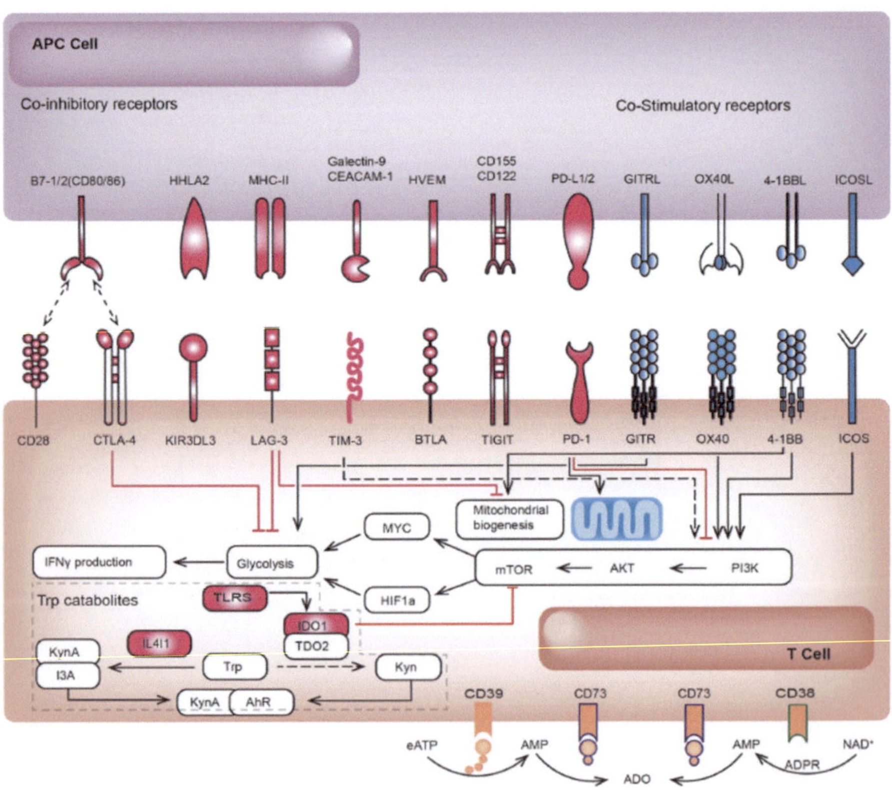

Fig. 6.2 Checkpoints and their interaction with their respective ligands. (Adapted from Sun et al. [2]. Permission to reuse under Creative Commons CC BY 4.0)

prevents autoimmune disease by suppressing effector T cells and secreting inhibitory cytokines [3].

6.3 Emerging Targets

Although immune checkpoint inhibitors have robust outcomes, as alluded to above, they meet with intrinsic and acquired resistance, which limit long-term responses and lead to disease progression. Neoantigen depletion can lead to immune resistance, faulty antigen presentation, and PD-L1 down regulation; extrinsic resistance is the result of the upregulation of inhibitory checkpoints related to T-cell exhaustion, a state of T-cell persistence featuring constant antigen exposure stimulation, leading to effector function loss and T-cell cytotoxicity (Fig. 6.2). To overcome resistance, a new generation of inhibitors was developed. According to Sun et al., "a comprehensive understanding of these new ICB targets" is needed, and the key signaling pathways and mechanisms forming the ICB treatment principles, side effects, resistance, and reactivity need to be revealed. Substantial variation in treatment exists among different tumors, which underlies the differences in patients' responses to treatment. Efficacy and feasibility are the goals because CTLA-4 and PD-1 inhibitors are not "sufficient to control tumor progression," and the elucidation of "diversified intervention pathways" is necessary [4].

LAG-3 or lymphocyte activation gene-3 is a coinhibitory receptor that is expressed on the surface of CD4 T cells, Treg cells and NK cells and consists of four Ig-like domains housed within a type I transmembrane protein. It negatively regulates T-cell proliferation and activation; ligands include MHCII and Gal-3. LAG-3's mechanism of action is to bind to a stable MHC II complex and the suppress antigen responsiveness of T cells. The ligand FGL-1–LAG-3 interaction achieved antitumor activity with CD8 and CD4 T cell dependence. Relatlinib is being evaluated by the US Food and Drug Administration (FDA) for treatment for melanoma in combination with nivolumab. In a phase II trial for microsatellite stability (MSS) CRC, favezelimab is another LAG-3 targeting antibody that is being evaluated that shows an objective response rate (ORR) of 6%. Leramilinab was combined with anti-PD-1 spartalizumab, which showed modest antitumor activity in patients with an ORR < 10% in RCC and 0% in NSCLC and triple-negative breast cancer (TNBC) [4].

TIM-3 is expressed on Treg, T helper, and CD8 T cells and is a cell surface receptor composed of a glycoprotein. It consists of a mucin stalk linked to a transmembrane-bound domain between an extracellular N-terminal V domain and an intracytoplasmic domain. Ligands include phosphatidylserine, Gal-9, the high-mobility group protein B1, and CEACAM. The binding of TIM-3 leads to the phosphorylation of Tyr256 and Tyr263, which competitively binds to both BAT3 and FYN, leading to T-cell inactivation via "an interaction with the phosphoprotein associated with the glycolipid enriched membranes and CSK tyrosine kinase," which leads to decreased T-cell signaling, inhibition, and genome/cell death.

Exhausted and regulatory T cells in tumors frequently express TIM-3. Preclinical models with anti-PD-1 and anti-TIM3 antibodies show evidence of tumor control. Sabatolimab is an anti-TIM3 antibody that has shown good safety profiles with grade 3–4 AEs only in 9% of patents, with disappointing ORR results (0%) and only five patients out of 133 showing partial response (PR).

The T-cell immunoglobulin and ITIM (TIGIT) domain is composed of an extracellular variable domain, an intracellular tail, and a transmembrane stalk and is a member of the immunoglobulin superfamily. With its ITIM domain and intention-to-treat (ITT)–like motif, it is implicated in regulatory signal transduction. In CD8 and CD4 T cell expression, its ligands include PVR, CD112, and CD113. PVR binding leads to p-ERK-mediated signaling in CD8+ T cells and decreased TCR expression, resulting in reduced T-cell activation and proliferation. Competitive binding between CD226, a costimulatory receptor, and PVR leads to decreased T-cell activation because PVR has a higher affinity. TIGIT has been observed to be expressed in NSCLC, melanoma, and colorectal cancers. In the phase II CITYSCAPE trial, the anti-TIGIT antibody tiragolumab when combined with atezolizumab demonstrated significant improvement in ORR (37% vs. 21%) and PFS (5.6 months vs. 3.9 months) compared to atezolizumab alone when evaluated in NSCLC alone. Comparable rates of AEs were observed. TIGIT expression also showed a predictive effect in a study of 105 patients, of whom 49 were defined as TIGIT high ($\geq$ 5% on immunohistochemistry (IHC)). TIGIT expression did not significantly affect PFS (HR 0.62, 95% CI 0.30–1.32). The SKYSCRAPER-01 trial was a follow-up to CITYSCAPE and investigated the regimen in first-line treatment in metastatic NSCLC with PD-L1 greater than 50%. No improvement was seen in progression-free survival (PFS) or overall survival (OS) from the combination; an ongoing SKYSCRAPER-06 phase III trial is being conducted. Other anti-TIGIT antibodies in the clinical stage include domvamalimab and ociperliamb. The former showed superior ORR and PFS versus the anti-PD1 agent zimberelimab in NSCLC. Other immune checkpoints include the glucocorticoid-induced TNF receptor family–related protein and the B7 H3 protein.

GITR is a costimulatory receptor that has constitutive expression on Tregs and high levels on T memory cells. Furthermore, the expression of 4-1BB and OX40, a member of the TNFR gene superfamily, increases T-cell activation. GITRL is a ligand of GITR that activates the NF-KB, resulting in a reduction in T-cell apoptosis and the expansion of T cells. B7 homolog 3 protein, or CD276, is a cell surface protein like most immune checkpoints and is expressed on NSCLC, prostate cancer, breast cancer, and CRC, with rare expression on normal tissues. In preclinical models, combining anti-B7-H3 and anti-PD1 was synergistic and led to increased antitumor immune response but was also associated with metastasis and tumor invasion, hallmarks of cancer [4].

The V-domain immunoglobulin suppressor of T-cell activation (VISTA) is also known as B7-H5, c10orf54, DD1α, Dies1, Gi24, PD-1H, SISP1, and VSIR and has the highest expression on myeloid cells, particularly neutrophils and microglia, but also CD4+ and Foxp3+ regulatory T cells in the lymphocyte compartment. Consisting of a stalk of 30 amino acids, it is a type I transmembrane protein with a single N-terminal (Ig) V domain and a transmembrane protein held by a 95-amino-acid cytoplasmic tail, of which the IgV domain possesses disulfide bonds. In terms of its structural comparison with other immune checkpoints, VISTA resembles CTLA-4 and CD28, but does not have the TIGIT motif, differentiating it from other B7 coreceptor molecules. It is able to bind to other STAT proteins through its conserved SRC homology 2 regions in the cytoplasmic tail that contains a proline-rich motif and protein kinase C binding sites. With its unique structure, VISTA is able to act as both a receptor and a ligand in its immune response. VISTA can act in melanoma models as an inhibitory checkpoint that has increased proportions of VISTA+ lymphocytes following anti-PD-1 treatment with or without ipilimumab. In the B16-BL6 melanoma model, investigators verified the function of VISTA as an inhibitory checkpoint by using VISTA inhibitors and additional evidence that melanoma survival is correlated with PD-L1/VISTA expression. Pancreatic tumors exhibit greater engagement from the VISTA inhibitory pathway, resulting in decreased CD8+ T-cell proliferation than the PD-L1 pathway and the inhibition of cytokine production by tumor infiltrating lymphocytes (TILs) with a significantly higher density of VISTA on CD68+ macrophages, providing evidence that both pathways are separate and independent in suppressing antitumor T-cell response in pancreatic cancer (PCa). In prostate cancer, VISTA has been identified as a target whereby combination therapies, including VISTA inhibitors, are showing efficacy and tolerability in early-phase trials. When prostate cancer was treated with ipilimumab, levels of VISTA inhibitory molecules increased on macrophages, particularly CD68+ macrophages, after treatment, which was recapitulated with PD-L1 treatment, possibly indicating that combination ICI treatment including VISTA functioning as an immunosuppressive checkpoint was promising. In RCC, VISTA was found expressed on CD45+ cells in tumor cells, especially hematopoietic tissues within the myeloid compartment, with VISTA identified as suppressing CD8+ T-cell response and tumor immunity. MDSCs in peripheral blood (PB) were highly expressed with VISTA, which was associated with PD-1 in AML patients. VISTA was also found to be an inhibitory checkpoint expressed on microsattelite instability (MSIh) CRCs at a higher level than that of MSS tumors. A similar observation was shown in high-grade serous ovarian cancer, where VISTA expression on ovarian tumor cells had good prognosis. VISTA also serves (unusually so) as a costimulatory checkpoint where, in certain solid tumors, positive staining VISTA in tumor cells but not immune cells showed prolonged OS that correlated with CD8 positive staining. An analysis of The Cancer Genome Atlas (TCGA) led to the elucidation of the expression profile of VISTA, demonstrating both its positive and negative roles and its clinical relevance. The results were that VISTA had higher expression in cholangiocarcinoma, glioblastoma (GBM), RCC, acute myeloid leukemia (AML), and pancreatic ductal adenocarcinoma (PDAC) compared to healthy tissue. Huang et al. conclude in their report that VISTA acts as an immune checkpoint in several tumor types, and according to the updated evidence from the literature, potential clinical performance, and in silico analysis, VISTA has a possible role as an immune checkpoint molecule [5].

The Noelle group has an account of the VISTA target as well, stating that VISTA expression is a poor prognostic indicator and that targeting it engages both innate and adaptive immunity. They also reiterate that the human VISTA protein has extracellular and cytoplasmic domains with a transmembrane protein, with no tyrosine-based signaling motifs but with protein kinase C sites. The VISTA ECD contains 10 beta strands, whereas the classical B7 family fold contain nine beta stands and a single IgV domain in lieu of the canonical IgV and IgC domains. VISTA has been shown to be both a receptor and a ligand, a characteristic of the B7 family, including CD80, PD-L1, and PD-L2. CD28, PD-1, CTLA-4, and ICOS function as receptors with their single IgV domains. An analysis of TCGA showed association with high VISTA expression and poor OS and was also associated with progression and increase in advanced disease in ovarian cancer. In melanoma patients after progression on anti-PD-1 treatment, VISTA-positive immune cells are increased, implicating VISTA expression in acquired resistance to anti-PD-1 therapy. VISTA expression is also upregulated after ipilimumab in prostate cancer and correlates with PD-1/PD-L1 expression in NSCLC and colon cancer. These data suggest that VISTA target could form a valuable immunotherapeutic strategy. As the authors state "[o]ur group and others have shown that VISTA deficiency or blockade can dramatically modulate the TME towards a more proinflammatory myeloid phenotype that favors the infiltration of tumor-reactive T cells." As they conclude, the blockade of VISTA enhances the activation of tumor-associated dendritic cells, leading to the release of inflammatory cytokines and the upregulation of APCs of these cells and other costimulatory molecules. Because anti-VISTA treatment is nonredundant with the PD-1/PD-L1 pathway, targeting VISTA to augment T-cell responses and remove restraints on exhaustion and priming are the most critical changes of anti-VISTA treatment [6, 7].

VISTA may correlate with disease progression and is indicative of poor survival in certain settings, particularly in melanoma, ovarian cancer, and other tumor types. The hypothetical model emerging is that VISTA promotes the migration of inhibitory myeloid cells that are part of exerting their immunosuppressive effects on the TME. In the CT26 model of CRC, the treatment of small tumors via single-agent anti-VISTA resulted in slowed tumor growth. Anti-VISTA therapy activated T-cell pathways, as revealed through the sequencing of tumor-specific CD8+ T cells, and these pathways are complementary and highly distinct from those activated via anti-PD-1 therapy, with VISTA-targeting therapy leading to a reduction in the regulators of T-cell quiescence [6] (Fig. 6.3).

An anti-VISTA antibody was constructed by a group led by Iadanato et al., and in vivo and in vitro models had antitumor efficacy. The monoclonal antibody KVA12123 served as a clinical candidate that was developed to show high affinity binding to VISTA with high specificity through a distinct epitope from other antibodies, which had no cross-reactivity against other B7 family members. Activity was shown as monotherapy at 100 mg/kg and in combination treatment with anti-PD-1 antibodies. As the authors reiterate, VISTA is expressed mainly on myeloid cells, Treg cells, and NK cells and plays a role in immune tolerance but leads to ineffective clinical response in response to tumors in the immunosuppressive TME, being a key driver in cold tumors where VISTA is highly expressed; T-cell infiltration is poor, and OS is poor. KVA12123 is a humanized IgG1-kappa mAB with a high half-life and reduced fragment crystallizable (Fc)-mediated immune effector

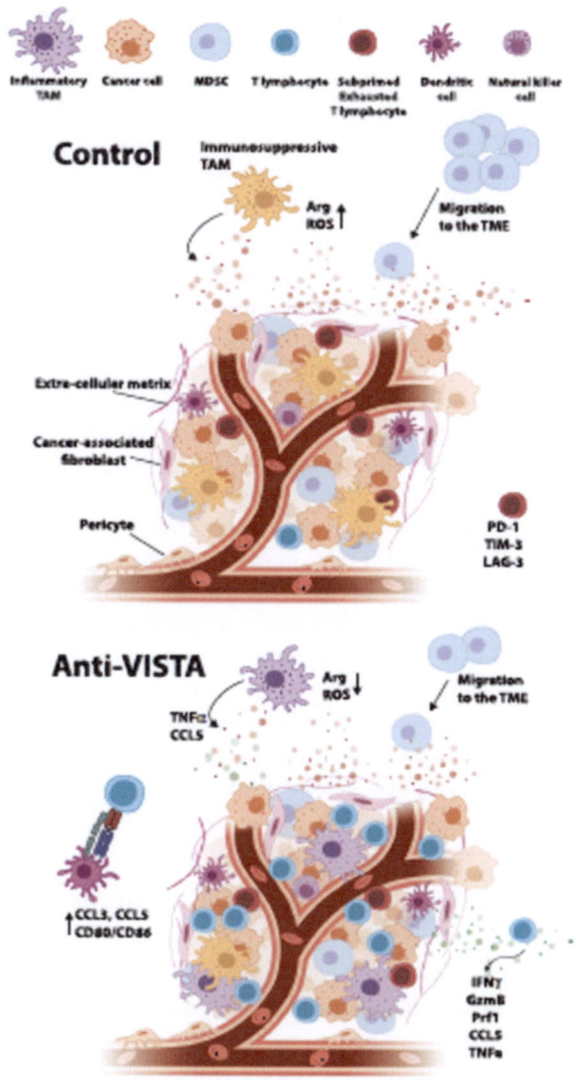

Fig. 6.3 VISTA blockade in the TME. (Adapted from ElTanblouy [7]. Permission to reuse under Creative Commons CC BY 4.0)

function that binds human VISTA at neutral and acidic pHs, and it blocks interaction with four known VISTA binding partners, namely LRIG1, VSIG3, VSIG8, and PSGL-1. "VSIG3, VSIG8, and LRIG1 bind to VISTA at neutral pH, while PSGL-1 binds only at acidic pH," with R54, F62, and Q63 being the relevant amino acids. Immune functions initiated on the binding of VISTA included increased IFN-gamma, TNFalpha secretion, and NK cell and monocyte activation. Statistically significant in CD4+ T-cell tumor infiltration was also observed and consistent with the induction of a long-lasting and strong antitumor response and the T effector memory phenotype (CD44+, CD62L-) results. VISTA blocking was also shown to reduce MDSCs, enrich M1 macrophages, and decrease immunosuppressive cells. As the investigators conclude, VISTA expression on innate cells, such as myeloid cells, interacts with the immune system toward homeostasis through mechanisms distinct from CTLA-4, PD-1, and LAG-3 (37). They show that VISTA strongly inhibits T-cell activation and the production of cytokines. They showed that the monoclonal antibody KVA12123 decreases myeloid-mediated immunosuppression and leads to NK cell activation and memory T-cell infiltration in the TME, "associated with a strong single-agent anti-tumor activity of KVA12123 in multiple tumor models, which is amplified in combination with an anti-PD-1 mAb" [8].

Other anti-VISTA antibodies include CI-8993, with a binding site at the C-C′ loop of VISTA blocking interaction with PSGL-1 and VSIG-3, construed with an active IgG1 FC domain that can interact with Fc gamma receptors and myeloid cells to support antibody-dependent cellular cytotoxicity (ADCC). In a phase I dose-escalation study, safety profiles were manageable with no dose-limiting (DL) side effects. A similar anti-VISTA antibody, HMBD-002, which is designed with an IgG4 Fc while not activating ADCC, is also being evaluated. It has been shown to led to a proinflammatory cytokine response and tumor growth inhibition in solid tumors and increased APCs and reduced MDSCs in the TME. The agent was combined with a pembrolizumab colon cancer model to determine synergy. As the authors conclude, with the emergence of adaptive resistance to common ICIs, anti-VISTA treatment becomes useful and will be explored in clinical studies. While VISTA-targeting antibodies are being clinically implemented, promising outcomes are becoming possible, but more assessment and development are required to gain a proper understanding of the how different Fc isotypes of antibodies have clinical consequences and TRAEs like cytokine release syndrome (CRS), beyond its role in tumor immunity regulation [6].

6.4 Clinical Studies and Solid Tumors

Immune checkpoint blockade inhibitors have made significant gains in the treatment of advanced and metastatic breast cancer. The KEYNOTE, CheckMate, and IMpower trials were pivotal in establishing pembrolizumab, nivolumab, and atezolizumab for early-stage, advanced, and metastatic breast cancer, with recent investigations into triple-negative breast cancer. One study found that according to clinicaltrials.gov, 745 immunotherapy trials were being conducted as of January 2022, both in adjuvant settings and in neoadjuvant settings, with new combination strategies being developed [9].

One study reported that mRNA binding proteins and their "functions and mechanisms" could play key roles in managing PD-1 checkpoint blockade for TNBC. RBMS1 binding protein was found to be prevalent in immune desert-rich regions in TBNC. An shRNA-mediated screen-depleted RBMS1 was increased in breast cancer, and when the mRNA binding protein was eliminated through the screen, the study investigators found that the level of PD-1 was correlated and cytotoxic T cells were stimulated. The study authors found that mechanistically,

"RBMS1 regulated the mRNA stability of B4GALT1, a newly identified glycosyltransferase of PD-L1" [10].

In the August 1, 2024, issue of *JCO*, the American Society of Clinical Oncology (ASCO) recommended the putative use of immunotherapy plus chemotherapy in the neoadjuvant setting for ER+/HER2- breast cancer, pointing to two large phase III clinical trials that investigated the addition of ICI to neoadjuvant chemotherapy, namely CheckMate-7FL and KEYNOTE-756; histologic grade and MammaPrint high-risk status served as inclusion criteria. In the PD-L1-positive subpopulations, the improved pathologic complete response (pCR) rate was most impressive; however, the positivity rates were reported as being dramatically different between both trials, as a result of different scoring methods and assay sensitivities.

CheckMate-7FL: 35% PD-L1 positive
Nivolumab: pCR increased from 20.2% to 44.3% (odds ratio (OR) 3.11)
KEYNOTE-756: 76% PD-L1 positive

For pembrolizumab plus T-AC versus placebo plus T-AC, pCR improved by 24.3% in the pembrolizumab arm and 15.6% in the control arm. The recommendations concluded that uncertainties and challenges remain, however, including "a lack of patient-level analysis" and "unequal sample sizes." The future of neoadjuvant immunotherapy depends on the "unanswered question [whether] improvements in the pCR rate will translate into improvements in RFS and EFS" [11].

The phase II DUO-E trial evaluated durvalumab plus carboplatin/paclitaxel followed by maintenance durvalumab with or without olaparib as first-line treatment for advanced endometrial cancer. Chemotherapy combined with immunotherapy has shown efficacy in endometrial cancer (EC), with greater benefit in MMR deficiency (MMR-D) than MMR proficiency (MRR-P), adding a PARPi that confers increased benefit. In this global phase III, double-blind, and placebo-controlled trial, patients were randomly assigned in 1:1:1 ratios to achieved the associated PFS:

- Carboplatin/paclitaxel plus durvalumab placebo followed by placebo maintenance (control)
- Carboplatin/paclitaxel plus durvalumab followed by maintenance durvalumab plus olaparib placebo (durvalumab arm); HR, 0.71 (95% CI 0.57 to 0.89); $p =$ 0.003 vs. control
- Carboplatin/paclitaxel plus durvalumab followed by maintenance durvalumab plus olaparib (durvalumab + olaparib arm); HR, 0.55 (95% CI 0.43 to 0.69)

The study investigators concluded that statistically significant and clinically meaningful PFS benefit in recurrent patients was demonstrated in the treatment of carboplatin/paclitaxel plus durvalumab followed by maintenance durvalumab [12].

Durvalumab plus carboplatin/paclitaxel followed by maintenance durvalumab with or without olaparib showed greater benefit in MMR-deficient than MMR-proficient advanced endometrial cancer. The addition of the PARPi olaparib was shown to possibly improve outcomes in this patient population. In a global phase III, double-blind, and placebo-controlled trial, 1718 patients with advanced or recurrent endometrial cancer were randomly assigned to receive the chemotherapy combination plus durvalumab placebo followed by placebo maintenance (control arm) or this regimen plus olaparib placebo (durvalumab arm) or followed by durvalumab plus olaparib (durvalumab + olaparib arm) in a 1:1:1 ratio. The primary endpoint was PFS in durvalumab versus control and durvalumab + olaparib arm versus control. Statistically significant benefit in PFS was seen in the ITT population (HR, 0.71 (95% CI 0.57 to 0.89)) and in the durvalumab arm (HR 0.555 (0.43 to 0.69)) versus control. PFS benefit was also seen in the dMMR subgroups and the pMMR subgroups.

Subgroup	Treatment	HR
dMMR	Durvalumab vs. control	0.42 (95% CI 0.22 to 0.80)
	Durvaluamb +olaparib vs. control	0.41 (95% CI 0.21 to 0.75)
pMMR	Durvalumab vs. control	0.77 (95% CI 0.60 to 0.97)
	Durvalumab + olaparib vs. control	0.57 (95% CI 0.44 to 0.73)

Safety profiles were consistent with individual agents. The investigators concluded that durvalumab followed by maintenance durvalumab with or without olaparib provided clinically meaningful PFS benefit [12].

In the MyPathway study was a tissue-agnostic basket study on human epidermal growth factor 2 (HER2), where pertuzumab + trastumuzumab were used to treat HER2 overexpression and amplification in solid tumors. HER2 amplification/overexpression is observed in 2–3% of all solid tumors. The MyPathway multiple basket study evaluated patients with advanced solid tumors who had potentially actionable alterations. Previous data suggested that in HER2-positive colon, salivary, and biliary cancers, the chemotherapy-free combination of P + T has activity that is not indicated for HER2-targeted treatment. KRAS and PIK3A activating mutations may influence EFGR-targeted therapy, necessitating analysis in larger populations and other tumor types, such as in the MyPathway basket trial. In this trial, 346 patients were enrolled, including 263 patients with HER2 overexpression and amplification. The ORR in entire HER2 patient cohort was 42.2, including five CRs (colon, $n = 1$; urothelial, $n = 2$; and salivary gland, $n = 2$), 62 partial responses (PRs), and 79 stable diseases (SDs) > 4 months. OS and PFS were 10.1 and 2.8 months, respectively [13].

Kidney transplant recipients are associated with malignancies such as advanced cutaneous cancers, including Merkel cell carcinoma (no immunosuppression), cutaneous squamous cell carcinoma (TACRO increase and pulse steroids), and melanoma (TACRO + pulse steroids) with 9.2 to 9.4 time-from-transplant years as a result of treatment- related allograft loss and immunosuppression. A prospective clinical trial evaluating the administration of ipilimumab + nivolumab + prednisone + tacrolimus was conducted on kidney transplant patients who possessed cutaneous cancers. Immunosuppression standardized with "TACRO (serum trough 2–5 mg/mL) + PRED 5 mg once daily received NIVO 480 mg IV once every week." CR or SD values were endpoints, along with values of PD. Dd-cfDNA was temporally measured as a potential predictor of allograft rejection once every 2 weeks. The results include the following: All eight patients achieved PD, and no trial endpoint was met. Six patients then received IP + NIVO + PRED +TACRO, with two CRs and four PDs resulting. Two of five NIVO biopsies demonstrated moderate immune infiltrates. In short, TACRO + PRED was shown to provide insufficient allograft protection and compromises immune-mediated antitumor growth in most kidney transplant recepient (KTR) and advanced cancers after NIVO administration with or without ipilimumab (IPI) [14].

Pembrolizumab was tested in resected stage IIB or IIC melanoma as adjuvant therapy in the final analysis of a phase III, double-blind, randomized KEYNOTE-716 study with significant RFS (HR 0.65, 95% CI 0.46 to 0.92) and distant metastasis-free survival (DMFS) observed (HR 0.64, 95% CI 0.47 to 0.88) compared with placebo, with FDA approval resulting. With a median follow-up of 39.4 months (range, 26 to 51.4 months), estimated DMSF was 84.4% and 74.7% in pembrolizumab and placebo, respectively (HR 0.59, 95% CI 0.44 to 0.79). Median RFS was not reached in either group; 36-month PFS was 76.2% and 63.4% in the treatment arm and placebo, respectively (HR 0.62, 95% CI 0.49 to 0.79). The values for relapse free survival (RFS) and DMFS were consistent across all subgroups among stage IIB and IIC melanoma, with manageable safety profiles [15].

The ATEZOTRIBE study showed that in the intention-to-treat (ITT) metastatic colorectal cancer population, median OS in patients receiving FOLFOXIRI/bevacizumab/atezolizumab in one cohort was 33 months compared to 27.2 months in the control group (HR 0.78). An interaction effect between Immunoscore (IS) and patients receiving atezolizumab was seen, with the Immunoscore high group showing higher benefit. Interactions between treatment group, Immunoscore, IC, and tumor mutational burden (TMB) were also seen [16].

Intratumoral *E. coli* was found to be associated with improved survival and a prognostic factor for ICI in advanced NSCLC. In one study, the intratumoral microbiome was mapped in 958 patients, in which unmapped NGS was queried with a bacterial genome database. *E. coli* FISH and transcriptome profiling were performed, which analyzed the expression signatures of *E. coli*. In that study, 1462 NSCLC patients received anti-PD-1 immunotherapy, and as prior evidence had indicated, intratumoral *E. coli* was associated with the TME; the study's primary goal was to determine whether intratumoral *E. coli* was associated with improved outcomes with ICI administration. In patients with intratumoral *E. coli*, PD-1 monotherapy was associated with significantly longer OS (16 vs. 11 months, HR 0.73 (95% CI 0.59 to 0.92)) and longer PFS (3.2 vs. 2.3 months, HR 0.82 (95% CI 0.66 to 1.01)), as shown by Kaplan–Meier survival curves. Negron-Figueroa et al. proposed that immunotherapy response may be potentiated by the intratumoral microbiome. One mechanism is that in the lung, epithelium *E. coli* can invade these epithelial cells, persist for a long period, and induce helper CD4 + T cell proliferation and *E. coli*-directed IgG to combat infections, suggesting that innate and humoral immune responses to pembrolizumab act cooperatively to recognize *E. coli* response [17].

6.5 Combination Therapies

The combination of bempegaldesleukin or BEMPEG, an engineered IL-2 cytokine drug with nivolumab and sunitinib or cabozanitib, is used as first-line treatment in untreated advanced RCC and was evaluated in the phase III randomized PIVOT-09 trial. OS and ORR served as the primary endpoints. In that trial, 623 intermediate/poor-risk patients were assigned randomly to BEMPEG plus NIVO or TKI. ORR in the experimental cohort was 23% (95% CI 18 to 28.7) versus 30.6% in the TKI cohort (95% CI 25.1 to 36.6). Median OS was 29.0 months versus nonestimable (HR 0.82). Adverse events (AEs) included pyrexia (32.6% vs. 2.0%) and pruritis (31.3% vs. 8.8%) [18].

In the phase III HIMALAYA trial, the anti-CTLA-4 inhibitor tremelimumab (300 mg) plus the anti-PD-L1 inhibitor durvalumab (1500 mg) regimen (STRIDE) was evaluated against hepatocellular carcinoma versus durvalumab monotherapy (1500 mg once every 4 weeks) and sorafenib (400 mg twice daily). The time to deterioration change from baseline, quality of life, functioning, and disease-related symptoms (including physical functioning, fatigue, and appetite loss) served as the primary endpoints.

STRIDE, $n = 393$; durvalumab, $n = 389$; and sorafenib, $n = 389$

According to the results, time to deterioration (TTD) with abdominal pain and nausea was numerically longer in the STRIDE arm (versus sorafenib), with disease-related symptoms, clinically meaningful improvement in GHS/QofL, and social and emotional functioning being greater in STRIDE and durvalumab versus sorafenib, where the assessment of PROs serves as a secondary objective. The authors conclude that the STRIDE regimen demonstrated that when compared with sorafenib, clinically meaningful improvements in quality of life and functioning with lower levels of symptom burden occurred in patients with unresectable HCC (uHCC). STRIDE also significantly improved OS (HR 0.78), with a 36-month rate of 30.7% versus 20.2% with sorafenib. The "incidence, frequency and severity of adverse events were consistent with known safety profiles of each agent" [19].

In previously treated mCRC, lenvatinib plus pembrolizumab was evaluated versus the standard of care in the randomized, open-label phase III LEAP-017 study. Patients with unresectable mCRC, regardless of MMR or MSI-high status, that had progressed on standard treatment were randomly assigned 20 mg of lenvatinib and 400 mg of pembrolizumab intravenously ($n = 241$) or SOC ($n = 239$) in a 1:1 ratio. Median OS was 9.8 versus 9.3 months (HR = 0.83; 95% CI 0.68 to 1.02) at a median follow-up of 18.6 months. Grade 3 or greater adverse events occurred in 58.4% versus 42.2% of patients. Two participants died in both groups. In pMMR or non-MSI-H mCRC patients who showed disease progression, the study authors found that the L + P treatment did not demonstrate statistically significant improvement in OS, with no new safety signals [20].

Immune checkpoint inhibitors durvalumab and tremelimumab, a novel anti-CTLA-4 inhibitor, with the best and proper supportive care was shown to be clinically effective over targeted therapy and cytotoxic chemotherapy in CRC patients with liver metastasis.

Key Results

- In the tremelimumab plus durvalumab group, mPFS was 1.82 months (90% CI 1.71–1.84) in patients with liver metastasis (LM) and 2.04 months (90% CI 1.87–3.71) among patients without LM. Best supportive care (BSC) resulted in an mPFS of 1.84 (90% CI 1.77–1.87) for patients with LM and 1.87 (90% CI 1.35–1.91) months for patients without LM.

Other Key Results

- In the durvalumab plus tremelimumab group, the median disease control rate (DCR) was 49% (90% CI 36%–62%), and in the BSC group, median DCR was 14% (90% CI 0–30%); it was 10% for patients without LM (90% CI 4%–16%) and 4% (90% CI 0–9%) for patients with LM.

Another significant aspect of this study was that plasma TMB was found to be higher in the LM group versus those not in the LM group (median, 19.2 (IQR, 11.5–30.6) vs. 12.3 (IQR, 7.7–20.6)) mutations/Mb; $p = 0.003$). Loss-of-function mutations associated with advanced CRC such as KRAS, BRAFV600E, and APC were also detected. The authors also posited that LM may confer resistance to immunomodulating agents such as ICIs, noted low statistical power with a relatively small cohort (58 patients), and concluded that LM was associated with lower OS in patients with advanced CRC [21].

ICI efficacy was shown to have efficacy in microsatellite stable CRC with liver metastasis in a secondary analysis. Prior studies have evaluated the efficacy of ICIs in MSI-high CRC, and authors in these studies hypothesized that LM might confer resistance to CRC. Patients randomly received durvalumab plus tremelimumab in a 2:1 fashion. Significantly improved PFS was seen in patients without LM (HR, 0.54 (90% CI 0.35–0.96)). The DCR was significant at 49%, also seen in patients without LM. Plasma TMB "was higher in patients with LM than in those without LM (median, 19.2 [IQR, 11.5–30.6] vs 12.3 [IQR, 7.7–20.6] mutations/Mb)" but was not associated with OS or PFS. APC, a common alteration in CRC, was also detected. With LM having a high incidence in CRC, the establishment of ICI efficacy has clinical relevance associated with unfavorable outcomes and may be included in the interpretation and design of trials [21].

Key Results

Treatment group	Cohort	Median PFS	Median DCR
Durvalumab and Tremelimumab group	Patients with LM	1.82 months (90% CI 1.71–1.84)	
Durvalumab and Tremelimumab group	Patients without LM	2.04 months (90% CI 1.87–3.71)	
Best and proper supportive care	Patients with LM	1.84 months (90% CI 1.77–1.87)	
Best and proper supportive care	Patients without LM	1.87 months (90% CI 1.35–1.91)	
Durvalumab plus tremelimumab group	Patients without LM		10% (90% CI 4%–16%)
	Patients with LM		4% (90% CI 0–9%)

Note: PFS = Progression Free Survival and DCR = Disease Control Rate

In a first-in-human (FIH) phase I study, the LAG-3 mAb fianlimab in combination with cemiplimab was shown to have a promising benefit–risk profile in advanced melanoma patients, including patients who underwent prior anti-PD-1 therapy in the adjuvant setting. ORR was 63% both for anti-PD-1-naive melanoma ($n = 40$) and for previous neo/adjuvant treatment melanoma ($n = 18$), and the median PFS was 13.3 months. In patients with prior anti-PD-1 treatment, the ORR was 61.5% and the mPFS 12 months. A waterfall plot showed a 72% response of patients, and a spider plot showed that in large proportion of patients, tumor responses were durable, deep, and rapid. Grade 3 events were reported in 44% versus 22% of patients, respectively, with only incidences of adrenal insufficiency. The negative results of this TKI plus ICI strategy "highlight the need for developing better immune-based combinatorial approaches" [20].

The adjuvant nivolumab and ipilimumab combination demonstrated less-than-optimal clinical results, not improving RFS (HR 0.92) and significantly resulting in grade 3 and 4 adverse events (43% vs. 23% for single agent), strongly suggesting that the intensification of therapy did not improve recurrence outcomes. A study on the neoadjuvant therapy of relatlimib and nivolumab demonstrated activity and feasibility in resectable melanoma and improved PFS in patients receiving two doses of 480 mg of nivolumab and 160 mg of relatlimib IV every 4 weeks, followed by ten doses of adjuvant combination therapy, with a 57% pCR and 70% pCR among 30 patients, which adds to the results of the RELATIVITY-047 trial [22].

Pembrolizumab in combination with a chemotherapy (carboplatin and paclitaxel) regimen was found in head and neck squamous cell carcinoma (HNSCC) to display antitumor activity with a tolerable safety profile in the KEYNOTE-B10 single-arm phase IV trial regardless of PD-L1 status as first-line treatment. This treatment was seen as a promising avenue because the standard of care, or fluorouracil, has a number of challenges associated with it, including continuous infusion, high costs, and the potential for adverse events, including cardiovascular and gastrointestinal toxicities. ORR according to response evaluation criteria in solid tumors (RECIST) was the primary endpoint. Also, 49 patients, or 49% of them, had an objective response, including seven complete responders. TRAES occurred in 76 patients, or 75% of them [23].

The United States had 465,000 cases of genitourinary cancer in 2023. Immunotherapy has now become the standard of care; however, considerable relapse and a lack of response occur. In a dose-escalation phase I study conducted by Apolo et al., cabozantinib and nivolumab (CaboNivo) was evaluated alone or with ipilimumab (CaboNivoIpi) and showed promising safety and efficacy in mUC, metastatic renal cell carcinoma (mRCC), and rare genitourinary tumors. ORR, PFS, and OS in seven expansion cohorts served as the primary endpoints. CaboNivo doublet therapies ($n = 64$) were administered to mUC, mRCC, and bladder adenocarcinoma patients, and CaboNivoIpi triplets ($n = 56$) were administered to mUC, mRCC, and squamous carcinoma patients.

Within 108 evaluable patients,

- mDOR: 20 months
- ORR: 38%; CR: 11%
- mUC: 42.4%; mRCC: 62.5%
- Bladder SCC: 85.7%; renal medullary carcinoma: 50%
- CaboNivo grade 3 TRAEs: 84%
- CaboNivoIpi grade 3 TRAEs: 80% [24]

The Targeted Agent and Profiling Utilization Registry (TAPUR) is a phase II basket trial that evaluates the clinical activity of cancer agents targeting genomic mutations and alterations. In a study reported in *JCO*, Cannon et al. evaluated pertuzamab and trastuzumab in advanced biliary tract cancer patients with ERBB2/3 amplification or overexpression. Patients received pertuzumab once every 3 weeks in IV infusion (840 mg followed by additional doses of 400 mg). Disease control served as the primary endpoint as an OR or SD of at least 16 weeks, as determined through response evaluation criteria in solid tumors (RECIST). The secondary endpoints were OR, PFS, and DOR, as determined through a radiographic assessment of target lesions until disease progression. The results included a CR = 1 and PR = 8 among 28 evaluable patients DC rate = 40%; 90% CI 27–100). Kaplan–Meier curves showed a median PFS of 11 weeks (95% CI 8 to 16) and a median OS of 30 weeks (95% CI 17 to 49). Additionally, 14% TRAEs were reported, including anemia, diarrhea, and fatigue. The authors concluded that pertuzumab and trastuzumab met prespecified criteria in biliary tract cancer (BTC) patients with ERBB2/3 mutation, amplification, or overexpression. Tumor-agnostic approvals also exist for this patient population, including dabrafenib and trametinib for BRAF V600E mutant tumors (3–4%), larotrectinb and entrecitinib for NTRK fusions (< 1%), selpercatinib (< 1%) for RET fusions, and pembrolizumab and dostarlimab for MSI-H tumors and high TMB [25].

A pivotal study was performed by Xia et al., as reported in the *JCO*, on the combination of short-course radiotherapy plus capecitabine and oxaliplatin along with toripalimab (single-agent PD-1 blockade) in pMMR/MSS locally advanced rectal cancer. CR and pCR served as the primary endpoints in a multicenter, randomized, open-label prospective, phase II TORCH trial. At a median follow-up of 19 months, pCR was 56.5% in group A that received short-course radiotherapy (SCRT) followed by consolidation immunochemotherapy and 54.2% in group B that received two cycles of immunochemotherapy followed by SCRT. Frequent grade 3 and 4 toxicities were hematologic. The results supported the added benefit of ICIs in the neoadjuvant treatment of pMMR/MSS locally advanced rectal cancer and remarkably improved outcomes in this patient population [26].

Anaplastic thyroid carcinoma harbors the BRAF mutation, for which treatment is generally well tolerated with good prognosis. Non-BRAF mutated tumors have poor prognosis, but no approved therapies are available. The authors state that "[p]rimary resistance to single-agent targeted therapy" is common in this tumor. One study reported a combination strategy of immune checkpoint inhibitor with small molecule inhibitors in three cohorts. Patients were divided into three cohorts:

Cohort 1 featured vemurafenib/cobimetinib plus atezolizumab for patients with mutated BRAF V600E tumors.
Cohort 2 featured cobimetinib plus atezolizumab for patients with mutated RAS (KRAS, HRAF, and NRAS) or NF1/2 tumors.
Cohort 3 featured bevacizumab and atezolizumab for patients without any of these variants.

Atezolizumab was administered to all patients; patients with BRAF V600E alterations in cohort 1 received vemurafenib/cobimetinib plus atezolizumab; patients in cohort 2 with RAS (NRAS, KRAS, or HRAS) or NF1/2 tumor alterations received cobimetinib plus atezolizumab. Patients in cohort 3 harboring actionable variants were assigned bevacizumab plus atezolizumab. All patients received atezolizumab. Driver mutations determined targeted therapy assignment: BRAF V600E mutations were assigned to vemurafenib/cobimetinib; RAS or NF mutations were assigned to cobimetinib; and non-BRAF/RAS-NF mutations were assigned to VEGF inhibitor.

Key Results

- For three cohorts, median OS was 19 months (95% CI 7.79–43.24).
  - Cohort 1 had a median OS and a median PFS of 43 months (95% CI 16–not estimable (NE)) and 13.9 months (6.6–64.1), respectively.
  - Cohort 2 had a median OS and a median PFS of 8.7 months (95% CI 5.1–37.0) and 4.8 months (1.8–14.7), respectively.
  - Cohort 3 had a median OS and a median PFS of 0.21 months (4.1–NE) and 1.3 months (1.3–NE), respectively.

Kaplan–Meier methods were used to assess OS and PFS, and the study found that PD-L1 inhibitors had increased OS in ATC [27].

Sun et al. conducted an evaluation on ICI rechallenge in R/M HNSCC patients. ICIs in KEYNOTE-048 were established as frontline therapy for R/M HNSCC; however, risks regarding rechallenge and the optimal duration of therapy remain unanswered. In a study on HNSCC patients, the survival was estimated for patients discontinued on ICI therapy at 1 or 2 years and after rechallenge, and the optimal duration of therapy was discussed.

Key Results

- Median (IQR) OS
  - In patients in frontline settings, it was 10.9 (4.1–29.1) months longer on ICI rechallenge (12.2 (4.8–32.0) vs. 8.7 (3.2–22.4) months).
  - In patients with Eastern Cooperative Oncology Group (ECOG) performance status of 0 or 1, it was 13.5 (5.2–33.9) vs. 5.5 (2.0–13.7) months).
  - In human papillomavirus (HPV)–positive cancer patients, it was 16.6 (6.5–43.9) vs. 8.8 (3.5–24.0) months.

- Median OS (IQR)
  - For patients who discontinued vs. continued at 1 year, it was 40.7 vs. 57.7 months (HR, 1.33 (95% CI 0.84–2.11)).
  - For the immediate ICI rechallenge group (n = 169), it was 6.4 (4.6–11.2) months after stopping the prior ICI-containing treatment.

The ICI agents administered were as follows:

- Pembrolizumab followed by pembrolizumab for 108
- Nivolumab first and then followed by nivolumab for 33
- Pembrolizumab followed by nivolumab for 12
- Pembrolizumab after nivolumab for 15

The study authors noted that the exploratory nature of the study was one of the limitations, and they concluded that ICI rechallenge can provide clinically meaningful benefit in recurrent HNSCC patients and that molecular profiling was worth considering [28].

PD-L1 expression was analyzed in NSCLC patients to determine the predictive value of ICI treatment monitored sequentially via liquid biopsy. A prospective single-blind study aimed to evaluate tumor-associated cells according to PD-L1 changes in expression in blood samples taken before (T0) or after treatment (T1) in rmNSCLC with or without IC (n = 41 both cohorts). Using the quantification method when applied to isolated tumor associated cells (TACs) for anonymized blood, high/low PD-L1 expression was measured, and (progression-free survival (PFS), overall survival (OS), and hazard ratio (HR) were evaluated at 18 and 24 months: No association was found in increased TAC PD-L1 in patients treated with ICI between T0 and TI and PFS or OS. However, significantly better PFS (HR, 3.49; 95% CI 1.5 to 8.3; $p = 0.0091$) and significantly better OS (HR, 3.058; 95% CI 1.2 to 7.9; $p = 0.0410$) were associated with increased TAC PD-L1 expression between patients who were not treated with ICI between T0 and T1. At 24 months, borderline significant OS (HR, 2.61; 95% CI 1.0 to 6.6; $p = 0.0716$) and PFS (HR, 3.49; 95% CI 1.5 to 8.3; $p = 0.0091$) were significantly improved with ICI and were associated with PD-L1 expression. At 18 months, significant OS was also shown for patients with increased PD-L1 expression (HR, 3.05; 95% CI 1.2 to 7.9). The study investigators concluded that rmNSCLC patients may benefit from ICI as determined through the blood-based monitoring of dynamic changes in PD-L1 in TACs [29].

The relationship between OS and immune related adverse events (irAEs) in mNSCLC was evaluated in one study where patients received immune checkpoint inhibitor therapies. The objective was to examined how irAEs were associated with OS severity in patients with NSCLC receiving ICIs, with toxicity leading to discontinuation or corticosteroid treatment after treatment exposure.

Key Results

- Median OS was associated with irAEs, where median OS with irAEs was 23.7 (95% CI 19.3–29.1) months.
- Median OS without irAEs was 9.8 (95% CI 8.7–11.4 months; $p < 0.001$).

- When comparing differences in OS for hospital treatment vs. outpatients, no association was seen for irAE: mOS, 20.8 (95% CI 11.7–30.6) vs. 25.6 (95% CI 20.1–29.8) months.
- Cox proportional hazards regression with known prognostic characteristics (HR, 0.53 (95% CI 0.40–0.70)) showed that OS remained associated with developing irAEs (HR, 0.53 (95% CI 0.40–0.70)).

High PD-L1 expression was also tested: 160 of 240 (66.7%) vs. 230 of 404 (56.9%) and $p = 0.05$.

Other patient characteristics

- Three or fewer (181 of 260 (69.6%) vs. 242 of 452 (53.5%)): derived neutrophil lymphocyte ratio (DNLR)
- 152 of 212 (71.7%) vs. 217 of 358 (60.6%): LDH
- 189 of 240 (78.8%) vs. 263 of 412 (63.8%): Albumin
- 215 of 296 (72.6%) vs. 322 of 503 (64.0%): no bone metastasis
- 175 of 265 (66.0%) vs. 264 of 457 (57.8%): levels within reference range for hemoglobin

A diagnosis of clinically meaningful irAEs of 37% was seen in 97 patients.

Common irAEs were dermatitis (63 [21.2%]), pneumonitis (82 [27.6%]), and colitis (42 [14.1%]), with a median time for developing an irAE of 3.4 (IQR, 1.4–8.4) months.

The authors concluded that in advanced mNSCLC patients, tumor histology, patient sex, tumor histology, and the presence of an underlying driver mutation were not associated with developing an irAE or with improved OS [30].

Choosing between anti-PD-1 monotherapy and anti-CTLA-4/anti-PD-1 combination therapy has been evaluated in advanced melanoma and found to be based on BRAF and NRAS mutational status, which determines clinical outcomes. While combination therapy is considered more toxic, one article showed that the outcomes of 2523 advanced melanoma patients were affected by BRAF and NRAS mutational status treated with nivolumab and ipilimumab, and their study remained significant in determining the effect of specific gene alterations on advanced melanoma patients. Advanced melanoma patients received either monotherapy or combination therapy, and ORR, PFS, and OS were shown to be associated with BRAF and NRAS status.

Key Results

- Median PFS BRAF-mutant melanoma was significantly higher in the ipilimumab–nivolumab cohort when compared to NRAS-mutant melanoma: 9.9 months (95% CI 6.8 to 17.2) versus 4.8 months (95% CI 3.0 to 7.5). Double wild-type mutants have an mPFS of 5.3 months (95% CI 3.6 to 7.1).
- A lower risk of PD and a lower risk of death were associated with BRAF-mutant melanoma in the ipilimumab–nivolumab cohort.
- When BRAF-mutant melanoma was compared with NRAS-mutant melanoma, mOS was significantly higher for double wild-type (WT) melanoma for both ICI treatments.

- When NRAS-mutant and double wild-type melanoma were compared with BRAF-mutant melanoma, improved OS and improved PFS were seen in patients with BRAF-mutant treated with ipilimumab–nivolumab.

The authors concluded that when choosing between mono checkpoint inhibition and dual checkpoint inhibition, BRAF mutation status may be a factor to consider, and when choosing between an ipi-nivo regimen and anti-PD-1 monotherapy, BRAF mutation status can also be taken into account [31].

High-risk resectable melanoma was found to be responsive to neoadjuvant anti-CTLA-4 and anti-PD-1 dual therapy versus monotherapy (anti-PD-1 therapy) in a study that analyzed the efficacy and safety data from multiple clinical studies (pooled analysis). The primary endpoint was the radiographic CR, and the secondary endpoints included radiographic pCR, the ratio of grade 3 or 4 toxicities, and surgical resection. Dual checkpoint inhibition (DCPI) was associated with grade 3 and 4 irAEs. Conventional dosing (51 patients) was distinguished from alternative dosing (129 patients). In 160 patients, radiologic response was reported, and in 173 patients, pathological response was reported; when compared with anti-PD-1 monotherapy, pathological response was associated with increasing odds of achieving rCR and pCR (OR, 2.55 (95% CI 1.10–5.93)) and pCR (OR, 3.87 (95% CI 2.34–6.40)). Also, 92 of 388 patients receiving neoadjuvant therapy experienced grade 3 and 4 events. As a result of the better survival among melanoma patients, this study was seen as validating neoadjuvant dual checkpoint inhibitor therapy, and it may be considered an optimal regimen [32].

Other predictors of ICB efficacy include the retinoblastoma gene, which was analyzed in small cell lung cancer (SCLC). When chemotherapy was combined with ICB, this regimen was demonstrated to be clinically effective for SCLC. Genomic alterations such as STK11 and KEAP1 are associated with ICB resistance in non-SCLC; however, in determining correlative genomic alterations, resistance to ICB in SCLC has not been investigated. A retrospective cohort study analyzed 42 SCLC patients who were treated with ICB monotherapy or ICB combination therapy and then validated in a large clinical study of 460 patients. DNA-seq and RNA-seq were performed. Treatment regimens included a "combination of ipilimumab (IPI, low dose) every 3 weeks and nivolumab (NIVO) every 3 weeks (19/42), and all but one patient received low-dose IPI with standard-dose NIVO every 2 weeks."

Key Results

- Patients harboring the RB1 WT treated with ICB had an mOS of 23.1 months (95% CI 9 to 37.5), whereas for patients harboring RB1 mutations, OS was 5 months (95% CI 2.5 to 26; $p = 0.04$).
- RB1 mutant and RB1 WT samples showed a differential gene analysis indicating the enrichment of downregulated immune-related genes and indicating among RB1 mutants an immune exclusion phenotype that did not exist in RB1 WT tumor samples.

In CheckMate 032, 460 patients were enrolled and assessed in a trial comparing NIVO or NIVO + IPI in SCLC.

- In this large cohort, RB WT patients on NIVO therapy had significantly better outcomes when compared with mutant patients. RB1 WT patients in this cohort had significantly improved outcomes (HR, 1.41; 95% CI 1.02 to 2.01).
- In the neuroendocrine subtypes (ASCL1 and NeuroD1), high RB1 LOSF signature scores had a significant association.
- Following treatment with NIVO, a longer OS was also seen in patients with lower RB1 LOF scores.

The authors concluded that ICB monotherapy administered to SCLC patients with RB1 WT status or lower RB1 LOF signature scores according to transcriptomics yielded better outcomes [33].

One study proposed that a "history of proton pump inhibitors" could predict the efficacy of ICIs and chemotherapy in a comparison of pembrolizumab monotherapy and combination therapy as first-line treatments. This study reported that clinical outcomes may be independent of PD-L1 Tumor Proportion Score (TPS) when comparing ICI and chemotherapy together and chemotherapy alone in NSCLC patients with targetable alterations. Long-term follow-up analysis showed that PD-L1 expression was associated with ICI and chemotherapy combination therapy, which would be more tolerable than cytotoxic chemotherapy. Baseline characteristics served as parameters for assessing clinical outcomes, including age, sex, smoking status, and ECOG scores.

Key Results

- In the first link settings, 425 NSCLC patients were enrolled, of whom 217 were treated with pembrolizumab monotherapy and 154 treated with ICI plus chemotherapy.
- ORR and DCR were 73.4% vs. 55.3% and 92.1% vs. 76.0%, respectively, and were significantly higher in the ICI plus chemotherapy group versus the pembrolizumab group.
- In the ICI plus chemotherapy group, HR was not statistically significant (HR, 0.77; 95% CI 0.59–1.00); the median (IQR) PFS was longer in the pembrolizumab monotherapy group than in the combination therapy group: 17.3 months (6.4 months to not reached) vs. 10.6 months (3.4 to 52.9 months).

Significantly, the authors also reported that a history of proton pump inhibitor (PPI) use was longer in the ICI and chemotherapy group than in the pembrolizumab monotherapy group.

Treatment group	Primary endpoints	Median IQROS
ICI chemotherapy group	5.7 [2.4 to 15.2] months; HR, 0.38; 95% CI 0.20–0.72	18.4 [10.5 to 50.0] months; HR, 0.43; 95% CI 0.20–0.92)
Pembrolizumab	19.3 months [9.0 months to not reached]	Reached [15.8 months to not reached]

Note: IQROS = Interquartile Range Overall Survival

The median interquartile range overall survival (IQROS) was significantly longer in the ICI plus chemotherapy group than in the pembrolizumab monotherapy group in patients with a history of PPI use. When comparing mPFS and mOS between the ICI plus chemotherapy group and the pembrolizumab monotherapy group, they were found to be similar in patients with a history of PPI use:

- 18.8 months (6.6 months to not reached) vs. 10.6 months (2.7 months to not reached); HR, 0.81; 95% CI 0.56 to 1.17
- 12.6 months vs. 29.9 (13.3 to 54.3) months; HR, 0.75; 95% CI 0.48–1.18

The study authors concluded that PPI was associated with worse clinical outcomes in NSCLC patients with PD-L1 TPS of 50% when comparing pembrolizumab with ICI and chemotherapy [34].

In the randomized phase III CONTACT-01 trial, mNSCLC patients who received ICI and chemotherapy, did not respond to immunotherapy, and experienced PD; atezolizumab + cabozantinib versus docetaxel were evaluated, where 186 patients received A + C, whereas 180 received docetaxel. Median OS was 10.7 months (95% CI 8.8 to 12.3) with A + C and 10.5 months (95% CI 8.6 to 13.0) with docetaxel. Median PFS was 4.6 months (95% CI 4.1 to 5.6) and 4.0 months (95% CI 3.1 to 4.4), respectively (stratified HR, 0.74 (95% CI 0.59 to 0.92)). Serious AEs occurred in 71 patients (38.4%) receiving A + C and 58 (34.7%) receiving docetaxel. Kaplan–Meier estimates displayed a decreasing response over time. Grade 3 or 4 events occurred in 73 (39.5%) of the A + C patients and 58 (34.7%) of the docetaxel patients. Grade 5 AEs occurred in 14 (7.6%) in the A + C arm and 10 (6%) in the docetaxel arm. The authors concluded that in this patient population with disease progression, combination regimen did not improve OS after anti-PD-L1/PD-1 immunotherapy with platinum chemotherapy even though consistent safety profiles were observed [35].

The prognostic classification of TNBC was proposed by one study identifying an immune signature that revealed that TNBC had high prognosis in an HRD and the DNA damage immune response (DDIR) signature, despite being an immune-depleted tumor microenvironment, because their combined assessment as simultaneously analyzed biomarkers would be prognostic. Both HRD and DDIR are considered clinically actionable biomarkers because DDR is associated with PD-1 upregulation and HRD stimulates interferon immune genes.

Key Results

- "HRD+ TNBCs exhibited significantly higher DDIR scores (Mann–Whitney: $p = 0.003$; odds ratio [OR], 3.26 [95% CI 1.42 to 7.49]; $p = 0.005$)."
- "The DFS HRs relative to the DDIR–/HRD– group:
  - DDIR+/HRD+ (HR, 0.36 [95% CI 0.20 to 0.63]); DDIR+/HRD– (HR, 0.46 [95% CI 0.23 to 0.89]); and DDIR–/HRD+ (HR, 0.46 [95% CI 0.25 to 0.83])."
  - Five-year OS was 87.5% (DDIR+/HRD+), 85.5% (DDIR+/HRD–), 83.1% (DDIR–/HRD+), and 69.1% (DDIR–/HRD–). There was a virtual absence of

IM signature in DDIR- tumors; PD-L1 in DDIR+ tumors showed upregulation. One of the findings is that the poor prognosis of DDIR-/HRD- is associated with tumor heterogeneity that contains a 3p21 expression profile with "exceptionally poor prognosis."

The study investigators concluded for heterogenous tumors that chemoimmunotherapy (CIT) would enhance chemoimmunosensitivity and the "tendency to use PD-L1 to suppress lymphocytes that are recruited after sustaining DNA damage from chemotherapy" and would support "classifying them as separate entities" [36].

The KEYNOTE-086 trial is an exploratory analysis of two cohorts (A and B) evaluating pembrolizumab monotherapy and their "prespecified association" with molecular biomarkers: PD-L1, CD8, stromal tumor lymphocytes, and TMB.

Key Results

- Of 254 patients enrolled in KEYNOTE-086,
  - Evaluable PD-L1 combined positive score (CPS) was observed in 253 patients (99.6%)
  - Evaluable CD8 was observed in 204 patients (80.3%)
  - Evaluable sTILs was observed in 228 patients (89.8%)
  - Evaluable TMB, HRD-LOH, and *BRCA1* and/or *BRCA2* mutation status was observed in 171 patients (67.3%)
  - Evaluable APOBEC Signature and Signature three were observed in 163 patients (64.2%)

Clinical associations include the following: CD8, sTILs, PD-L1 CPS, and TMB were associated with ORR. When the cohorts were combined, CD8 and TMB were significantly associated with PFS, whereas PFS, CD8, and stromal tumor infiltrating lymphocytes (sTILs) were significantly associated with OS.

- TMB, sTILs, and PD-L1 CPS were significantly associated with ORR when evaluated as continuous variables in the combined cohort. TMB and Signature 3 were significantly associated with PFS and CD8, whereas TMB was significantly associated with OS.

The study authors concluded that when cohorts A and B were combined, pretreatment tumor PD-L1 CPS, CD8, sTILs, and TMB as continuous variables were significantly associated with response to pembrolizumab [37].

An ultrasensitive ctDNA analysis, or target digital sequencing (TARDIS), distinguished between PR and CR in patients treated with immune checkpoint inhibitor in mRCC patients in a study conducted by Cherazi-Raffle et al.

Key Results

- In patients who received either nivo at 50% or nivo + ipi at 50%, of the 12 analyzed, nine (75%) achieved PR.
- Through ctDNA analysis, average coverage depth was 103,342 reads per target of an incorporated average of 30 patient-specific mutations (range, 19–35). PR and CR showed a significant difference in variant allele frequencies (VAFs):

median, 0.181% (IQR, 0.077%–0.420%) vs. 0.007% (IQR, 0.0%–0.028%), respectively, as was quantified via TARDIS ($p = 0.014$).
- On ctDNA assessment, 6/12 patients in the series demonstrated subsequent radiographic progression. Significantly higher ctDNA levels were identified in patients who progressed on subsequent scans versus those who maintained their response: median 0.362% (IQR, 0.181%–2.71%) vs. 0.033% (IQR, 0.007%–0.077%), respectively.

This study concluded that TARDIS led to a significant difference in VAF between CR and PR in mRCC patients receiving immunotherapy, with the capability of being an "efficacious platform" for detecting minimal residual disease (MRD) and relapse, overcoming some of the challenges in the clinical application of liquid biopsy for achieving sensitivity and precision when encountering low blood volumes. Tumor genomic profiling was also conducted, with the "most frequently altered genes [being] VHL (67%), SMARCA4 (25%), BAP1 (17%), PBRM1 (17%), SETD2 (17%), and TSC1 (17%)" [38].

A similar study showed that in phase I/II clinical studies, 162 plasma samples were collected from 81 patients treated with PD-1/PD-L1 inhibitor harboring 27 tumor types, with tumor-naive ctDNA serving as an early response biomarker.

Key Results
- In 24 patients, a decrease in mean variant allele frequency (mVAF) from baseline to precycle 2 was observed (37.5%) and was associated with longer PFS (1.8 months (95% CI 1.6 to 1.9) versus 2.7 months (95% CI 1.9 to 5.6); HR, 0.43; (95% CI 0.24 to 0.77)) and OS (10.8 months; 95% CI 9.53 to NR (HR, 0.54; 95% CI 0.3 to 0.96)) when compared with an increase.

In early-phase clinical trials, decreases in ctDNA level were shown within the early days of immuno-oncology (IO)–based therapy to be associated with responses in PFS and OS, with the implication that ctDNA kinetics is an early pharmacodynamic marker "providing proof-of-mechanism readouts of biological activity for investigational IO agents." However, ctDNA was unable to differentiate hyperPD from pseudoPD, and the retrospective study analyzed a heterogenous cohort, with further validation studies and real-time analysis required before routine clinical use [39].

Gastrointestinal (GI) cancers were subject to an analysis investigating PD-1/PD-1 inhibitor plus chemotherapy versus PD-1/PD-L1 monotherapy in advanced MSI/MMRh mutated tumors, with OS, PFS, DCR, and ORR as the primary endpoints, which was the first analysis of its kind, being a multicenter retrospective cohort study. The study was motivated by resistance to ICI monotherapy, lending itself to finding dual combination therapies that may work.

Key Results
- Of 256 evaluable patients, 68 and 188 received chemo-anti-PD-1/PD-L1 and anti-PD-1/PD-L1, respectively.

- When comparing the chemo-anti-PD-1/PD-L1 group with the anti-PD-1/PD-L1 group, significant improvements were seen in ORR (61.8% vs. 38.8%), DCR (92.6% vs. 74.5%), PFS (NR vs. 27.9 months), and OS (NR vs. NR).
- When comparing chemo-anti-PD-1/PD-L1 with anti-PD-1/PD-L1 after overlap weighting, ORR was 62.5% vs. 38.3%; DCR was 93.8% vs. 74.2%; PFS was NR vs. 26.0 months; and OS was NR vs. NR.

Sensitivity analysis corroborated these results, with gastroesophageal junction/gastrointestinal cancer (GEJ/GC) and dMMR being the most prevalent biomarker, showing that dual chemo-anti-PD-1/PD-L1 therapy is superior to monotherapy, improving efficiency and prognosis and further establishing MSI-H/MMR as a "pan-cancer biomarker for ICI therapy" [40].

Resistance and response to immune checkpoint inhibitors were also further analyzed for melanoma due to progression on anti-PD-1 therapies and BRAFV600E targeted therapies, which when compared to clinical studies offers further insights into how the mechanisms of resistance directly lead to less-than-effective clinical outcomes. One review posited that resistance to ICBs was the result of neural crest stem cells (NCSC)-like subpopulations in melanocytes and wild-type antigen loss due to intrinsic resistance factors such as interferon-γ (IFNγ) signaling driven by melanoma dedifferentiation to an NCSC-like (NGFRhi) cell state. T-cell exclusion becomes predominant in the tumor microenvironment. Lineage plasticity is also implicated. A review in *JCO* implicated tumor-intrinsic pathways such as aberrations in signaling pathways as a result of mutations in JAK1 and PTEN that regulate the IFN-gamma response. The increased infiltration of immunosuppressive cells such as MDSCs, TAFs, M2 macrophages, and regulatory T cells is also thought to drive ICB resistance in the TME. In this context, ICI rechallenge showed both in the first-line setting (50% SD, 33.3% objective response) and second-line setting (35.7% SD, 42.9% partial response), with nivolumab rechallenge being less effective [41, 42].

A biomarker study was also conducted on pancreatic ductal adenocarcinoma cancers, a tumor seen as nonimmunogenic; however, some tumors were surmised to potentially harbor MMRd/MSI-H or TMB biomarkers that may be predictive of response to ICI therapy (a combination of tremelimumab and durvalumab, and durvalumab monotherapy in one phase II trial and ipilimumab in another phase II trial); the study analyzed outcomes of identified pathogenic alterations and high-TMB patients who underwent comprehensive genomic profiling in a harsh tumor microenvironment possibly due to the tumor's dense stroma and high percentage of immunosuppressive cellular components. OS served as the primary endpoint, and time-to-treatment discontinuation was the secondary endpoint.

Key Results

- Of 21,932 PDAC patients, 21,639 (98.7%) had available comprehensive genomic profiling (CGP) data, including 293 (1.3%) with high TMB and 293 with low TMB (1.3%).
- Among high-TMB patients, a greater number of alterations were identified in BRAF, BRCA2, PALB2, and MMRP genes, whereas fewer alterations were identified in KRAS, with longer survival being observed in high-TMB patients

(25.7 vs. 5.2 months; HR 0.32; 95% CI 0.11 to 0.91), supporting the role of high-TMB as a biomarker predicting the efficacy of ICI.
- Targetable fusions such as ROS1, ALK, NTRK1/2/3, NRG1, RET, and FGFR2 were not associated with high TMB (1.4% vs. 0.7%) and were overall rare (0.7%).
- Finally, 60%, or 6/10, of high-TMB patients when receiving an ICI had longer mOS compared with patients receiving "first-line line preferred chemotherapy (gemcitabine + paclitaxel or FOLFIRINOX) or ≥ 2 line chemotherapy," showing that in a tumor type with 1% high TMB, longer OS is predictive of efficacy when compared to chemotherapy regimens and low-TMB tumors [43].

A systematic review was performed on stage I-III CRC patients with dMMR receiving neoadjuvant immunotherapy (NIT), with CR and pCR serving as the primary endpoints. Systematic review criteria included the following:

- First, "37 publications that included 423 patients with colon ($n = 326$, 77%) and rectal ($n = 97$,23%) cancers aged 19–82 years; most patients had stage III CRC (88%)."
- Second, 67% were administered monotherapy with anti-PD-1 agents, with the remainder receiving ipi-nivo. The CR rate (pCR + cCR) in the overall population was 72% (305 of 423), with only four patients (0.9%) having primary resistance to neoadjuvant immunotherapy, demonstrating that NIT is associated with high response rate and low resistance. The authors also found that NIT did not delay surgery, with an extremely low rate of "delayed surgery," with no cancer recurrence after surgery. Also, 15 studies reported irAEs, with grade 3 being the most common and with disease progression during the administration of treatment being the prevailing concern but showing excellent tolerability [44].

A pilot study on genitourinary (GU) cancers was conducted to determine whether the longitudinal monitoring of ctDNA could improve the prognosis and prediction of ICI therapies and showed the value of ctDNA monitoring in prospectively enrolled and histologically confirmed advanced GU malignancies.

Key Methods and Results
- For at least 12 weeks, all eligible patients received ICI treatment, followed by the serial collection of blood samples every 6–8 weeks and conventional scans approximately every 12 weeks until PD.
- For 20 patients (15 renal, four urothelial, and one prostate), 98 banked plasma samples had ctDNA analysis conducted.
- ORR was the reported primary endpoint and was 70%.
- PD occurred in eight patients. An overall concordance between radiographic response and ctDNA dynamics was revealed for 15/18 (83%) of patients.
- CR and PR occurred in three and 11 patients, respectively, with SD in six and a CBR of 100%.

ICIs Regimens Utilized
- Pembrolizumab plus axitinib ($n = 7$)
- Pembrolizumab monotherapy ($n = 4$)

- Nivolumab plus cabozantinib ($n = 1$)
- Ipilimumab plus nivolumab followed by nivolumab monotherapy ($n = 6$)
- Durvalumab/gemcitabine/cisplatin followed by durvalumab monotherapy ($n = 1$)

Although this proof-of-concept study recommended that larger prospective studies be carried out to validate the clinical utility of ctDNA monitoring to ICI response, it successfully monitored ICI treatment response in patients with metastatic GU tumors [45].

In one study, CNTN1 immunotherapy and EMP1 immunotherapy were evaluated as key molecules with prognostic value for determining efficacy in bladder cancer (BCa) patients. Immunotherapy responsiveness was determined to assess the prognosis and prediction of therapy in bladder cancer to improve immunotherapy sensitivity, remaining an unmet need. Five key genes, namely PTGIS, MFAP5, CNTN1, MAP 1A, and EMP1, which were significantly related to immune checkpoint molecules and prognosis and immune checkpoint molecules of patients, were screened out, and CNTN1 and EMP1 were "further experimentally confirmed for their significant tumor-promoting effects." Risk scores were constructed to predict immunotherapy efficacy in patients with BCa on the basis of five key genes, and the study showed that high-risk patients have less sensitivity to ICIs and less efficacy and worse prognosis than low-risk patients, as shown by the risk scores. The risk scores that they determined may contribute to the development of personalized treatment for BCa. The expression of EMP1 and CNTN1 was shown to lead to the proliferation of BCa cells with proproliferative and antiapoptotic effects. TME immune cells were also enriched in high-grade tumors, suggesting that the ability to present antigens and eradicate tumors is shown by the CIBERSORT algorithm that determined that M2 macrophages, M0 macrophages, and CD4 memory T cells are the most prevalent immune cell types and suggesting the antiapoptotic effects and proproliferative effect of CNTN1 and EMP1 on tumor cells. The study authors concluded that risk scores were significantly associated with immune checkpoint expression, immune cell infiltration, prognosis, and immunotherapy response in BCa and fully confirmed that the differences in immune cell infiltration are more likely to be inherent characteristics of individual differences in molecular alteration profiles and risk score efficacy [46].

Platelets were found to predict PD-L1 response in NSCLC and inhibit CD4+ and CD8+ T cells. The quantification methods significantly showed that platelets predicted ICI therapy better than PD-L1 expression through a study on the interaction of platelets with lung cancer cells through direct imaging. Consistent with other studies, platelets were found to re-enter the bloodstream after tumor cell attachment, and because protein translation is possible in platelets, a strong positive correlation with PD-L1 expression was shown through flow cytometry analysis and GFP data, showing the expression of PD-L1 on platelet cells mediated by fibronectin. Vδ1+ T cells, distinct from CD8+ T cells, also predicted PD-1 ICI response, with distinct, functional states defined. CD8+ T-cell cytotoxic activity was also observed as distinct from T-cell exhaustion, which PD-L1 expression is associated with, leading to the "derepression" of ICIs [47, 48].

GBM, a tumor associated with poor prognosis, has been studied in preclinical models, and recent clinical trials have evaluated ICIs for this tumor. GBM has shown resistance to immune checkpoint inhibitors, having an immunosuppressive environment as a result of the presence of Tregs and inhibitory M2 macrophages, leading to reduced CD8+ T-cell activity. GITR is an immune checkpoint blockade that leads to increased tumor-infiltrating CTL proliferation and effector function and decreases the suppressive function of Treg cells. Anti-PD-1 does not exhibit activity in GBM but leads to T-cell anergy, and a mice model showed that anti-PD-1 and anti-CTLA-4 did not alleviate this resistance to tumor burden. GITR is selectively expressed in GBM, and it has been found to be lower in spleen and blood, whereas Treg cells express glucocorticoid-induced tumor necrosis factor-related protein. An antibody blocking GITR was administered to mice and led to fewer Treg cells, mediated by MHC1 recognition and IFN-gamma. The investigators showed that the identified mechanism was the conversion of Treg cells and the reactivation of CD8 T cells after αPD1+ αGITR treatment. MHC upregulation on tumor cells allows for recognition and tumor cell killing, overcoming the immunosuppressive environment [49].

A genetic ablation of the IL-6 GBM model combined with pharmacological inhibition led to the discovery of the synergy of anti-PD-1 and anti-CTLA-4 immunotherapy through the dual targeting of IL-6 and CD40. The study authors "identified a Stat3/HIF-1α-mediated axis, through which IL-6 executes an antitumor role to induce CD40 expression" in inhibitory macrophages that are present in the immunosuppressive TME. The combination targeting led to tumor cell killing and extended animal survival through the stimulation of CD40 expression, even though immunosuppressive macrophages were induced. Notably, ICIs combined with the dual targeting led to a complete therapeutic response, with all treated animals surviving with no detectable tumors. In short, "IL-6 neutralization and CD40 stimulation plus immune checkpoint blockade synergistically reduces Mϕ-mediated immune suppression and enhances T-cell infiltration and activation in GBM" [50].

A significant finding also in a GBM model showed that Siglec-9 is also an immune checkpoint molecule, and expression led to decreased T-cell priming and immunosuppression. Unique monocyte-derived TAM subpopulations possessing functional plasticity were identified, and this led to the high expression of the immunosuppressive SIGLEC9 gene and preferential accumulation in nonresponders to anti-PD-1 treatment. Tumor growth was controlled, and prolonged survival and CD4+ and CD8+ T cell activation through the deletion of SIGLEC-9 were observed. Anti-inflammatory and angiogenesis-related genes, such as SLC40A1, FOLR2, IL10, VEGFB, and CSF1R; antigen presentation; and phagocytosis-related genes C1QA/C1QB/C1QC were upregulated with the increased expression of CD80 and MHCII activation markers, further suggesting the clinical application of combination therapies featuring T-cell and macrophage inhibition [51].

However, limited clinical benefit has been shown with anti-PD-1 inhibitors combined with other checkpoint inhibitors,, with researchers evaluating TIM-3, TIGIT, and LAG-3 antibodies in ongoing studies. The CheckMate-498, CheckMate-543, and CheckMate 143 (combined with bevacizumab) did not prolong PFS or OS for nivolumab. Furthermore, 35 recurrent GBM patients underwent treatment with neoadjuvant pembrolizumab that prolonged survival when compared to adjuvant postsurgical treatment (mOS, 13.7 vs. 7.5 months; mPFS, 3.3 vs. 2.4 months) [51].

Three clinical trials evaluated ICIs for hepatocellular carcinoma in various settings and stages. Before the emergence of ICIs, unresectable or metastatic HCC had poor prognosis, with 5-year survival rates of 10–18%. The phase 3 IMbrave150 trial evaluated bevacizumab and atezolizumab; significant OS and PFS benefits were observed; and improved ORR was also reported in the combination therapy compared with sorafenib. This combination was shown to have substantial synergistic efficacy in HCC. In Study 22, a phase II trial, the efficacy and safety of durvalumab plus bevacizumab was demonstrated, with an ORR of 21.3%. This was also demonstrated in the phase III IMbrave 150 trial evaluating atezolizumab plus bevacizumab versus sorafenib in the systemic treatment of advanced HCC, with an mPFS of 6.9 versus 4.3 months (HR, 0.59), a treatment regimen that was selected as preferred first-line treatment. The primary endpoints included ORR, safety, and tolerability, as assessed through RECIST. Chen et al., as reported in Clinical Cancer Research, conducted a prospective single-arm phase II trial evaluating anti-PD-1 inhibitor toripalimab (a humanized IgG4K antibody specific for PD-1) plus bevacizumab in treatment-naive advanced HCC. Here, 54 patients were enrolled and received 240 mg of toripalimab with 15/mg/kg of bevacizumab every 3 weeks. ORR was 31.5% (95% CI 19.5–45.6) and mOS was not reached. The 12-month and 24-month OS values were 77.3% and 63.5%, respectively. Grade 3 TEAEs occurred in 27 patients, including hypertension (38.9%), increased AAT (33.3%), amylase (29.6), and decreased platelet count (27.8%). Six patients (11.1%) achieved the best overall response of CR and PR, with an ORR of 46.3% (95% CI 32.6–60.4). DCR was 92.6% (95% CI 82.1–97.9). As the investigators assessed, 33 patients had disease progression, and four patients died without disease progression. Median PFS was 8.5 months (95% CI 5.5–11.0). Additionally, 53 patients (98.1%) reported at least one TEAE; 20% or more of patients reported elevated levels of ASP, bilirubin, decreased lymphocyte count, and increased C-reactive protein; 37% experienced SAEs, and TEAE leading to death was reported in one patient that was not related to the study treatment. Also, irAEs were evaluated by the investigators and were found to be greater than grade 3 in 10 patients (18.5%), including proteinurea, decreased platelet count, increased amylase, and increased blood CPK, the most common being decreased platelet count. As the study authors concluded, promising antitumor activity was achieved in the toripaliumab plus bevacizumab combination treatment, which was also well tolerated and safe, supporting further clinical study of this duo therapy in patients with untreated advanced hepatocellular carcinoma; the results compared favorably with the ORIENT-32 sintilimab–bevacizumab biosimilar (20% and 73%, respectively) cohort and the IMbrave150 atezolizumab–bevacizumab (25.6% and 74.1%, respectively) cohort, with comparable safety profiles [52].

MORPHEUS-Liver evaluated tiragolumab, an anti-TIGIT antibody, with atezolizumab and bevacizumab versus the latter two agents alone in mHCC in a randomized phase 1b/2 study. The addition of this antibody to the combination regimen was evaluated for clinical activity and safety, the rationale being that TIGIT is a novel immune checkpoint antibody present on exhausted, activated, and regulatory T cells in HCC. Tiragolumab is a human anti-TIGIT monoclonal antibody that might synergize with atezolizumab plus bevacizumab to improve T-cell activation as well as their effectiveness and natural killer cell activity to enhance antitumor response. The phase 2 CITYSCAPE trial described earlier enrolled chemotherapy-naive PD-L1 positive recurrent or mNSCLC patients administered tiragolumab plus atezolizumab, leading to clinically meaningful improvement in ORR and PFS when compared to placebo. The MORPHEUS-Liver trial is a global multicenter trial that investigated this regimen versus the standard of care with the hypotheses that tiragolumab when added to atezolizumab and bevacizumab could lead to a better tumor response and to an improved and more-durable clinically benefit for locally advanced, metastatic unresectable patients. Eligible patients were Child-Pugh class A disease, ECOG scores of 0–1, and a life expectancy of at least 3 months. Permuted block randomization 2:1 was applied: Patients received tiragolumab 15 mg/kg plus 1200 mg atezolizumab and bevacizumab 15 mg/kg versus 1200 mg atezolizumab plus 15 mg/kg bevacizumab. ORR was the primary endpoint, and treatment continued until toxicity or the loss of clinical benefit. In the TAB group, ORR was 20.6 months and 14 months in the dual therapy. Confirmed ORR was 43% (95% CI 27–59, *n* = 17) and 11% in the tiraglobumab group versus the atezolizumab plus bevacizumab group.

Key results included a population of 58 efficacy evaluable patients who showed as per RECIST v11 an investigator-assessed ORR that was recorded in 17 patients with a 31% confirmed ORR (95% CI 6–57) found in the tiragolumab plus atezolizumab plus bevacizumab group (*n* = 40) versus 11% (1–35) in the atezolizumab plus bevacizumab (*n* = 18). Ongoing responses were experienced in 59% (10/17) in the tiragolumab plus atezolizumab plus bevacizumab cohort and 100% (*n* = 2) of the atezolizumab plus bevacizumab cohort, and PR was evident in all patients in both treatment responses. Moreover, mPFS was found to be longer in the tiragolumab plus atezolizumab plus bevacizumab cohort than in the atezolizumab plus bevacizumab cohort (median 12.3 months (95% CI 8.2–17.5)) versus (4.2 months (1.6–7.4); (HR 0.51, 95% CI 0.27–0.95)). Median DOR was not evaluable in either cohort, and the PFS rate "continued to be higher in the tiragolumab plus atezolizumab plus bevacizumab group at 6 months (75% [95% CI 62–88] vs. 41% [18–65]) and 12 months (50% [35–65] vs. 24%)."

- Hypertension was reported in 15% of patients, or 40 patients, in the tiragolumab plus atezolizumab plus bevacizumab cohort and 2/18 patients (11%) in the atezolizumab plus bevacizumab group. Other common AEs were ALT increases in three (8%) of 40 patients versus one (6%) of 18 patients, and proteinuria was reported in two (5%) of 40 patients versus two (11%) of 18 patients.
- TRAEs were reported in 39 (98%) of 40 patients in the tiragolumab plus atezolizumab plus bevacizumab cohort and 15 (83%) of 18 patients in the atezolizumab plus bevacizumab cohort. Pruritus was reported in 17 (43%) of 40 patients, proteinuria in 15 (38%) patients, fatigue in 11 (28%) patients, rash in ten (25%) patients, hypertension in ten (25%) patients, and arthralgia in nine (23%) patients, which accounts for the most common adverse events. TRAEs were seen in 13 (33%) of 40 patients in the tiragolumab plus atezolizumab plus bevacizumab

cohort, and eight (44%) of 18 patients in the atezolizumab plus bevacizumab cohort who experienced grade 3–4 events.
- When TRAEs were divided according to system organ class, they were all GI disorders with three (8%) in 40 patients in the tiragolumab plus atezolizumab plus bevacizumab cohort and three (17%) of 18 patients in the atezolizumab plus bevacizumab cohort.
- At clinical cutoff, 45% of 40 patients in the tiragolumab plus atezolizumab plus bevacizumab cohort and 14 (78%) of 18 patients in the atezolizumab plus bevacizumab cohort had died.

As the study authors concluded, the anti-TIGIT mAb tiragolumab when added to atezolizumab and bevacizumab showed superior outcomes and might be more efficacious than the combination of atezolizumab and bevacizumab treatment for patients with unresectable HCC, with comparable safety profiles and positive benefit–risk ratios reported, providing a basis for further investigation into tiragolumab additive therapy using atezolizumab and bevacizumab as a novel first-line treatment option for unresectable HCC [53].

SAFFRON-104 is a phase Ib/II study evaluating the combination therapy of the anti-PD-1 ICI tislelizumab and the TKI sitravatinib in advanced HCC patients, the rationale being that the combination of ICI with an immunomodulatory agents can overcome resistance and enhance antitumor activity. Tislelizumab is engineered to reduce antibody-reduced phagocytic resistance pathways because it reduced Fc gamma receptor binding to macrophages and was shown to have efficacy as monotherapy versus sorafenib in a phase III trial and in combination with chemotherapy in the RATIONALE-305 study. In a phase I study on NSCLC patients, the combination of sitravatinib and tislelizumab showed clinical and antitumor activity in both treatment-naive and treatment-experienced patients and in patients with PD-L1-treated disease with "no new safety signals identified." Phase I determined the RP2D of sitravatinib with or without tislelizumab and phase II evaluated the sitravatinib monotherapy in pretreated HCC patients and sitravatinib plus tislelizumab in anti-PD-L1-naive HCC patients. The primary endpoints were safety and tolerability in phase I and ORR in phase II. Grade 3 or greater AEs were 14 (51.9%) or 42 (50%) patients, respectively. In pretreated HCC receiving sitravatinib monotherapy, the ORR was 25% (95% CI: 8.7–49.1); with patients receiving sitravatinib plus tislelizumab, the ORR was 11.5% (95% CI 2.4–30.2); with anti-PD-(L)1–naive HCC, the ORR was 9.5% (95% CI 1.2–30.4); and with anti-PD-(L)1–treated HCC, the ORR was 16.1% (95% CI 5.5–33.7) in anti-PD-(L)1–naive GC/GEJC patients. Safety and tolerability were phase I endpoints, and ORR, DCR, and PFS served as the secondary endpoints. Investigator-assessed ORR was the primary endpoint of phase II, and investigator-assessed DCR and PFS were the secondary endpoints. No DLTs were reported in the DLT-evaluable set (n = 22) or in the cohort receiving sitravatinib monotherapy at 80 mg or 120 mg. The majority of patients (n = 81/84) in the dual therapy cohort experienced a TRAE, of which 82.7% were related to the ICI. Also, 50% of the dual therapy cohort reported grade 3 or greater TRAEs related to sitravatinib and 28.4% (n = 23/81) related to tislelizumab, with 11 (13.6%)

serious TRAEs related to this agent. Eight (9.9%) TRAEs led to treatment discontinuation. The most common TRAEs were proteinuria, AAT increase, hypertension, and diarrhea. Furthermore, 35.7% ($n = 30/84$) of patients receiving the dual agents reported imAEs related to the dual agents that led to treatment discontinuation in two patients. Four fatal treatment-related TEAEs were reported. The confirmed ORR was 25% and 11.5% in the monotherapy and dual therapy cohorts, respectively, in the anti-PD-L1 treated group. Median OS was 26.7 months (95% CI 9.1 to NE) in the phase II safety analysis set, and median PFS was 6.8 months (95% CI 4.0–7.4) in phases I and II combined. In the phase II set, mOS was 20.5 (95% CI 7.4 to NE) and 12.4 months (95% CI 7.0 to 14.1), respectively. The authors discuss how recent advances in immunotherapy have led to significant clinical benefit; however, an unmet medical need remains for "greater tumor control without significantly compromising treatment tolerability and … SAFFRON-104 showed the combination therapy to have promising efficacy and managing tolerability" in anti-PD-L1-naive and anti-PD-L1-treated HCC patients. Phase I RP2D of sitravatinib was 120 mg of QD in monotherapy and combination with tislelizumab. No new safety signals were observed, and grade 3 or greater TRAEs occurred in 50% of combination therapy patients, but only 10.7% led to treatment discontinuation, with a higher median OS and moderate ORR observed in anti-PD-L1-naive HCC patients (11.5%% and 20.5 months, respectively) compared with anti-PD-L1-treated HCC patients (9.5% and 12.4 months, respectively). As the study authors conclude, the results from this study show clinical evidence supporting the addition of tislelizumab to sitravetinb in advanced HCC patients [54].

The ipi-nivo regimen was investigated in 5-year follow-up results from the CheckMate 040 study treating cohorts with HCC previously treated with sorafenib. Ipi-nivo demonstrated "promising clinical activity and durable responses in sorafenib treated patients." Patients were randomized 1:1:1, and the primary endpoints were safety, tolerability, and ORR.

- ORR in arms A, B, and C was 4% ($n = 17$), 27% ($n = 13$), and 29% ($n = 14$), respectively.
- Median OS in arms A, B, and C was 22.2 months (34/50; 95% CI 9.4–54.8 months), 12.5 months (38/49; 95% CI 7.6–16.4 months), and 12.7 months (40/49; 95% CI 7.4–30.5 months), respectively.

No new safety signals were identified, and no new discontinuations due to imAEs were reported. The study authors concluded that their primary analysis revealed that the arm A regimen of ipi-nivo showed "clinically meaningful responses and long-term survival benefit, with no new safety signals in patients with advanced HCC following sorafenib treatment, further supporting its use as a second-line treatment in these patients" [55].

Akula et al. discussed the benefits of neoadjuvant immunotherapy for HCC and hypothesized that increased antigen release and T-cell expansion in the neoadjuvant setting could enhance immunotherapy and eliminate micrometastasis, which has been supported by preclinical models and some prospective trials. "PD-1 attenuates CTL while CTLA-4 downregulates tumor antigen-presenting cells," and previously published retrospective cohort and case reports have shown that neoadjuvant monotherapy ICIs can lead to CRs and PRs in solid tumors such as HCC (Fig. 6.4). The following are some example studies:

- Neoadjuvant nivolumab with or without ipilimumab had similar PRs and was generally well tolerated in monotherapy versus combination therapy, with 3/9 vs. 3/11 patients showing major pathologic response (MPR), respectively. Nivo alone, however, had a better side effect profile (23% with grade 3–4 TRAEs vs. 43%). Five patients experienced pCR, with one demonstrating MPR with > 70% necrosis, where the pathology of the response was associated with brisk T-cell response.
- PR in resectable HCC receiving neoadjuvant cemiplimab, an anti-PD-1 mAb was 1. Here, 7/20 patients had 50% or greater tumor necrosis, with three displaying complete tumor necrosis histopathology. Increased TILs were shown by an analysis of post-treatment lesions with 50% or greater necrosis compared to < 50% necrosis with higher CD8 T-cell infiltration in tumors when compared with the surrounding tissue.
- Neoadjuvant administration of tislelizumab in recurrent HCC was shown in the phase 2 TALENT trial, and of the 11 patients enrolled, one achieved CR, one achieved PR, and four experienced AEs (none were severe), with ORR being 18.2% and where PD = 1. Two patients had an MPR, with an 85% response and where CR = 1. Recurrence was seen in two patients at 1 year. The safety and modest efficacy of neoadjuvant tislelizumab for rHCC patients were demonstrated.
- The superiority of anti-PD-1 treatment over other options in the neoadjuvant treatment of HCC patients was supported by a meta-analysis of five phase 1/2 studies in 96 patients, who showed that adding TKIs to anti-PD-1 therapy does not improve ORR or pathological outcomes. Single anti-PD-1 therapy when compared with combination treatment with anti-CTLA-4 mAb showed no difference in pCR rates.

Combination Therapy

- A phase 1b clinical trial, PRIME-HCC evaluated the safety and efficacy of ipi-nivo combination as neoadjuvant therapy in patients with early-stage HCC prior to liver resection, whose primary objective was to evaluate the safety outcomes of combination treatment and assess the secondary endpoints of RR, OS, and PFS. This study included data from an abstract of the 2023 ASCO meeting that included 25 patients, of whom 21 were assessed for radiological response and underwent surgical resection. MPR was observed in 56% (9/16) of evaluable patients, with an ORR of 29%. Also, pCR was observed in 38% (6/16) of evaluable patients, with the combination well tolerated and 24% experiencing grade ≥ 3 AEs [56]

Childs conducted a review of ICIs in HCC and described how the tumor's immunotolerance leads to limitations in autoimmunity but predisposes the liver to immune evasion by cancer cells. Augmented immune suppression causes hepatocytes to avoid immune clearance (Fig. 6.4). The balance between immune

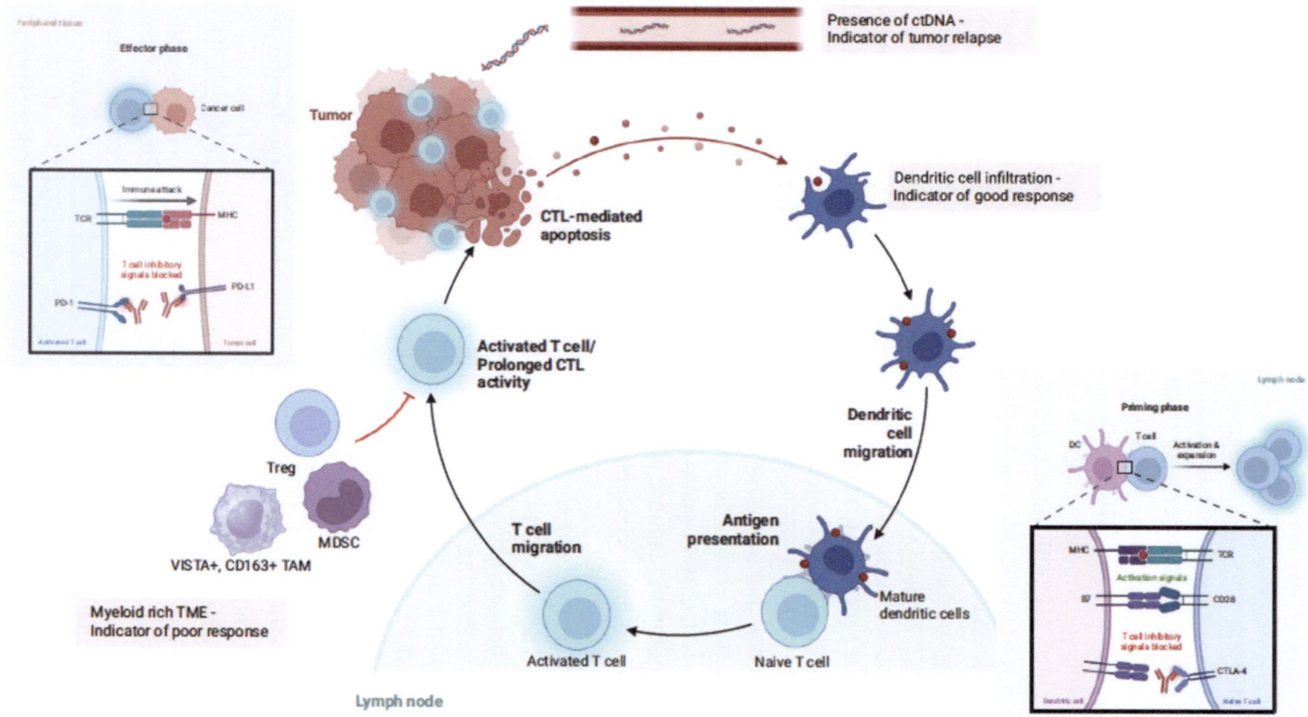

Fig. 6.4 TME interaction with ICIs. (Adapted from Akula et al. [56]. Permission to reuse under Creative Commons CC BY 4.0)

activation and evasion is "determined by the opposing action of these cellular components and their soluble mediators, and their relative composition within the tumor microenvironment (TME) has been used to denote four subclasses of HCC with distinct clinical outcomes." Immune suppressors in the HCC TME include Tregs, TAMs, and MDSCs. Tregs are present in higher numbers within the TME of HCC when compared to the healthy liver, which corresponds to lower OS and DFS and to higher-grade tumors. TAMs further lead to immunosuppression through the production of immunosuppressive cytokines such as IL-10, the expression of PD-L1, and the downregulation of MHCII and recruit Tregs via the production of chemokines. The downregulation of MHC II is especially significant because "the costimulatory molecules required for successful CD8+ T cell activation are inhibited." When skewed toward the M2 phenotype, the presence of TAMs correlates with worse prognosis. MDSCs also promote Tregs and inhibit CD8+ T cells and NK cell activation through mediators such as TGF-β. CD8+ T cells are highly dysfunctional in the HCC TME, leading to further immunosuppression, with single-cell studies showing a reduction in these cells and more-pronounced exhaustion phenotypes that express PD-L1, CTLA-4, TIM-3, LAG3, and TIGIT. Gamma-delta T cells and NK cells also display an exhausted functional profile. Inflammatory cytokines such as TGF-beta, IL-10, and IL-16 secreted by various cells in the TME also promote immunosuppression and are secreted by tumor cells, CAFs, and TAMs. TGF-β is associated with poor prognosis and poorer response to sorafenib and pembrolizumab. However, IL-2, IFN-gamma, CXCL-10, and CXCL9 attract effector cells that mount an antitumor response where IFN drives PD-L1 that predicts a favorable response to ICIs. Immune checkpoint inhibition was also described for advanced-stage and early-stage HCC, in both adjuvant and neoadjuvant settings as single agents in both first-line and second-line settings and in combination with other targeted agents. The phase III CheckMate 459 and KEYNOTE-240 failed to demonstrate an OS benefit when compared to sorafenib. KEYNOTE-394 evaluated pembrolizumab in first-line settings versus in second-line settings in an Asian population and showed a statistically significant improvement in median OS (14.6 vs. 13 months; HR 0.79; 95% CI 0.63–0.99) and with an ORR of 12.7 vs. 1.3%. The HIMALAYA trial showed the safety and efficacy of single-agent ICI in terms of OS for durvalumab monotherapy, which was shown to be noninferior to sorafenib. RATIONALE-301 showed "a non-inferiority of tislelizumab with sorafenib in the first-line setting" (HR 0.85, 95% CI 0.71–1.02). A median DOR for the immunotherapy arm (36.1 months, 95% CI 18.8 to not evaluable, vs. 11 months, 95% CI 6.2–14.7) and a higher ORR rate of 14.3% versus 5.4% were observed. The phase III IMbrave-150 study, as alluded to earlier, determined in the first-line setting that superior clinical benefit was observed with the dual therapy of atezolizumab and bevacizumab when compared to sorafenib, and this has become the standard of care. In the atezolizumab/bevacizumab arm, an mOS of 19.2 months (95% CI 17–23.7) vs. 13.4 months (95% CI 11.4–16.9; stratified HR (0.66, 95% CI 0.52–0.85)) in the sorafenib arm was demonstrated. Also, the ORR (30% vs. 11%) and mDOR (18.1 months (95% CI 14.6–not evaluable) vs. 14.9 months (95% CI 4.9–17.0)) were shown to be significantly improved with this combination for atezolizumab–bevacizumab when compared to sorafenib. However, for improved OS, the LEAP-002 trial did not meet prespecified significance for pembrolizumab plus lenvatinib. In the treatment of HCC in first-line settings, the anti-PD-1 antibody camrelizumab plus rivoceranib demonstrated an OS of 22.1 months, the longest for a systemic therapy, with statistical superiority to sorafenib (22.1 months, 95% CI 19.1–27.2, vs. 15.2 months, 95% CI 13.0–18.5; HR 0.62, 95% CI 0.49–0.80). Combining ICIs was explored in the phase III CheckMate 9DW (ipi-nivo) and STRIDE (tremelimumab and durvalumab), both showing OS benefit. For early-stage disease in the adjuvant setting, the IMbrave-050 trial showed improved RFS with atezolizumab/bevacizumab treatment, with an HR of 0.72 (95% CI 0.53–0.98). Additionally, 61% of the surveillance arm crossed over to the therapy. In neoadjuvant settings, early-phase trials have shown MPR rates of 17.6% and 33%. In a phase II study on neoadjuvant nivo or ipi-nivo, six of the 20 patients who underwent resection had an MPR with no recurrence at 26.8 months of follow-up. Despite grade 3 adverse events occurring, surgery was not delayed for the patients. The multicenter PRIMER-1 trial is an example featuring the randomization of participants to 6 weeks of neoadjuvant treatment consisting of pembrolizumab/lenvatinib, pembrolizumab, or lenvatinib with subsequent treatment with adjuvant pembolizumab given postoperatively. These studies will further explain in the neoadjuvant or perioperative setting the role of immunotherapy in the context of biomarkers. TMB and PD-L1 expression have been studied, and HCC was shown to be on the lower end of the spectrum (0.42 to 65.6 Mut/Mb). An analysis in the IMbrave 150 study identified no relationship between response and TMB. CheckMate 459 showed similar results, with a significant difference between OS and low or high TMB. Studies have also shown that PD-L1 expression does not correlate with tumor PD-L1 expression. With regard to mutations, randomized trials have failed to confirm that CheckMate 459 and IMbrave 150 have no survival difference on the basis of Wnt/beta-catenin pathway activity or CTNNB1 mutations, as was shown in the ICI-containing cohorts. As the review authors conclude, in the appropriate management of advanced HCC, ICIs have proved transformational, with data emerging for new roles in early-disease-stage settings. However, as shown in the phase III IMBRAVE 251, the data require robust evaluation to be reliably indicated for therapy at later stages of advanced disease, including in the sequencing of treatment and the continuation of ICIs beyond disease progression for patients to show clinical benefit. Resistance to ICIs has emerged in monotherapy and combination treatments in first-line settings and novel combinations, and alternate immunotherapy strategies are being developed in ongoing studies to answer questions to determine how to improve survival benefit in advanced disease stages, necessitating patient recruitment and embedded translational research to build on already-required data to improve patient outcomes [57].

A meta-analysis and a systematic review were conducted by Maiorano et al. to determine the putative predictive significance of PD-L1 in mUC, and they stated that the association of PD-L1 with response and survival in patients treated with ICIs is controversial. This association was evaluated in the study between "ORR, OS and PFS in patients with PD-L1 positive and PD-L1 negative tumors." For mUC, nivolumab and pembrolizumab as well as atezolizumab, durvalumab, and avelumab are approved for treating these cancers.

Key Results

PD-L1 expression	ORR	Median OS	PFS
Positive	13.8%–78.6%	8.4 to 24.1 months	HR, 0.55; 95% CI 0.44–0.69; $p < 0.001$
Negative	5.1% to 63.2% (HR, 1.94, 95% CI 1.47–2.56)	6.0 to 19.1 months HR, 0.71; 95% CI 0.57–0.89	

An association was shown between PD-L1 status and ORR that favored positive expression levels, and pooled HR indicated a significant reduction in risk in PD-L1 positive tumors versus PD-L1 negative tumors. PD-L1 positive tumors had improved PFS when compared to PD-L1 negative tumors. As the authors conclude, their results show that ORR, mOS, and PFS in mUC patients had a positive association with PD-L1 status, with the caveat that PD-L1 cannot serve as a valid predictive biomarker for tumor type patient selection and further cannot serve to guide ICI administration in mUC [58].

Prostate cancer is characterized by a strong immunosuppressive environment with few TILs, abundant immunosuppressive cells, and low immunogenicity, rendering the potential effectiveness of ICIs very low in terms of overcoming immunosuppression and activating the immune system. Low expression levels of neoantigens and tumor-associated antigens make them immune-resistant cold tumors. The malignancy of prostate cancer leads to adverse consequences for T-cell function, leading to immune evasion and the expression of coinhibitory molecules that induce cytotoxicity and inhibit proliferation. CTLA-4, PD-1, and LAG-3 that suppress T-cell function are also expressed. PD-L1 binds to PD-1 on T cells, inhibiting their activation and promoting tumor progression. T-cell exhaustion that are driven by immunosuppressive metabolites in the tumor and compounded by large levels of cytokines, chemokines, and other cells lead to immunosuppression, leading to the reduced recruitment of cytotoxic cells and ineffective tumor eradication. Prostate cancer has many immunosuppressive cells, such as TAMs, MDSCs, and Tregs. Prostate cancer cells induce the expression of CD163, CD206, and B7-H3, which are immunosuppressive markers in macrophages that reprogram tumor-eradicating M1 macrophages into immunosuppressive M2 macrophages while losing antitumor proliferative abilities. TAMs promote prostate cancer invasion and metastasis as a result of cell proliferation through the release of CCL5 and CCL6. Through perforin and granzyme release and CTLA-4 and PD-L1 expression, Tregs directly suppress effector cells. The indirect inhibition of T-cell activation is the result of CTLA-4 expression on Tregs that bind costimulatory CD80/86 on antigen-presenting cells. In terms of tumor neoantigens, prostate cancer has a mutation frequency that is seven to 15 times lower than that of lung cancer and melanoma. The immune system also has issues with recognizing tumor cells given the fewer neoantigens present, leading to tumor escape. The cross-presentation between APCs and CLTs leads to a noninflammatory TME as a result of a lack of these neoepitopes and low infiltration at the tumor site of immune cells and mitigated pMHC presentation. As a result of all of these interacting factors, ICI monotherapy has limited success in PCa treatment. Monotherapy with ICIs has limited success in the treatment of prostate cancer. A phase 3 clinical trial in which a cohort treated with ipilimumab was compared to placebo showed no change in OS, with adverse actions such as diarrhea being present. In KEYNOTE-028, pembrolizumab treated PD-L1 positive prostate cancer patients, with an ORR of 17% (4/356) and with no CR observed. In KEYNOTE-199, the ORR in PD-L1 positive patients was 5%, with a 7.9–14.1-month survival period. Dual therapy with ipi-nivo shows an ORR of 25% and 10% in chemotherapy refractory patients. However, with increased dMMR, MSI-H, and TMB, the ICI combination has potentially good therapy outcomes. Four out of 90 mCRPC patients with high TMB had complete tumor regression and durable clinical response with the ipi-nivo regimen. In MSI-H/dMMR patients, pembrolizumab treatment elicited favorable treatment outcomes, with decreased PSA levels in 6/11 patients (54.6%) showing response, whereas the MSI-H/dMMR molecular phenotype though uncommon (3.1% of cases) enhanced the efficacy of pembro in mCRPC, with better survival outcomes coinciding with increases in TMB, but without MSI-H co-occurring, TMB presence elicited no response. The CDK12 gene leads to gene fusion, increased T-cell infiltration, and neoantigen load, and patients harboring CDK12-mutated cancers clinically benefit from ICI treatment, which has therapeutic significance [59].

Wu et al. also note how the low immunogenicity of prostate cancer leads to the lack of robust clinical outcomes in prostate cancer, in which most cases progress to metastatic resistance prostate cancer attendant with the lack of predictive biomarkers to personalized treatment. The authors highlight five potential biomarkers, including dMMR, MSI, PD-L1 expression levels, CDK12 deficiency, and TMB. Tumors such as prostate cancer exploit mechanisms designed to maintain immune homeostasis and immune tolerance with the TME to evade immune surveillance. Tumor cells that express PD-L1 and T-cell immune response are suppressed, and tumor growth and dissemination are permitted. KEYNOTE-028 and KEYNOTE-199 evaluated pembrolizumab for PD-L1 positive mCRPC patients, and in the former, 23 patients who were pretreated elicited a 17% ORR, a 30% DCR, and a 37% 12-month OS, whereas in the second trial, three cohorts of mCRPC patients treated with docetaxel (n = 133,66,59) received 200 mg, eliciting a 5% ORR and a 3% ORR, respectively; DCRs of 10%, 9%, and 22%, respectively,; and median OS values of 9.5 months, 7.9 months, and 14.1 months in each of the cohorts, respectively. Checkmate 650 evaluated pembro-ipi in 90 mCRPC patients who were enrolled, of whom 63 patients possessed an evaluable tumor with status-assessing PD-L1 expression.

In those patients, PD-L1 $\geq$ 1% vs. PD-L1 < 1% had ORRs of 36.4% (10.9–69.2) vs. 12.1% (3.4–28.2), respectively, with confirmed PSA response rates of 25.0% (5.5–57.2) vs. 7.7% (1.6–20.9), with median rPFS (95% CI) of 5.6 (1.9–NE) vs. 3.9 (2.7–5.5) months, and where OS (95% CI) was not reached (7.7–NE) vs. 15.2 (8.4–19.0) months—showing that PD-L1 positivity allowed patients to benefit from higher treatment levels with pembro-ipi treatment. In determining the safety and efficacy of a treatment regimen of mCPRC, the Imbassador250, a concurrent, randomized phase 3 trial, evaluated atezolizumab plus enzalutamide versus enzalutamide monotherapy, and in PD-L1 < 1%, PD-L1 ≥ 1%, or PD-L1 ≥ 5% status patients, the subanalysis showed that a longer PFS was associated with atezolizumab administration in the presence of PDL1 IC2/3 expression and increased levels of CD8+ T cells.

In prostate cancer, the MSI-H/dMMR rate is low, with an occurrence of 1–3%. In one study that consolidated 65 prostate cancer patients with dMMR, 19 patients received anti-PD1 treatment; a mPFS of 24 weeks resulted. This reflected the results of Graham et al., where 17 men received pembrolizumab, and out of 15 evaluable patients, eight had a 53% response, with seven showing a PSA90 decline. CDK12 loss-of-function mutations have one of the highest prevalence in mCRPC, and inactivation and the loss of CDK12 results in a unique genomic instability with focal tandem duplications present in coding regions, resulting in gene fusion and induced neoantigens. Nine men were identified with at least one CDK12 alteration and received PD-1 inhibitor. In another study, 46 patients had CDK12 mutations, of which 34 patients (79%) had biallelic CDK12 loss. Five out of 46 CDK12 patients (10.9%) received at least one dose of anti-PD-1 checkpoint inhibitor immunotherapy, with 2 of them having achieved a PSA50 response, when receiving at least one dose of anti-PD-1 inhibitor monotherapy. The authors conclude that larger samples sizes are necessary to confirm the predictive efficacy of ICB therapy for mCRPC. Although TMB tumors respond better to ICIs because their high mutational burden confers more neoantigens, triggering an immune response when the immune system has been recognized, the predictive value of TMB-H for ICI therapy in mCRPC patients needs further investigation, being controversial [60].

Velho conducted a study with similar implications for determining predictive biomarkers for mCRPC when administering nivolumab in patients with or without DNA repair defects. They showed through an evaluation of PSA(50) response that DNA repair defects did not predict response to nivolumab. The study was a phase II multicenter single-arm trial on patients with prior docetaxel therapy. DRD was assessed by using ctDNA, with PSA response being the primary endpoint and ORR, rPFS, and OS serving as the secondary endpoints. PD-L1 expression evaluation along with CGP via whole-exome sequencing (WES) took place. The authors note that despite the ICI benefit in tissue-agnostic tumors with MSI-H and dMMR defects, no pathologic or clinical characteristics, such as PD-L1 expression, visceral metastasis, disease burden, or de novo disease, assist in selecting patients with mCRPC to receive ICIs, even though Wnt/b catenin, CDK12 inactivation, and T-cell dynamics were evaluated in preclinical and clinical studies. Still no specific biomarker has been shown to reliably identify patients with mCRPC who benefit from ICIs. DRD has been shown to be present in 23–33% of patients with mCRPC, and its presence in somatic and germline mutations has important prognostic and predictive implications given that TMB, TIL, and PD-L 1 expression and genomic scars suggest that genomic alterations in HRD tumors may be associated with PD-1/PD/L1 blockade and may contribute to immune response. Nivolumab was administered

IV at 3 mg/kg for 60 minutes over 2 weeks until "disease progression or unacceptable toxicity." Before the study, prior therapy for 63.1% of patients was administered with four or more lines of treatment, with most (80%) having an ECOG performance status of 0 to 1. Furthermore, 10 out of 38 patients had observed decreases in PSA levels, and the PSA(5) response was achieved in 10.5% of patients; 63.1% had received four or more lines of therapy before the study; most (80%) had an ECOG performance status of 0 to1; 10 of 38 patients (26%) had PSA decline; and PSA(50) response was achieved in 10.5% of patients. Median PFS was 4.3 months (95% CI 2.8–10.4), and mOS was 14.12 months (95% CI 10.21–18.9). TP53, PTEN, and BRCA2 along with CDK12 were the most common pathogenic alterations found, with germline alteration in ATM, TP53, and ERCC3. Mean TMB was 9.51 mutations per megabase. The final result was that patients with combination treatment identified with DRDs did not have superior PSA(5) response compared to patients with genomic alterations (18.2% versus 8%), respectively, showing that PD-L1 status was not indicative of PSA or radiographic response. Finally, mPFS was shown as 1.9 vs. 2.8 months, and rPFS was 3.4 vs. 5.5 months, with very little statistical difference between patients with or without DRD, and little evidence supported the clinical benefit of nivolumab demonstration, as determined by using ctDNA [61].

6.6 Immune-Related Adverse Events and Management (Figs 6.5 and 6.6)

Adverse events, or toxicities, for immune checkpoint inhibitors are common clinical presentations in patients, which are present as cutaneous, cardiac, neurologic, pulmonary, and endocrine and can be acute or chronic. Patients should remain cognizant of the potentialities of toxicities as ICBs and for survivorship. These adverse events are treatment-related adverse events that should raise suspicion for the clinician or are immune-related side effects for the close monitoring of laboratory values relevant for each toxicity. ASCO guidelines published in 2021 recommend that organ-based toxicity presenting with grades 1, 2, and 3 toxicities warrant corticosteroids (an initial dose of 0.5–1 mg/kg/d of prednisone or equivalent) tapered after 4–6 weeks and close monitoring, except for neurologic, hematologic, and cardiac adverse events. Immunosuppressive agents are usually required for cases resistant to treatment. Treatment discontinuation is generally recommended for grade 4 toxicities, except for endocrinopathies that should be addressed with hormone replacement therapy. The presence of adverse events usually affects ICI prognosis. Mechanisms of action underlying irAE are hypothesized to be related to activated T cells, T-cell reactivity against unaffected organs, and a loss of peripheral tolerance.

Cutaneous irAEs as described in detail in a review by Watanabe and Yamaguchi are among the first to present and include maculopapular rash, treated with corticosteroids (0.5–1 mg/kg/day); pruritus is often seen on the trunk and scalp as erosions and hyperpigmentation, and in severe cases, itchiness that requires discontinuation occurs. Psoriasis typically manifests as scaly plaques on the trunks and extremities

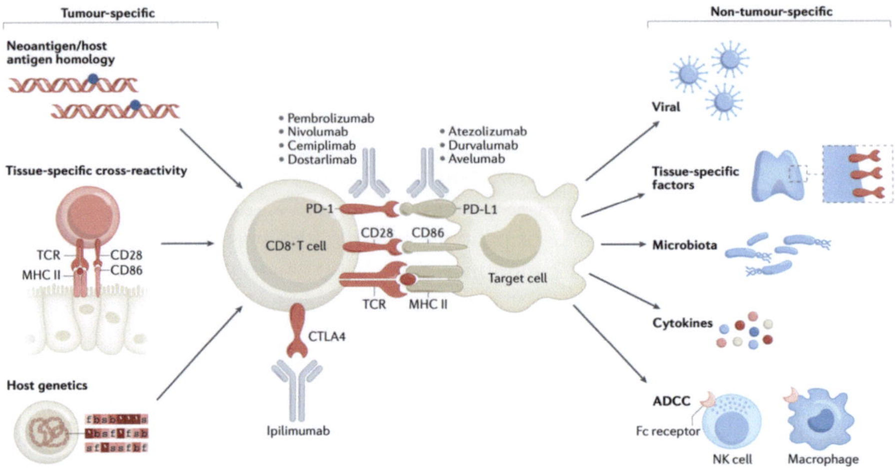

Fig. 6.5 The mechanism of adverse effects associated with ICIs. (Adapted from Johnson [62]. Permission to reuse under Creative Commons CC BY 4.0)

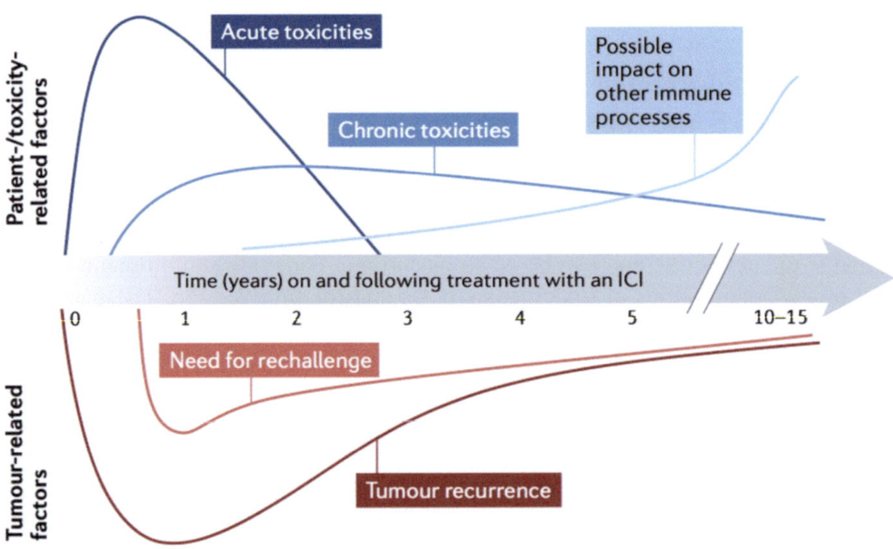

Fig. 6.6 The time course of treatment issues associated with ICIs. (Adapted from Johnson [62]. Permission to reuse under Creative Commons CC BY 4.0)

and small rashes. Bulbous disease also manifests on the extremities and as eruptions on the skin. Stevens–Johnson syndrome also presents rarely, and treatment with high-dose corticosteroids (0.5–1.0 mg/kg/day of prednisone) "is recommended because the mechanism of adverse events involves T-cell immune-directed toxicity." Each of these cutaneous events is associated with distinct histopathological features evidenced by the appearance of inflamed immune cells.

Hypotheses for the mechanism of action of cutaneous AEs include the following:

- The first explanation is that T-cell activation against antigens on normal tissue leads to the release of inflammatory cytokines as a result of immune stimulation and cross-reactivity with normal melanocytes.
- The second explanation is that inflammatory cytokines demonstrate increased release via Th17 activation and immune-related effects associated with antigens in specific tissues and organs.
- The third explanation is the association between specific HLA variants and organ-specific irAEs: "Among cutaneous irAEs, 102 patients with metastatic cancer who received ICIs treatment were significantly associated with HLA-DRB1*11:01 and pruritus (OR = 4.53, X2 1,95 = 9.45, $p < 0.01$)."

A review on the neurological complications of ICI treatment was conducted by Haugh et al. Neurologic events as a result of ICI administration involve either the central nervous system or the peripheral nervous system. Central nervous system neuropathies that are idiopathic are encephalitis, aseptic meningitis, and (uncommonly) multiple sclerosis. Often presenting as an altered mental state, fatigue, headache, and weakness, encephalitis is typically diagnosed with lumbar puncture and treated with inpatient monitoring and IV-administered steroids. Aseptic meningitis and encephalitis come with diagnostic challenges present with similar symptoms. More common with ipilimumab, ICI-related meningitis typically resolves by itself following treatment discontinuation and steroid therapy. ICI rechallenge may be necessary during the monitoring of treatment. PNS involvement includes peripheral neuropathy and myasthenia gravis. Myasthenia gravis, an autoimmune disorder, is a great challenge to diagnose because AChR antibodies are fewer than they are in traditional myasthenia gravis when compared to non-ICI-related myasthenia gravis. Respiratory involvement, life-threatening bulbar, and ocular symptoms such as ptopsis and diplopia are indications of ICI-related myasthenia gravis. A serious complication, a myasthenic crisis requires hospitalization and also frequently requires ventilation. Other guidelines include steroid therapy. The typical timeframe is 29 days of onset, much earlier than the time of onset of other toxicities, namely 61–80 days. The presence of AChR antibodies is highly specific for myasthenia gravis. Myositis, myocarditis, and myasthenia gravis usually present simultaneously, reported in 8% of patients.

Endocrinopathies usually manifest as hypothyroidism in 10% of patients receiving anti-PD-1 therapy and in up to 20% receiving ipi-nivo. Hypophysitis is managed with hydrocortisone 20–30 mg or prednisone 5–7.5 mg daily (as two divided daily doses) and presents with headache, nausea, and diplopia [62].

ICI-associated myocarditis usually presents as cardiac arrhythmia, and the troponin biomarker usually is involved in diagnosis, although 50% of patients lack it. Combination ipilimumab and pembrolizumab is a high-risk factor (4.74 risk) compared with nivolumab alone. Myositis, colitis, and pneumonitis are other AEs that present with ICIs.

Hepatoxicity is a common adverse event associated with ICIs in HCC, which is posited to be due to the loss of T-cell inhibition and T-cell exhaustion due to complement activation and impaired self-tolerance, leading to T-cell-mediated cholangitis, hepatitis, and hepatocyte injury. According to one report, ipilimumab is associated with a higher incidence of immune checkpoint inhibitor–induced hepatotoxicity when compared to nivolumab and pembrolizumab, and when used synergistically, it has higher rates. In the IMBrave150 trial, the "overall incidence of a grade 3/4 increase in ALT and AST was slightly higher in the atezolizumab-bevacizumab group" versus the sorafenib group. Symptoms include fever, nausea, rash, and general malaise, with laboratory elevation of AST, ALT, and alkaline phosphatase [63].

Curkovic and Johnson reiterate many of the common adverse events that present with ICI administration, including cutaneous toxicities, endocrine toxicities, gastrointestinal toxicities, pneumonitis, rheumatological toxicities, and myocarditis. The etiology of ICI adverse events is a result of the mechanism of action of immune checkpoints. PD-1 is expressed on activated T cells, B cells, and myeloid cells, whereas CTLA-4 is expressed on T cells. "CTLA-4 binds to CD80 and prevents interaction between CD80 and the costimulatory receptor CD298 regulating priming of naive T cells while interaction between PD-1 and PD-L1 dampens activity of effector T cells to maintain peripheral tolerance." Checkpoint blockade promotes the loss of self-tolerance and subsequent exposure to self-antigens, which manifest as irAEs, potentially affecting any organ and more commonly occurring in cases of combination therapy and ipilimumab alone rather than monotherapy with anti-PD-1 immunotherapy. As the authors state, identifying "reliable biomarkers to predict which patients will experience severe toxicities remains an urgent need." Cutaneous irAEs include pruritis and dermatitis. One study showed that 76 ICI-treated melanoma patients "experienced a flare," with longer PFS in those patients. In advanced melanoma patients receiving CTLA4 agents, Vitiligo has been associated with survival benefit in patients. Mild inflammatory dermatitis can be treated with topical steroids if it is mild to moderate. Common endocrine toxicities include thyroiditis, insulin-deficient diabetes, hypothyroidism, and primary adrenal insufficiency. The development of hypophysitis when PD-1 agents are administered has significant differences from the hypophysitis that develops due to ipilimumab, which develops as a result of the ectopic expression of CTLA4 on pituitary cells. Adrenal insufficiency that is mild to moderate is treated with steroids. The most common endocrine irAE is thyroiditis; it is most frequently reported with combination PD-1/CTLA4 blockade and may progress to hypothyroidism. Gastrointestinal toxicities present themselves as colitis and diarrhea, are frequently encountered, and can be serious and life-threatening. Mild diarrhea occurs in half of all patients, and severe colitis occurs in 15–20% of patients receiving combination therapy. Mild diarrhea can be managed with agents such as loperamide. ICI therapy is withheld, and corticosteroids are given for grade 2 or higher colitis, with immune suppression in some cases being warranted. Pneumonitis occurs more commonly in PD-1/PD-L1 monotherapy and more frequently in NSCLC and RCC patients. Though it more commonly presents as mild to moderate, it can be fatal and causes the most fatalities. Patients with higher grades should begin corticosteroids and have ICI treatment withheld. Myositis is a rheumatological toxicity that is treated with steroids and can be found in isolation, with myasthenia gravis, or with myocarditis, which doubles the fatality rate. Myocarditis is rare and presents with left ventricular dysfunction, arrythmias, and acute coronary syndromes and presents with congestive heart failure, and it should be monitored when shortness of breath, chest pain, or syncope is presented. Neurological toxicities include peripheral neuropathy, cranial nerve palsy, and myasthenia gravis–like symptoms. They are rare and commonly occur with combination ICI treatment when compared with PD-1 monotherapy. Evaluation includes imaging when encephalitis and meningitis are suspected and management with corticosteroids and immunomodulatory therapies. Hematological toxicities are common and include hemolytic anemia and immune thrombocytopenia, with bone marrow failure, thrombosis, heme irAE spectrum occurring [62].

ICIs are among the first innovative treatments in the immunotherapy field. They have had remarkable outcomes and in the clinical setting have proven invaluable in the treatment of recalcitrant solid tumors, usually associated with poor prognosis. This chapter presents guidelines and demonstrates the unique complexity behind this treatment in terms of the emergence of new checkpoints, mechanisms of action, clinical studies conferring novel roles for older treatments, and adverse events and their management.

References

1. Sharma P, Goswami S, Raychaudhuri D, Siddiqui BA, Singh P, Nagarajan A, et al. Immune checkpoint therapy-current perspectives and future directions. Cell. 2023;186(8):1652–69.
2. Sun Q, Hong Z, Zhang C, Wang L, Han Z, Ma D. Immune checkpoint therapy for solid tumours: clinical dilemmas and future trends. Signal Transduct Target Ther. 2023;8(1):320.
3. Liu Q, Guan Y, Li S. Programmed death receptor (PD-)1/PD-ligand (L)1 in urological cancers: the “all-around warrior” in immunotherapy. Mol Cancer. 2024;23(1):183.
4. Borgeaud M, Sandoval J, Obeid M, Banna G, Michielin O, Addeo A, et al. Novel targets for immune-checkpoint inhibition in cancer. Cancer Treat Rev. 2023;120:102614.
5. Huang X, Zhang X, Li E, Zhang G, Wang X, Tang T, et al. VISTA: an immune regulatory protein checking tumor and immune cells in cancer immunotherapy. J Hematol Oncol. 2020;13(1):83.
6. Noelle RJ, Lines JL, Lewis LD, Martell RE, Guillaudeux T, Lee SW, et al. Clinical and research updates on the VISTA immune checkpoint: immuno-oncology themes and highlights. Front Oncol. 2023;13:1225081.
7. ElTanbouly MA, Schaafsma E, Noelle RJ, Lines JL. VISTA: coming of age as a multi-lineage immune checkpoint. Clin Exp Immunol. 2020;200(2):120–30.
8. Iadonato S, Ovechkina Y, Lustig K, Cross J, Eyde N, Frazier E, et al. A highly potent anti-VISTA antibody KVA12123 - a new immune checkpoint inhibitor and a promising therapy against poorly immunogenic tumors. Front Immunol. 2023;14:1311658.
9. Debien V, De Caluwe A, Wang X, Piccart-Gebhart M, Tuohy VK, Romano E, et al. Immunotherapy in breast cancer: an overview of current strategies and perspectives. NPJ Breast Cancer. 2023;9(1):7.
10. Zhang J, Chadha JS. Developmental therapeutics in metastatic prostate cancer: new targets and new strategies. Cancers (Basel). 2024;16(17):3098.
11. Rios-Hoyo A, Cobain E, Huppert LA, Beitsch PD, Buchholz TA, Esserman L, et al. Neoadjuvant chemotherapy and immunotherapy for estrogen receptor-positive human epidermal growth factor 2-negative breast cancer. J Clin Oncol. 2024;42(22):2632–6.

12. Westin SN, Moore K, Chon HS, Lee JY, Thomes Pepin J, Sundborg M, et al. Durvalumab plus carboplatin/paclitaxel followed by maintenance Durvalumab with or without Olaparib as first-line treatment for advanced endometrial cancer: the phase III DUO-E trial. J Clin Oncol. 2024;42(3):283–99.
13. Sweeney CJ, Hainsworth JD, Bose R, Burris HA, Kurzrock R, Swanton C, et al. MyPathway human epidermal growth factor receptor 2 basket study: Pertuzumab + Trastuzumab treatment of a tissue-agnostic cohort of patients with human epidermal growth factor receptor 2-altered advanced solid tumors. J Clin Oncol. 2024;42(3):258–65.
14. Schenk KM, Deutsch JS, Chandra S, Davar D, Eroglu Z, Khushalani NI, et al. Nivolumab + tacrolimus + prednisone +/− Ipilimumab for kidney transplant recipients with advanced cutaneous cancers. J Clin Oncol. 2024;42(9):1011–20.
15. Luke JJ, Ascierto PA, Khattak MA, de la Cruz Merino L, Del Vecchio M, Rutkowski P, et al. Pembrolizumab versus placebo as adjuvant therapy in resected stage IIB or IIC melanoma: final analysis of distant metastasis-free survival in the phase III KEYNOTE-716 study. J Clin Oncol. 2024;42(14):1619–24.
16. Antoniotti C, Rossini D, Pietrantonio F, Salvatore L, Lonardi S, Tamberi S, et al. Upfront fluorouracil, Leucovorin, Oxaliplatin, and Irinotecan plus bevacizumab with or without Atezolizumab for patients with metastatic colorectal cancer: updated and overall survival results of the ATEZOTRIBE study. J Clin Oncol. 2024;42(22):2637–44.
17. Negron-Figueroa D, Colbert LE. Mechanisms by which the Intratumoral microbiome may potentiate immunotherapy response. J Clin Oncol. 2024;42(28):3350–2.
18. Tannir_CheckMate 214.pdf.
19. Sangro B, Galle PR, Kelley RK, Charoentum C, De Toni EN, Ostapenko Y, et al. Patient-reported outcomes from the phase III HIMALAYA study of Tremelimumab plus Durvalumab in Unresectable hepatocellular carcinoma. J Clin Oncol. 2024;42(23):2790–9.
20. Kawazoe A, Xu RH, Garcia-Alfonso P, Passhak M, Teng HW, Shergill A, et al. Lenvatinib plus Pembrolizumab versus standard of Care for Previously Treated Metastatic Colorectal Cancer: final analysis of the randomized, open-label, phase III LEAP-017 study. J Clin Oncol. 2024;42(24):2918–27.
21. Chen EX, Loree JM, Titmuss E, Jonker DJ, Kennecke HF, Berry S, et al. Liver metastases and immune checkpoint inhibitor efficacy in patients with refractory metastatic colorectal cancer: a secondary analysis of a randomized clinical trial. JAMA Netw Open. 2023;6(12):e2346094.
22. Amaria RN, Postow M, Burton EM, Tetzlaff MT, Ross MI, Torres-Cabala C, et al. Neoadjuvant relatlimab and nivolumab in resectable melanoma. Nature. 2022;611(7934):155–60.
23. Dzienis M, Cundom J, Fuentes CS, Spreafico A, Nordlinger M, Pastor AV, et al. Pembrolizumab plus carboplatin and paclitaxel as first-line therapy for recurrent/metastatic head and neck squamous cell carcinoma (KEYNOTE-B10): a single-arm phase IV trial. J Clin Oncol. 2024;42(25):2989–99.
24. Apolo AB, Girardi DM, Niglio SA, Nadal R, Kydd AR, Simon N, et al. Final results from a phase I trial and expansion cohorts of Cabozantinib and Nivolumab alone or with Ipilimumab for advanced/metastatic genitourinary tumors. J Clin Oncol. 2024;42(25):3033–46.
25. Cannon TL, Rothe M, Mangat PK, Garrett-Mayer E, Chiu VK, Hwang J, et al. Pertuzumab plus Trastuzumab in patients with biliary tract cancer with ERBB2/3 alterations: results from the targeted agent and profiling utilization registry study. J Clin Oncol. 2024;42(27):3228–37.
26. Xia F, Wang Y, Wang H, Shen L, Xiang Z, Zhao Y, et al. Randomized phase II trial of immunotherapy-based Total Neoadjuvant therapy for proficient mismatch repair or microsatellite stable locally advanced rectal cancer (TORCH). J Clin Oncol. 2024;42(28):3308–18.
27. Cabanillas ME, Dadu R, Ferrarotto R, Gule-Monroe M, Liu S, Fellman B, et al. Anti-programmed death ligand 1 plus targeted therapy in anaplastic thyroid carcinoma: a nonrandomized clinical trial. JAMA Oncol. 2024;10(12):1672–80.
28. Sun L, Cohen RB, D'Avella CA, Singh AP, Schoenfeld JD, Hanna GJ. Overall survival, treatment duration, and Rechallenge outcomes with ICI therapy for recurrent or metastatic HNSCC. JAMA Netw Open. 2024;7(8):e2428526.

29. Moran JA, Adams DL, Edelman MJ, Lopez P, He J, Qiao Y, et al. Monitoring PD-L1 expression on circulating tumor-associated cells in recurrent metastatic non-small-cell lung carcinoma predicts response to immunotherapy with radiation therapy. JCO Precis Oncol. 2022;6:e2200457.
30. Cook S, Samuel V, Meyers DE, Stukalin I, Litt I, Sangha R, et al. Immune-related adverse events and survival among patients with metastatic NSCLC treated with immune checkpoint inhibitors. JAMA Netw Open. 2024;7(1):e2352302.
31. van Not OJ, Blokx WAM, van den Eertwegh AJM, de Meza MM, Haanen JB, Blank CU, et al. BRAF and NRAS mutation status and response to checkpoint inhibition in advanced melanoma. JCO Precis Oncol. 2022;6:e2200018.
32. Mangla A, Lee C, Mirsky MM, Wang M, Rothermel LD, Hoehn R, et al. Neoadjuvant dual checkpoint inhibitors vs anti-PD1 therapy in high-risk Resectable melanoma: a pooled analysis. JAMA Oncol. 2024;10(5):612–20.
33. Dowlati A, Abbas A, Chan T, Henick B, Wang X, Doshi P, et al. Immune checkpoint blockade outcome in small-cell lung cancer and its relationship with retinoblastoma mutation status and function. JCO Precis Oncol. 2022;6:e2200257.
34. Kawachi H, Yamada T, Tamiya M, Negi Y, Goto Y, Nakao A, et al. Concomitant proton pump inhibitor use with Pembrolizumab monotherapy vs immune checkpoint inhibitor plus chemotherapy in patients with non-small cell lung cancer. JAMA Netw Open. 2023;6(7):e2322915.
35. Neal J, Pavlakis N, Kim SW, Goto Y, Lim SM, Mountzios G, et al. CONTACT-01: a randomized phase III trial of Atezolizumab + Cabozantinib versus docetaxel for metastatic non-small cell lung cancer after a checkpoint inhibitor and chemotherapy. J Clin Oncol. 2024;42(20):2393–403.
36. Stecklein SR, Barlow W, Pusztai L, Timms K, Kennedy R, Logan GE, et al. Dual prognostic classification of triple-negative breast cancer by DNA damage immune response and homologous recombination deficiency. JCO Precis Oncol. 2023;7:e2300197.
37. Loi S, Salgado R, Schmid P, Cortes J, Cescon DW, Winer EP, et al. Association between biomarkers and clinical outcomes of Pembrolizumab monotherapy in patients with metastatic triple-negative breast cancer: KEYNOTE-086 exploratory analysis. JCO Precis Oncol. 2023;7:e2200317.
38. Chehrazi-Raffle A, Muddasani R, Dizman N, Hsu J, Meza L, Zengin ZB, et al. Ultrasensitive circulating tumor DNA pilot study distinguishes complete response and partial response with immunotherapy in patients with metastatic renal cell carcinoma. JCO Precis Oncol. 2023;7:e2200543.
39. Sanz-Garcia E, Genta S, Chen X, Ou Q, Araujo DV, Abdul Razak AR, et al. Tumor-naive circulating tumor DNA as an early response biomarker for patients treated with immunotherapy in early phase clinical trials. JCO Precis Oncol. 2023;7:e2200509.
40. Chen M, Wang Z, Liu Z, Deng T, Wang X, Chang Z, et al. PD-1/PD-L1 inhibitor plus chemotherapy versus PD-1/PD-L1 inhibitor in microsatellite instability gastrointestinal cancers: a multicenter retrospective study. JCO Precis Oncol. 2023;7:e2200463.
41. Robertson BM, Fane ME, Weeraratna AT, Rebecca VW. Determinants of resistance and response to melanoma therapy. Nat Cancer. 2024;5(7):964–82.
42. Passaro A, Attili I, de Marinis F. Neoadjuvant chemotherapy plus immunotherapy in early-stage Resectable non-small-cell lung cancer. J Clin Oncol. 2022;40(25):2871–7.
43. Quintanilha JCF, Storandt MH, Graf RP, Li G, Keller R, Lin DI, et al. Tumor mutational burden in real-world patients with pancreatic cancer: genomic alterations and predictive value for immune checkpoint inhibitor effectiveness. JCO Precis Oncol. 2023;7:e2300092.
44. Chakrabarti S, Mahipal A. Circulating tumor DNA-guided recurrence risk assessment in esophageal and gastric cancer: assay holds the key. JCO Precis Oncol. 2023;7:e2200710.
45. Jang A, Lanka SM, Jaeger EB, Lieberman A, Huang M, Sartor AO, et al. Longitudinal monitoring of circulating tumor DNA to assess the efficacy of immune checkpoint inhibitors in patients with advanced genitourinary malignancies. JCO Precis Oncol. 2023;7:e2300131.

46. Zhou T, Chen H, Wang Y, Wen S, Dao P, Chen M. Key molecules in bladder cancer affect patient prognosis and immunotherapy efficacy: further exploration for CNTN1 and EMP1. JCO Precis Oncol. 2023;7:e2200630.
47. Hinterleitner C, Strahle J, Malenke E, Hinterleitner M, Henning M, Seehawer M, et al. Platelet PD-L1 reflects collective intratumoral PD-L1 expression and predicts immunotherapy response in non-small cell lung cancer. Nat Commun. 2021;12(1):7005.
48. Davies D, Kamdar S, Woolf R, Zlatareva I, Iannitto ML, Morton C, et al. PD-1 defines a distinct, functional, tissue-adapted state in Vdelta1(+) T cells with implications for cancer immunotherapy. Nat Cancer. 2024;5(3):420–32.
49. Amoozgar Z, Kloepper J, Ren J, Tay RE, Kazer SW, Kiner E, et al. Targeting Treg cells with GITR activation alleviates resistance to immunotherapy in murine glioblastomas. Nat Commun. 2021;12(1):2582.
50. Yang K, Halima A, Chan TA. Antigen presentation in cancer – mechanisms and clinical implications for immunotherapy. Nat Rev Clin Oncol. 2023;20(9):604–23.
51. Mei Y, Wang X, Zhang J, Liu D, He J, Huang C, et al. Siglec-9 acts as an immune-checkpoint molecule on macrophages in glioblastoma, restricting T-cell priming and immunotherapy response. Nat Cancer. 2023;4(9):1273–91.
52. Chen Y, Du C, Shen S, Zhang W, Shan Y, Lyu A, et al. Toripalimab plus bevacizumab as first-line treatment for advanced hepatocellular carcinoma: a prospective, multicenter, single-arm, Phase II Trial. Clin Cancer Res. 2024;30(14):2937–44.
53. Finn RS, Ryoo BY, Hsu CH, Li D, Burgoyne AM, Cotter C, et al. Tiragolumab in combination with atezolizumab and bevacizumab in patients with unresectable, locally advanced or metastatic hepatocellular carcinoma (MORPHEUS-liver): a randomised, open-label, phase 1b-2, study. Lancet Oncol. 2025;26(2):214–26.
54. Li J, Bai Y, Chen Z, Ying J, Guo Y, Fang W, et al. SAFFRON-104: a phase Ib/II study of sitravatinib alone or with tislelizumab in advanced hepatocellular carcinoma and gastric cancer/gastroesophageal junction cancer. Cancer Immunol Immunother. 2024;73(11):219.
55. Melero I, Yau T, Kang YK, Kim TY, Santoro A, Sangro B, et al. Nivolumab plus ipilimumab combination therapy in patients with advanced hepatocellular carcinoma previously treated with sorafenib: 5-year results from CheckMate 040. Ann Oncol. 2024;35(6):537–48.
56. Akula V, Chen L, Acikgoz Y, Klein K, Yavuz BG, Cevik L, et al. Neoadjuvant immune checkpoint inhibitors for hepatocellular carcinoma. NPJ Precis Oncol. 2025;9(1):60.
57. Childs A, Aidoo-Micah G, Maini MK, Meyer T. Immunotherapy for hepatocellular carcinoma. JHEP Rep. 2024;6(10):101130.
58. Maiorano BA, Di Maio M, Cerbone L, Maiello E, Procopio G, Roviello G, et al. Significance of PD-L1 in metastatic urothelial carcinoma treated with immune checkpoint inhibitors: a systematic review and meta-analysis. JAMA Netw Open. 2024;7(3):e241215.
59. Liu D, Wang L, Guo Y. Advances in and prospects of immunotherapy for prostate cancer. Cancer Lett. 2024;601:217155.
60. Wu Z, Zhang J, Li L, Wang Z, Yang C. Biomarkers in metastatic castration-resistant prostate cancer for efficiency of immune checkpoint inhibitors. Ann Med. 2025;57(1):2426755.
61. Isaacsson Velho P, Bastos DA, Saint'ana PT, Rigatti B, da Costa ET, Muniz DQB, et al. Nivolumab in patients with metastatic castration-resistant prostate cancer with and without DNA repair defects. Clin Cancer Res. 2024;30(23):5342–52.
62. Curkovic NB, Johnson DB. Updates in toxicities associated with immune checkpoint inhibitors. Expert Rev Clin Immunol. 2023;19(9):1117–29.
63. Ruli TM Jr, Pollack ED, Lodh A, Evers CD 3rd, Price CA, Shoreibah M. Immune checkpoint inhibitors in hepatocellular carcinoma and their hepatic-related side effects: a review. Cancers (Basel). 2024;16(11):2042.

Chapter 7
Bispecific Antibodies and Immune Cell Engagers

Bispecific antibodies (BsAbs), also called bispecific T-cell engagers, are constructed from fragments (Fc and Fab), merging CD3 and CD19 epitopes to direct cytotoxic T cells to cancer cells [1]. Specific BsAbs or BiTEs form a distinct class of immunotherapies to treat hematologic malignancies such as acute lymphoblastic leukemia, non-Hodgkin lymphoma (NHL), multiple myeloma, and acute myeloid leukemia. Emerging treatments are actively being investigated and developed for solid tumors in preclinical models, and some have been approved by the US Food and Drug Administration (FDA) [2].

Bispecific antibodies have a unique mechanism of action with their clinical efficacy and favorable toxicity profiles resulting from low immunogenicity and MHC-independent cytotoxic activity as a result of their construction. An FDA-approved BsAb is blinatumomab for B-cell Ph+ ALL, and recent clinical data for the B-cell maturation antigen (BMCA)–directed teclistamab for multiple myeloma have emerged. Unlike CAR T-cell therapies, which require a complex manufacturing process, bispecific T-cell engagers are produced through an off-the-shelf allogeneic process. CD16a is an epitope that serves as the target for natural killer (NK)–redirected cell engagers. Also under preclinical study and clinical development are other types of bispecific engagers, such as innate immune cell engagers (including NK cell engagers), armed engagers, and T-cell-secreting engagers. Neurotoxicity and cytokine release syndrome (CRS) are serious adverse events (AEs) resulting from the administration of bispecific antibodies in the clinic [2] (Table 7.1).

P. Hays, *Personalized Medicine in Oncology*,
https://doi.org/10.1007/978-3-032-14437-9_7

Table 7.1 Prophylaxis and the management of toxicities from bispecific antibodies

Category	Recommendations	Comments
Cytokine release syndrome	Grade 1—acetaminophen +/– tocilizumab or dexamethasone Grade ≥ 2—tocilizumab or dexamethasone, supportive care CRS refractory to tocilizumab and dexamethasone—recommend anakinra Additional options*: high-dose steroids, siltuximab, etanercept, sarilumab, ruxolitinib, cyclophosphamide, etoposide, and emapalumab	Tocilizumab 8 mg IV Dexamethasone 10 mgPO//IV Anakinra 100–200 mg PO Q8H
Immune effector cell–associated neurotoxicity syndrome (ICANS)	Grade 1—supportive care, dexamethasone if prolonged Grade 2—dexamethasone, neurologic evaluation Grade ≥ 3 or refractory grade 2 ICANS—dexamethasone, neurologic evaluation, consider anakinra and antiseizure prophylaxis, escalate steroids to methylprednisolone 1 g BID for 1–3 days	Dexamethasone 10 mgPO//IV Q6H Anakinra 100–200 mg PO Q8H
Neutropenia	Filgrastim for ANC < 1000 Avoid during step-up dose(s) and during active CRS/ICANS	
Anemia	Transfusions as needed for Hgb < 7 or symptomatic Consider the use of ESAs for persistent Hgb < 10	
Thrombocytopenia	Use transfusions as needed for Plt < 10 or symptomatic Consider use of TPO-mimetics for persistent high-grade thrombocytopenia	
Hypogammaglobulinemia	Recommend primary infectious prophylaxis with IVIG 0.4 mg/kg q 3–4 weeks May need to delay initiation of IVIG in the setting of high burden IgG myeloma to avoid hyperviscosity	
Infection Prevention	HSV/VZV—prophylaxis with acyclovir or valacyclovir HBV—in patients at risk for reactivation, prophylaxis with entecavir or tenofovir alafenamide PJP—prophylaxis with trimethoprim/ sulfamethoxazole, dapsone, atovaquone, or pentamidine Up-to-date on vaccinations—annual influenza, COVID-19, pneumococcus, VZV, RSV	Influenza—consider 2 doses 1 month apart given impaired immunologic response

Adapted from Pan and Richter [31]

7.1 The Properties of Bispecific Engagers

Bispecific engagers (Figs 7.1 and 7.2) are distinguished from monoclonal antibodies by being engineered constructs that have one binding site that recognizes a tumor-associated antigen and an immune effector cell that consists of an activating cell surface. Their development was closely related to their immunogenicity in that murine-derived constructs evaluated in preclinical models had increased immunogenicity. Humanized constructs led to decreased immunogenicity and allowed for the clinical translation of bispecific engagers. The Fc fragment conferred a unique pharmacokinetic profile and mechanism of action, whereas engagers lacking this domain are smaller, use a single chain variable fragment (scFv), and have shorter half-lives. Fc-mediated responses mimic the cytotoxicity of monospecific antibodies, and those lacking this fragment initiate immune-mediated cytolytic responses between the cancer cell and immune cell and lead to the release of perforin and granzyme B. Bispecific engager designs are based on antigen selection in choosing antigens present on the tumor cell but not healthy cells, maximizing cytolytic activity and limiting on-target and off-target toxicity [2].

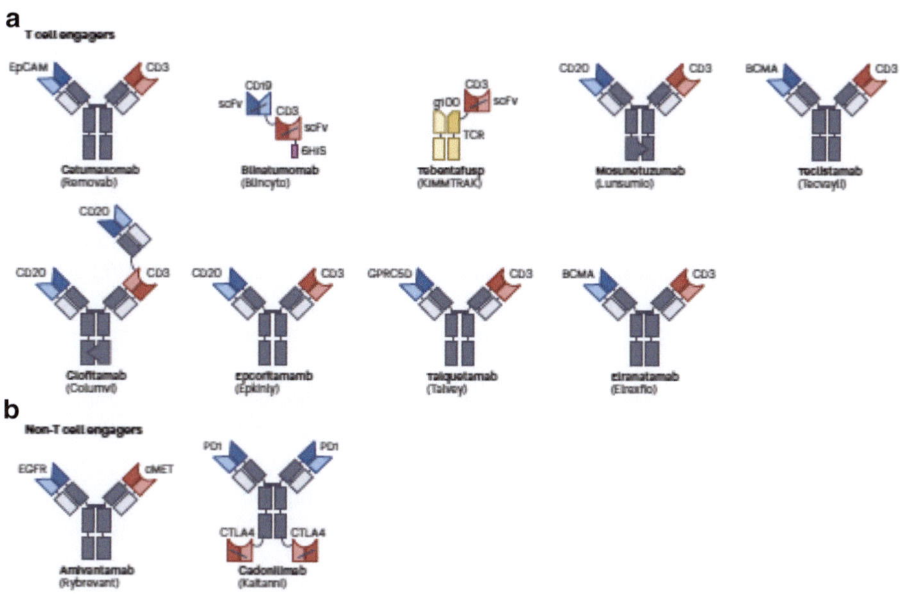

Fig. 7.1 (**a**) T-cell engagers and (**b**) non-T-cell engagers. (Adapted from Klein [32])

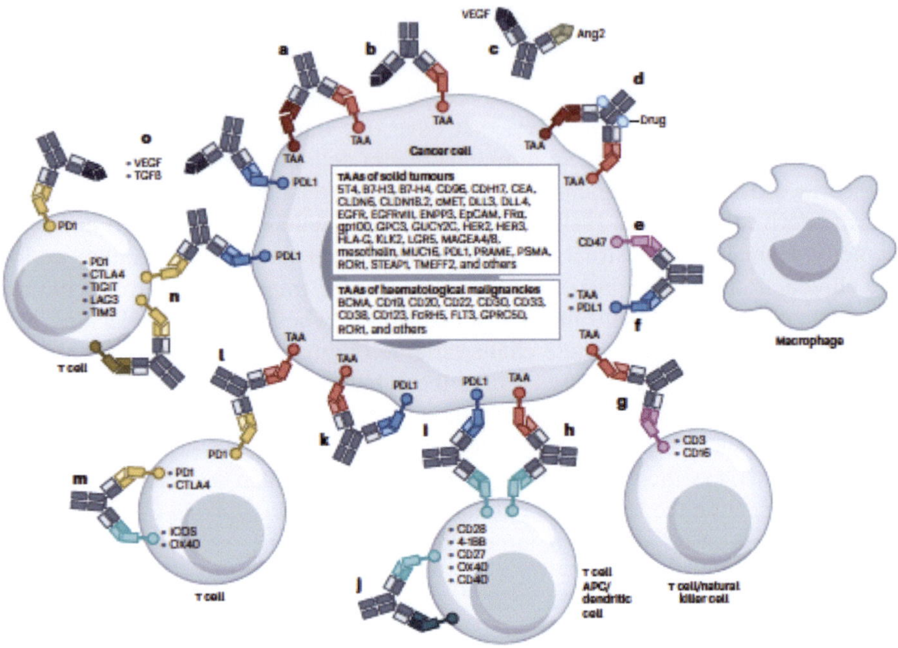

Fig. 7.2 Bispecific antibodies undergoing clinical trials. (Adapted from Klein [32])

7.2 Hematologic Malignancies

Natural killer (NK) cells are innate immune cells having both stimulatory and inhibitory receptors that lead to the tumor-directed specificity of cytolytic activity in that healthy cells have inhibitory receptors, whereas tumor cells possess stimulatory receptors. BiKEs, TriKEs, and TetraKEs have been generated in this context.

According to Epperly et al., NK engagers in hematological malignancies that focus on CD19 and CD22 B-cell malignancies and CD33, CLEC12A (or two antigens CD19 × CD22 × CD16), MDS, and AML have been investigated in preclinical and clinical studies and have shown activity in acute lymphoblastic leukemia (ALL) and chronic lymphocytic leukemia (CLL) through direct CD16 signaling [2].

Ongoing phase I and phase II studies evaluating NK cell engagers include GTB-3550, a CD33 × CD16 × IL15 TriKE, and the TriKE involving the CLEC12A antigen for AML. Hodgkin lymphoma patients demonstrated a favorable safety profile for the single-agent AFM13, a CD30 × CD16 NK cell engager, and when combined with pembrolizumab, has entered phase II studies. Multiple myeloma (MM) showed preclinical antitumor responses when administered CS1 × NKG2D and BCMA × NKG2D bispecific antibodies, also mediated through NK cell activation. AML/MDS has shown responses to CD33 × XCD16 NK cell engagers with antitumor activity that improved with the addition of IL15. An NKG2D receptor against a CD19 target has also been constructed [2].

Another category of bispecific engagers under development and evaluation for hematological malignances are T-cell-secreting bispecific engagers. Created from lentiviral or retroviral transduction or the electroporation of RNA encoding the bispecific engager, and after expansion and evaluation, the infused construct allows for the constant exposure of the small molecule secreted by T cells without the need for continuous infusion. The small molecules generated have longer half-lives and lead to a local inflammatory response at the site of action. Both the secreting antibody T cells and the augmenting bystander T cells are involved in the antitumor response and have shown in vivo and in vitro cytolytic activity in CD19XCD3 ALL and CD123XCD3 AML with limited systemic toxicity. One limitation of this technology is its lack of costimulation, which typically characterizes CAR T-cell therapy and is overcome through the expression of the CD28 or 4-1BB56 costimulatory ligands on T cells for improved antitumor response that prevents the dampening of the antitumor response. An example of T-cell-secreting bispecific engagers has been observed in AML models, where a "dual antigen-specific effect" was generated through "T cells secreting a CLEC12A × CD3 engager, [which] was enhanced by the addition of a chimeric CD123. IL7Rα receptor, with a dual antigen-specific effect" [2].

7.3 Multiple Myeloma

7.3.1 Teclistamab

Teclistamab is a bispecific T-cell engager that targets CD3 antigen on T cells and BCMA on multiple myeloma cells. The relapsed or refractory (R/R) multiple myeloma standard of care includes immunomodulatory agent, proteasome inhibitors, and anti-CD38 monoclonal antibody.

Prior to teclistamab's evaluation in the MajesTEC-1 trials for demonstrating the efficacy of the agent for R/R multiple myeloma, Mateos et al. conducted a long-term follow-up study on teclistamab in which four trials of daratumumab were analyzed for comparison: the APOLLO (daratumumab and pomalidomide and dexamethasone versus pomalidomide and dexamethasone alone), CASTOR (daratumumab and bortezomib plus dexamethasone vs. bortezomib plus dexamethasone alone), EQUULEUS (daratumumab and other combinations), and POLLUX (daratumumab and lenalidomide plus dexamethasone vs. lenalidomide plus dexamethasone alone) trials on triple-class exposed relapsed or refractory multiple myeloma (RRMM). The study authors showed that teclistamab was superior to physician's choice of therapy in triple-class exposed RRMM patients through an indirect comparison involving a comparative efficacy analysis. Outcomes were ORR, OS, PFS, and very good partial response (VGPR) or better.

7.3.1.1 Key Results

- The primary analysis of comparative effectiveness revealed that patients receiving teclistamab were 2.41 times more likely to have an objective response and 5.56 times more likely to have a ≥ VGPR versus physician's choice with ORR, with the rate of ≥ VGPR being significantly greater with teclistamab than with physician's choice.
- Median OS was 18.3 months with teclistamab and 9.4 months (HR 0.54; (95% CI 0.40–0.73)) with physician's choice.
- Median PFS was 11.3 months with teclistamab and 5.7 months (HR 0.59 (95% CI 0.46–0.78)) with physician's choice.

The study authors concluded that when comparing clinical outcomes between teclistamab and physician's choice, teclistamab demonstrated a statistically significant improvement in effectiveness. ORR was 63%versus 26.2% for teclistamab and physician's choice, respectively, and the rates of very good partial response were similarly higher among patients receiving teclistamab (58.8% vs. 10.6%) [3].

On the basis of the MajesTEC-1 study, teclistamab was approved for RRMM as an off-the-shelf BCMAXCD3 bispecific antibody with deep, durable, and rapid responses after a median follow-up of 14.1 months.

- ORR: 63%
- CR rate: 39%
- Median DOR: 18.4 months
- Median PFS: 11.3 months

With a cohort of 165 patients and a median follow-up of 22 months, a CR of 43%, an mDOR of 24 months (95% CI 16.2–not estimable (NE)), an mOS of 21.9 months (95% CI 16.0–NE), and an mPFS of 12.5 months (95% CI 8.8–17.2) were achieved. Adverse events included hematologic ones (neutropenia (72% versus 65%); lymphopenia (35% versus 33%); and thrombocytopenia (42% versus 22%)) and infections (78%, 52% grade 3/4; COVID-19 infections (27%), other viral infections (10%), fungal infections (5%), and respiratory infections (56%)). Furthermore, 72% of patients experienced CRS: 0.6% were grade 3, none were grade 4/5, and five patients reported nine immune effector cell–associated neurotoxicity syndrome (ICANS) events, all grade 1.2 and resolved. Six treatment-related deaths occurred, and three were due to COVID-19; five (3%) patients reported nine ICANS events (all grade 1/2 and all resolved) [4].

In 2022, a phase 1/2 study enrolled R/R patients after three therapy lines.

7.3.1.2 Key Results

- Of the 165 patients who received teclistamab, 77.6% had triple-class refractory disease and a median of five previous lines of therapy.

- ORR was 63% with 65 patients (39.4%) having a CR at a median follow-up of 14.1 months.
- And 44 patients (26.7%) experienced minimal residual disease (MRD) negativity.

Teclistamab received FDA approval in 2022 for patients receiving four lines of therapy; soluble BCMA was the biomarker for tumor burden. Serum levels were found to decrease in responders, and an 82% reduction was seen in 27 patients with sCR and an 87% reduction in eight patients experiencing complete response (CR). Soluble BCMA served as the biomarker for tumor burden for response. Dosing is initial SC injection at 0.03 mg/kg on day 1 and increased to 1.5 mg/kg on day 5 after receiving corticosteroids for CRS, neurotoxicity, infectious diseases, and hematologic disease prophylaxis. Treatment discontinuation occurs with disease progression or unacceptable toxicity [5].

7.3.2 *Erlanatamab*

In the ongoing phase 2 MagnestiMM-3 study, an open-label, single-arm, multicenter trial enrolling RRMM refractory patients with measurable disease according to the International Myeloma Working Group using one proteasome inhibitor, one immunomodulatory drug, and one anti-CD38 antibody, erlanatamab, a humanized BCMA-CD3 BsAb, was found to be a novel agent. In this trial, 97 patients constituted the primary efficacy population with at least four lines of prior therapy. Key results included an ORR of 57.7% at the recommended dose at a median follow-up of 11.1 months among responders, mDOR not reached (NR), and a DOR rate at 12 months of 75.3% and PFS at 12 months of 56.6% [6].

According to a study published in *Nature Medicine*, patients subcutaneously received the agent once weekly after six cycles; a durable, deep response was observed in cohort A ($n = 123$), who did not receive any prior BCMA-directed treatment, with 50 responders switching to biweekly dosing. ORR served as the primary endpoint and was reported at 61.0% (75/123 (95% CI 51.8–69.6)), as well as a 35% CR rate with a maintenance period of 6 months consistent across high-risk subgroups, including cytogenetics and 50% bone marrow plasma cells at baseline. A VGPR of 56.1% was also shown and nine patients (7.3%) achieved CR while remaining on treatment. The time to response to DOR, PFS, OS, and MRD negativity served as the secondary endpoints. Adverse events included grade 3–4 CRS (57.7%), infections (69.9%, 39.8%), and hematologic side effects such as anemia (48.8%, 37.4%) and neutropenia (48.8%, 48.8%), with higher grade events experienced when patients switched to biweekly dosing. PFS and OS were not reached after a median follow-up of 14.7 months (range, 0.2–25.1 months). Of the patients who achieved CR, 89.7% were MRD negative and "were evaluable for MRD (n = 29), corresponding to 60.5% of patients with ≥ CR." The study authors concluded that a deep and durable response was elicited for elranatamab with a good safety profile and that elranatamab induced deep and durable responses with a manageable safety profile. "Switching to biweekly dosing may improve long-term safety without compromising efficacy" [7].

MagnetisMM-5 was a phase 3, open-label clinical trial conducted to confirm the antitumor activity and tumor regression of preclinical studies, and the ongoing (at the time) phase 1 MagnetisMM-1 study also evaluated subcutaneous (SC) elranatamab as monotherapy versus in combination with SC daratumumab in RRMM who received proteasome inhibitor and lenalidomide. MagnetisMM-5 was proposed to determine guidelines for optimal dosing for the priming duration (14 d) and the first cycle (28 d) of the subcutaneous administration of the combination therapy and dose-limiting toxicities in the first part.

The study consisted of a second part in which patient stratification would occur, where 450 patients were grouped in a 1:1:1 ratio to receive elranatamb SC or SC elranatamab+ SC daratumumab or SC daratumumab + oral pomalidomide + oral dexamethasone "by prior lines of therapy (1 vs 2–3 vs ≥ 4) and prior treatment with anti-CD38 therapy (yes vs no)." PFS according to International Myeloma Working Group (IMWG) response criteria and PFS according to investigator assessment served as the primary and secondary endpoints, respectively. OS, CR rates, DOR, the duration of CR, the time to response, MRD rates, safety profiles, quality of life, immunogenicity, and the evaluation of pharmacokinetics were reported as secondary endpoints for subsequent evaluation [8].

Elranatamab for RRMM patients was granted approval with the following dosing schedule: "'step-up dose 1' of 12 mg on Day 1, 'step-up dose 2' of 32 mg on Day 4, followed by the first treatment dose of 76 mg on Day 8, and then 76 mg weekly, thereafter, through week 24," with a dose interval transition to a 2-week schedule continued until unacceptable toxicity and disease progression [6].

7.3.3 Linvoseltamab

Linvoseltamab, a BCMA-CD3 bispecific antibody, was evaluated in the LINKER-1MM trial in RRMM patients who had received proteosome inhibitor, anti-CD38 antibody, and an immunomodulatory drug. Patients had progressed on these prior lines of therapy. In this phase I/II trial, 117 MM patients receiving a 200 mg dose were enrolled, of whom 39% had high-risk cytogenetics and 28% penta-refractory disease. The clinical outcomes were positive, with ORR being 71% and with 50% achieving CR. For patients receiving a 50 mg dose, the ORR was 48%, with 21% achieving CR. Hematologic side effects such as anemia (3.4% grade 1, 4.3% grade 2, and 30.8% grade 3) and neutropenia (0.9% grade 2, 18.8% grade 3, and 23.1% grade 4) were the most common, along with incidences of CRS and immune effector-associated neurotoxicity syndrome, occurring in 7.7% of patients; mostly grade 1 infections were reported in 74.4% of patients. The authors concluded that at the 200 mg dose, patients experienced deep, durable responses and had an mDOR of 29.4 months, with tolerable safety profiles representing another option for MM treatment. The authors also suggested that CAR T-cell therapy could be considered an optimal approach in sequential treatment [9].

7.3.4 *Talquetamab*

Talquetamab is a bispecific T-cell engager directed toward G-protein coupled receptor (GPRC5D), an orphan receptor expressed in malignant plasma cells. The agent's toxicity profile (the primary endpoint) and clinical response were evaluated in a study by Chari et al., reported in *NEJM* as a phase 2 study; also, in heavily pretreated multiple myeloma patients (six lines of prior therapy); grade 1 or 2 CRS (70% and 80% of patients) and skin-related reactions (63% and 57%) developed from SC doses of 405 μg per kilogram weekly (30 patients) and 800 μg per kilogram every other week (44 patients), respectively, which were the most common side effects. However, the one dose-limiting toxicity of a grade 3 rash was reported in a patient at the 800-μg dose level. Supportive therapy and "tocilizumab [were] administered to 63% of the patients who had received talquetamab at the 405-μg dose level and to 54% of those who had received it at the 800-μg dose level" for managing side effects. Moreover, 70% of the responses (21/30) were observed in the cohort receiving a dosage of 405 ug/kg every 2 weeks and 64% (28/44) in the cohort receiving a dosage of 800 ug/kg every 2 weeks. The detection of mRNA GPRC3D served as a biomarker of response, being variable in skin samples. The authors concluded that potential delays, attrition, and burden, which are associated with CAR T-cell therapy, could be avoided with talquetamab treatment, leading to responses in patients typically exhibiting poor response to other previous T-cell-redirecting BCMA targets [10].

After FDA and European Medicines Agency approval of talquetamab at the recommended dosages, a comparative effectiveness study was reported in *CLML* that showed that talquetamab after indirect treatment comparisons was superior to real-world treatment options ($n = 1169$), including triple-class exposed patients, according to data culled from a deidentified database (Flatiron Health).

7.3.4.1 Dosing and Administration Schedules

Dosing Cohort	mPFS	mOS	TTNT
0.4 mg/kg QW	7.5 (95% CI 5.72–9.43), HR 0.56	Not reached	> 4.0 months
RW	4.0 (95% CI 3.52–4.57), > 3.5 months	16.8 (13.9–22.3) months	> 8.2 months

Note: median progression-free survival (mPFS); median overall survival (mOS); time to next treatment (TTNT) every one week (QW; real world (RW)

However, after adjustment, mOS showed no improvement (NR for each cohort) in comparison to the mOS in the RW cohort: "16.5 months in the RW cohort vs. NR in the talquetamab 0.4 mg/kg QW cohort and 15.9 months in the RW cohort vs. NR in the talquetamab 0.8 mg/kg Q2W cohort." The study authors stated that the single-arm MonumenTAL-1 trial was potentially limited due to lower incidences of extramedullary disease (which serve as a prognostic factor) and unavailable CR rates as a result of prior treatment and might be a factor in their analysis, and on the basis of these results, talquetamab was shown to be superior and clinically meaningful for RRMM patients when compared to the standard of care [11].

7.3.5 Teclistamab–Talquetamab Combination Treatment

Dose-limiting toxicities for treatments administered subcutaneously, adverse events, and the initial efficacy of the combination treatment of approved teclistamab and approved talquetamab bispecific antibodies that both target CD3 on T cells, leading to cytotoxic activity in triple-class exposed RRMM, were shown in a recent phase 1b-2 study published by *NEJM* in 2025. Phase 1 consisted of dose escalation (five levels in 28-day cycles), and phase 2 consisted of talquetamab at 0.8 mg per kilogram body weight plus teclistamab at a dose of 3.0 mg per kilogram every other week. The total cohort was 94 patients, and 44 patients received phase 2 dosing, with a median follow-up of 20.3 months.

The five dose levels of talquetamab plus teclistamab that were investigated are as follows:

- Talquetamab at 0.2 mg per kilogram plus teclistamab at 0.75 mg per kilogram weekly (dose level 1)
- Talquetamab at 0.2 mg per kilogram plus teclistamab at 1.5 mg per kilogram weekly (dose level 2)
- Talquetamab at 0.4 mg per kilogram plus teclistamab at 1.5 mg per kilogram weekly (dose level 3)
- Talquetamab at 0.8 mg per kilogram plus teclistamab at 1.5 mg per kilogram every 2 weeks (dose level 4)
- Talquetamab at 0.8 mg per kilogram plus teclistamab at 3.0 mg per kilogram every 2 weeks (dose level 5)
- Dose level 5 selected as the recommended phase 2 regimen

The phase 1 endpoint was dose-limiting toxicity, and ORR was the secondary endpoint, along with the evaluation of likely long-term responders.

7.3.5.1 Key Results

- The most common AEs were CRS, dysgeusia, neutropenia, and skin events, with grade 3 or 4 being hematologic side effects (96%) and infections (64%). Cycle delays or dose adjustments (87 or 93%) primarily due to infections occurred in 68% of patients. Dose-limiting toxicities were reported in three patients, including grade 4 thrombocytopenia ($n = 1$).

- Dose-limiting toxic effects occurred at doses of 0.2 mg of talquetamab and 0.75 mg of teclistamab ($n = 3$; oral herpes and increased ALT and AST) and at Recommended Phase 2 Dosage (RP2D) (grade 4 thrombocytopenia).
- Discontinuation as a result of one or both agents due to adverse events occurred in 15 patients; these adverse events were investigator related in 7% of cases and also due to infections.

In this study, 14 patients (15%) died due primarily to infections such as pneumonia, COVID-19, adenovirus, cytomegalovirus (CMV)–associated pneumonia, respiratory tract pneumonia, sepsis and septic shock, cardiac arrest, and respiratory failure. The adverse events in this category were high, with 11 patients (12%) experiencing a grade 3 or higher AE across all dose levels, which was higher in the first 6 months of study and plateaued (antiviral prophylaxis (77 of 94, or 82%)), and antibacterial prophylaxis against *Pneumocystis jirovecii* pneumonia (46, or 49%) was given; COVID-19 vaccine was given to 59 patients (63%). Among the 38 patients (40%) who had COVID-19, 17 (18%) had grade 3 or 4 events and two (2%) died. Opportunistic infections occurred in 10 patients (11%).

The investigators reiterated the adverse events of CRS and ICANS typically associated with bispecific antibodies in that 74 patients (79%) experienced CRS (duration of onset: 2 days) that was of grade 1 or 2 during the early stages of treatment that led to cycle delays and dose adjustment in 14 patients (15%). Only two patients (2%) experienced grade 3 CRS; both cohorts received supportive therapy (61, or 65%) and tocilizumab (24, or 26%), with a 98% recovery rate. Events of ICANSs (four) also occurred during the step-up phase, with a median duration of 3 days, and two patients experienced concurrent CRS and ICANS. Grade 3 tumor flare occurred in one patient with taste changes occurring in 61 patients that also led to dose adjustments in five patients (5%) and treatment discontinuation of talquetamab in one patient. Grade 3 events of skin rashes occurred during phase 2 dosing levels, with lower grades in 37 patients (39%) and nonrash events in 57 patients (61%). Efficacy across all clinically relevant subgroups was shown and consisted of 80% response with 77% VGPR and 52% CR or better, including those in high-risk categories according to cytogenetic profiles and instances of extramedullary disease (20 of 34 patients, or 59%). Additionally, 70 patients (74%) had a VGPR or better, and 45 (48%) had a CR or better. At R2PD, at 12 months and 18 months after treatment, likely responders occurred in 91% (95% CI 75 to 97) and 86% (95% CI 66 to 95), respectively, and at 86% (95% CI 75 to 92) and 77% (95% CI 64 to 85), respectively, across all dose levels. At R2PD, 12-month and 18-month responses were 82% (95% CI 45 to 95) at both time points, and across all dose levels, they were 70% (95% CI 45 to 85) at 12 months and 52% (95% CI 25 to 74) at 18 months. The study authors concluded that the responses were deep, durable, and maintained in all 28 patients who transitioned from monthly dosing to R2PD, with the incidence of grade 3 or 4 infections higher in the combination treatment than observed with each therapy alone. Deep, durable responses were also seen across all dose levels, providing strong evidence for further studies evaluating the combination treatment, with possible approval [12].

7.4 Lymphoma

7.4.1 Glofitamab

Glofitamab (Fig. 7.3) is a CD3-CD20 bispecific antibody that targets CD3 on T cells and CD20 on B cells and is approved for R/R diffuse large B-cell lymphoma (DLBCL) and R/R large B-cell lymphoma (LBCL) arising from follicular lymphoma (FL) in a pretreated patient population receiving two or more lines of systemic therapy. Glofitamab has a "novel 2:1 tumor T-cell binding configuration" that is bivalently oriented to CD20 and monovalently oriented in a way that leads to the elimination of malignant plasma cells R-CHOP is considered the standard of care for DLBCL; however, a large percentage of patients relapse. An early phase I study providing support for this approval, which was reported in *NEJM*, evaluated patients with B-cell non-Hodgkin lymphoma (B-NHL) who typically have poor prognosis and are not amenable to intensive measures such as hematopoietic stem cell transplantation (HSCT) or CAR T-cell therapy. To prevent CRS, pretreatment obinatuzumab was also given. Efficacy was attributed to durable response rates and positive safety profiles. All patients had CRS (one grade 3 or grade 4). In total, 171 patients began enrollment, with 35 continuing to recommended phase 2 dosing (2.5/10/30 mg). Also, 98% ($n = 168$) of patients had adverse events related to glofitamab, and 83% of patients had experienced AEs as a result of obinutuzumab, with five withdrawals of glofitamab. Neutropenia ($n = 43$), anemia ($n = 13$), and thrombocytopenia ($n = 14$) were reported. Furthermore, 100 patients had serious side effects from glofitamab ($n = 77$); 88 events occurred in 61 patient due to CRS.

7.4.1.1 Key Efficacy Results

- "Aggressive B-NHL (DLBCL, trFL, PMBCL, MCL, and Richter's transformation), the ORR and CR were 48.0% (61 of 127) and 33.1% (42 of 127), respectively, including 41.1% (30 of 73) and 28.8% (21 of 73) in patients with

Fig. 7.3 Glofitamab. (Adapted from Klein)

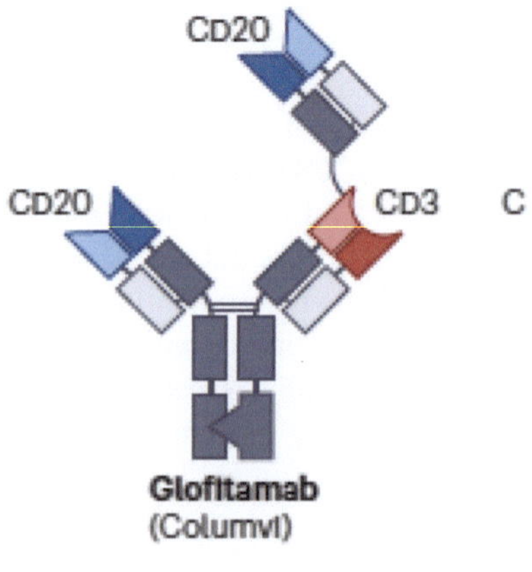

DLBCL. At the recommended phase 2 dosing, ORR and CR were 71.4% (10 of 14) and 64.3% (9 of 14), respectively."

Pharmacodynamic data showed rapid significant cytotoxic T-cell activity with long-term T-cell activation and less activity in peripheral circulation. The study authors concluded that glofitamab effected a T-cell response and had manageable CRS, along with other measures, leading to a favorable safety profile in B-NHL with a high response rate [13].

In a study confirming efficacy results, a CR of 39% (95% CI 32 to 48) was achieved, which was ongoing for 78% after 12 months. The 12-month mPFS was 4.9 months (95% CI 3.4 to 8.1), and a DOR of 18.4 months was reported. Grade 3 or 4 AEs were experienced by more than 50% of patients (CRS being the most common); 108 patients discontinued therapy at data cutoff; and 34 patients completed the full course of therapy. Most patients were at late- or advanced-stage disease and refractory to treatment (58%) and to last treatment (86%). OR was achieved in 52% of patients (95% CI 43 to 60).

7.4.1.2 Key Safety Results

- Five patients (5 3%) experienced a treatment-related AE that led to treatment discontinuation as a result of myelitis ($n = 1$), GI hemorrhage ($n = 1$), or neutropenia ($n = 2$).
- Fatal grade 5 events (no progressive disease) that were due to sepsis ($n = 2$), delirium ($n = 1$), or COVID-19-related pneumonia ($n = 5$) occurred in eight patients.
- CRS presented as the most common adverse event.

The study authors stated that glofitamab in R/R DLBCL led to deep, durable responses at the early stages of treatment, with 78% of patients experiencing CR and remission extending to 12 months. An OS of 50% was reported at 12 months, and the poor prognosis on chemotherapy was considered meaningful. Long-term follow-up data from the supporting arm had a complete remission at lower doses, confirming deep and durable complete remissions as well on the agent at fixed doses, with ICANS not being commonly reported [14].

Glofitamab received accelerated approval from the FDA thanks on results from the NP30179 trial for R/R LBCL (80% of the patient population with at least two prior lines of systemic therapy, with central nervous system (CNS) lymphoma disease patients excluded). ORR was 56% (95% CI 47–65), with a 43% CR rate. Boxed warnings included serious adverse events such as fatal CRS (70%, grade 3 or higher 4.1%), ICANS (4.8%), infection (18%), and tumor flare (12%). The most common adverse events were CRS, rash, fatigue, and musculoskeletal pain, with laboratory tests revealing abnormal lymphocyte and neutrophil counts; phosphate and fibrinogen; and increases in uric acid. Intravenous administration is prescribed according to a step-up dosing schedule (2.5 mg on Day 8 (Cycle 1); 10 mg on Day 15 (Cycle 1); 30 mg on Day 1 (each subsequent cycle for 12 cycles)), with a cycle length of 21 days, where hospitalization is recommended for CRS risk for the first 24 hours [15].

7.4.2 Epcoritamab

A preclinical study in 2021 showed that epcoritimab (Fig. 7.4) (GEN3013), a CD3-CD20 bispecific engager, induced T-cell cytotoxicity in the allogeneic setting, activating T cells from peripheral blood mononuclear cells (PBMCs) (n = 24) and lymph nodes (n = 15) obtained from a healthy donor, providing proof-of-concept evidence for its further clinical study. Tumor biopsies were obtained from both newly diagnosed and R/R B-NHL patients, showing significant tumor lysis in 65%, 74%, and 84% of DLBCL (n = 16), FL (n = 15), and MCL (n = 8) samples, respectively, even in patients with prior rituximab and obinutuzumab therapy. The study also reported that T-cell-mediated cytotoxicity was not correlated with the killing of malignant plasma cells, showing that intrinsic resistance was a factor in epcoritamab-induced cytotoxicity and could not be accounted for by the results given that granzyme B release took place. T-cell activation was found not be associated with PD-L1 expression; however, the low expression of herpes virus entry mediator (HVEM) was correlated with the activation of allogeneic CD4+ and CD8+ T cells. In fact, LN T cells were found to induce epcoritamab-induced cytotoxicity in the autologous setting: "low to moderate levels of cytotoxicity in DLBCL (median 20%; range 0–46%; n = 15), FL (median 17%; range 0–46%; n = 15) and MCL (median 0%; range 0–11%; n = 8)." Overall lower response levels than in the allogeneic setting were observed in T cells from PBMCs. The study authors state that preclinical proof of concept was established for epcoritamab for patients relapsing after prior monoclonal antibody treatment and indicate no apparent intrinsic dysfunctions in LN-derived T cells and peripheral blood in B-NHL patients that could adversely affect the efficacy of epcoritamab [16].

A dose-escalation study involving the "escalation of the priming, intermediate, or full dose (0.0128–60 mg) administered in 28-day cycles" established standard

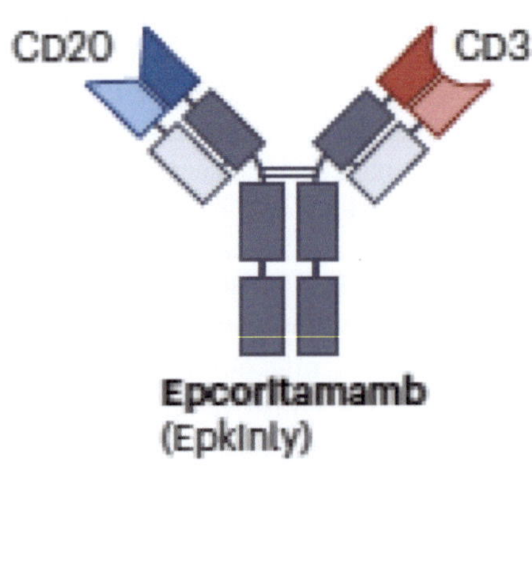

Fig. 7.4 Epcoritamab. (Adapted from Klein)

criteria for recommended and maximum tolerated dosages for epicoritamab, as reported in the *Lancet* in 2021 in a cohort of patients with R/R CD20+ B-cell malignancies. Although the maximum tolerated dose was not reached, the recommended full phase 2 dosage was reported as 40 mg. Common adverse events were reported as pyrexia (47 patients, or 69%), CRS (40, or 59%, grades 1 and 2), and grade 1 injection-site reactions (32, or 47%). No treatment-related discontinuations or treatment-related deaths occurred [17].

A phase I/II study also evaluating epicoritamab administered SC in a dose-expansion cohort further established evidence for the bispecific antibody as reported in *JCO*, and the authors confirmed the relevance of the value of bispecific antibodies in this setting. Durability and high response rates in refractory LBCL treated with epcoritamab were observed further positing its clinical use in earlier lines of treatment. The patients included those who received prior anti-CD20 therapy. Median follow-up was 10.7 months, with 106 patients discontinuing treatment due to disease progression (83, or 52.9%), AEs (11, or 7%), and patient decision for allogeneic transplantation (seven, or 4.5%), with one patient deciding to continue with chimeric antigen receptor (CAR) T-cell therapy.

7.4.2.1 Key Results

- ORR, the primary endpoint at a median follow-up of 10.7 months, was 63.1% (95% CI 55.0 to 70.6), and the CR rate was 38.9% (95% CI 31.2 to 46.9).
- TEAEs were pyrexia (23.6%), CRS (49.7: 47.1% were grade 1 or 2; 2.5% were grade 3), and ICANs (6.4%, one fatal event).

Median PFS was 4.4 months (95% CI 3.0 to 7.8); the PFS rate was 43.9% (95% CI, 35.7 to 51.7) at 6 months. 107 patients were MRD evaluable, and MRD-negative patients had a longer PFS, as shown by ctDNA analysis. Common treatment-related AEs, which occurred in the first 12 cycles, were CRS, injection-site reaction, and neutropenia (49.7%, 19.7%, and 17.8%, respectively). Nine patients (5.7%) had fatal AEs as a result of COVID-19 ($n = 2$), MI, hepatoxicity, progressive multifocal leukoencephalopathy, and ICANS (one of 10 patients, or 6.4%). Grade 1 and grade 2 events occurred in seven and two patients, respectively. The investigators concluded that "[s]ubcutaneous epcoritamab achieved rapid, deep, and durable responses, including CRs and MRD negativity, in this cohort of patients with challenging-to-treat and highly refractory LBCL" [18].

Epcoritamab received approval for R/R follicular lymphoma on the basis of data in the NHL-1 trial and for patients with greater than two lines of systemic therapy on the basis of the EPCORE NHL-1 study. A three-step dosage was recommended for CRS prophylaxis on the basis of the efficacy results of an ORR of 82% (95% CI

74.1–88.2) with a CR of 60% and similar ones reported in the step-dosing regimen. Common AEs were injection-site reactions, CRS, cough, pyrexia, and COVID-19. Common laboratory abnormalities were decreased neutrophile and decreased lymphocyte count. A boxed warning was included as prescribing information for CRS (49%), ICANS (6%), cytopenia, and serious infections (40%). Dosing instructions included 0.16 mg on Day 1, 0.8 mg on Day 8, 3 mg on Day 15, and 48 mg on Day 22 (Cycle 1); 48 mg on Days 1, 8, 15, and 22 (Cycles 2 and 3); 48 mg on Days 1 and 15 (Cycles 4 to 9); and 48 mg on Day 1 (Cycle 10) [19].

7.4.3 Mosunetuzumab (Fig. 7.5)

Accelerated approval for mosunetuzumab, a CD3/CD20 BsAb for R/R FL, was granted on FL after two or more lines of systemic therapy on the basis of the GO29781 trial, which enrolled 90 patients receiving anti-CD20 Mab and an alkylating agent. ORR according to an independent review of standard criteria for NHL was the primary endpoint; at a median follow-up of 14.9 months, mDOR was 22.8 months (95% CI 10–not reached); and the estimated DOR rate at 12 months was 62% and at 18 months was 57%. A boxed warning for CRS was included, along with warnings and precautions for infections, tumor flare, neurologic toxicity, and cytopenia. Among 218 patients, CRS occurred in 39% (grade 2 in 15%; grade 3 in 2%; grade 4 in 0.5%), neurologic toxicity in 39%, and serious infections in 17%. Common AEs were CRS, fatigue, headache, and pyrexia. Grade 3 and 4 laboratory abnormalities (> 10%) were decreased phosphate, increased glucose, decreased neutrophil and lymphocyte count, increased uric acid, decreased platelets, decreased hemoglobin, and decreased white blood cell (WBC) count. The recommended dose

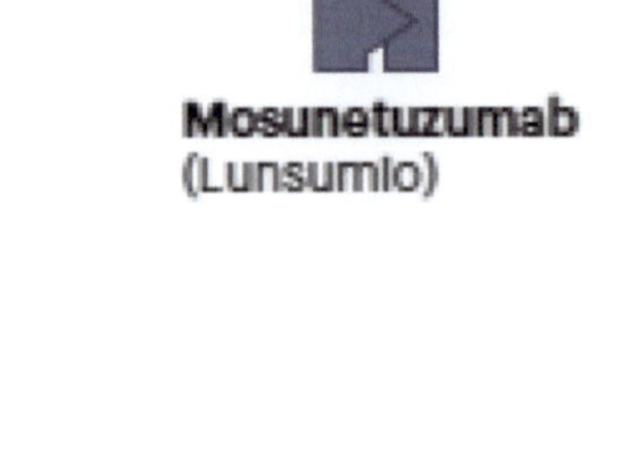

Fig. 7.5 Mosunetuzumab. (Adapted from Klein [32])

is 1 mg on Cycle 1 Day 1, 2 mg on Cycle 1 Day 8, 60 mg on Cycle 1 Day 15, 60 mg on Cycle 2 Day1, and 30 mg on Day 1 on subsequent cycles for a treatment cycle of 21 days up to eight cycles until acceptable toxicity or decreased progression. Treatment should be discontinued upon complete response. Patients experiencing PR or SD should continue treatment up to 17 cycles unless disease progression or unacceptable toxicity occurs [20].

A pivotal phase I/II dose-escalation study performing a comprehensive safety analysis, published by Matasar et al. in *CLML*, evaluated mosunetuzuamb and showed a favorable safety profile supporting its use in the outpatient setting, demonstrating a ORR of 80% (95% CI 70–88) and, a CR of 60% (95% CI 49–70). An estimated 57% (95% CI 44–70) of patients remain in remission 18 months after achieving first response.

In the dose-escalation phase, step-up dosing took place in the following regimen: Cycle (C) 1 (C1 Day 1 (C1D1), 1 mg; C1D8, 2 mg; C1D15/C2D1, 60 mg; and C3D1 and onwards, 30 mg). CRS was the most serious AE, occurring in 39.4% of NHL and 44.4% of FL patients, managed with tociluzumab, steroids, and supportive care. ICANS was reported in 0.9% of NHL and 1.1% of FL patients. Mosunetuzuamb targets CD20 on B cells and CD3 on T cells and leads to T-cell activation and proliferation and "the potent T-cell-directed killing of B cells via the granzyme-perforin pathway."

7.4.3.1 Key Results (R/R NHL)

Summary of Adverse Events

Serious adverse events (AEs)	Grade 3/4 AEs	Mosunetuzumab-related serious adverse events (SAEs)	Dose modification	Interruption of mosunetuzumab due to AEs	Neurologic toxicity	HLH	Hematologic toxicity	Serious infections
114/218 (52.3%)	75 (34.4%)	103 Sepsis ($n = 1$)	73 (33.5%)	Neutropenia (25) and CRS (17; grade 1 or 2 maximum severity (grade 1, 22.5%; grade 2, 14.2%); grade 3 events: 5/218 patients (2.3%) and 1 patient (0.5%))	Grade 3 events in 6/218 (2.8%); most frequent neurologic events included headache (20.2%), insomnia (10.6%), dizziness (9.6%), and peripheral neuropathy (6.4%).	HLH (grade 4 SAE; study Day 8), leading to mosunetuzumab treatment interruption. The HLH did not resolve, and the patient eventually died from disease progression on study day 17.	82/21; bone marrow assessment at baseline: 64/82 (78.0%); bone marrow involvement: 23/64 (35.9%); neutropenia: 123; decreased neutrophil count: 60/128 (27.5%); grade 3/4 neutropenia events: 53/218 patients (24.3%); Two SAEs of neutropenia ($n = 1$ grade 3; $n = 1$ grade 4).	82/218 patients (37.6%) in the R/R NHL cohort experienced hematologic events; of these, 64/82 (78.0%) had a bone marrow assessment at baseline, and 23/64 patients (35.9%) had bone marrow involvement. In total, 123 neutropenia events (including decreased neutrophil count) were reported in 60/218 patients (27.5%). Grade 3/4 neutropenia events were reported in 53/218 patients (24.3%). Two SAEs of neutropenia ($n = 1$ grade 3; $n = 1$ grade 4) were reported.

Note: *HLH* hemophagocytic lymphohistiocytosis

As the study authors concluded, a manageable safety profile was demonstrated, and with IV monotherapy, low grades of CRS events occurred. These safety results were consistent with the agent's mechanism of action and its outpatient administration [21].

A *JCO* study reiterated the treatment's use as an off-the-shelf treatment being administered in the outpatient setting in R/R FL patients receiving two or more previous lines of therapy. The agent is "undergoing further development for the treatment of both indolent and aggressive B-cell non-Hodgkin lymphoma (iNHL and aNHL), respectively." A dose-escalation phase I/II study showed in R/R indolent NHL (iNHL) or aggressive NHL (aNHL) a 65.7% response with iNHL and a 36.4% response with aNHL. Median DOR in iNHL patients for all responders was reported as 23.2 months (95% CI 13.8–not estimable (NE)), but not in complete responders (95% CI 21.0 to NE); however, after a median time on study of 38.9 months, no relapses were observed in complete responders beyond 26 months. Also, aNHL patients had a median DOR of 7.8 months (95% CI 4.6 to 22.8) for all responders. Patients with progression after treatment and then retreated ($n = 12$) had an OR of 83.3% and a CR of 58.3% achieved with a second CR. The study authors concluded that BsAbs for NHL demonstrate that "mosunetuzumab can mediate durable remissions with time-limited treatment" [22]. h

7.4.4 *Odronextamab*

Odronextamab is a CD20XCD3 BsAb that was evaluated in the phase II ELM-2 study ($n = 128$) in R/R FL patients after two or more lines of therapy with ORR through an independent central review. ORR was reported as 80%, and the CR rate was 73.4%. Median PFS was 20.7 months, and mOS was not reached. TEAEs included CRS (56%; grade 3 or greater 1.7%; 1/60), neutropenia (39%), and pyrexia (38%). The study results are significant in FL, an indolent NHL, because chemoimmunotherapy with a CD20 monoclonal antibody inevitably results in relapse with outcomes worsening after successive relapses. Odronextamab is an off-the-shelf bispecific T-cell engager that targets CD3 and CD20 to effect cytotoxic killing by engaging T cells and malignant B cells. In the phase 1 dose-escalation/dose-expansion ELM-1 study in B-NHL patients, ORR was 91%, and the CR rate was 72%. In ELM-2, > 90% of responders achieved CR. By week 12, 91/103 (88%) achieved a PR, with five converting to CR (two at SD) and one patient achieving SD that converted to CR by 28 weeks of treatment. The probability of maintaining CR for 12 months was 75%.

7.4.4.1 Key Results

- Median PFS: 20.7 months
  - 12: 66.2%
  - 18: 57.5%
  - 24: 46.1%
- Median OS: not reached
  - 12: 86.2 months
  - 24: 70.1 months

MRD-negative patients experienced PFS, and 118 experienced one treatment-related TEAE, including common ones such as pyrexia (38%), CRS (56%), and neutropenia (39%), which led to dose interruption and delay in 107 patients and treatment discontinuation in 20 patients, due primarily to infection. One grade 2 ICANS was observed (07/4/20 mg step-up regimen). As the study authors conclude, in a heavily pretreated population, the agent had deep and durable responses with a demonstrated manageable safety profile [23].

7.5 Acute Myeloid Leukemia

A novel BiTE construct was developed for AML targeting the GRP78 tumor-associated antigen and evaluated in vitro and in vivo. Constructed by using a peptide of 13 amino acids (Pep42) instead of two scFv fragments, this novel bispecific engager targeting csGRP78 and CD3 has a relatively long half-life and leads to the T-cell activation and cytotoxicity of tumor cells in csGRP78-expressing cells and primary AML cells, as shown through in vitro experiments and in xenograft mouse models. Cell lines expressing csGRP78 (U937 and KG-1a) were found to exhibit T-cell cytotoxicity, which was not observed in csGRP78-negative K562 cells but which was observed in the treatment group in primary AML cells. Cytokines such as TNF-alpha were also present, and this immune-mediated event was only against csGRP78-expressing AML cells. The BiTE also eliminated human AML cells in human mouse models at a dose of 0.2 mg/kg or higher and led to tumor clearance, higher survival rates, and increases in TNF-alpha, which was higher in the negative control, where mice were injected with T cells with the negative control CD19-CD3 BiTE. As the study investigators concluded, "we have developed a bispecific cell engager targeting CD3+ T cells and csGRP78+ leukemia AML cells. Instead of using conventional scFv structures to target csGRP78, we utilized a small molecular weight cyclic peptide" [24].

7.6 Solid Tumors

Tarlatanib is an immunotherapy in the BiTE class that redirects cytotoxic T cells to tumor cells that express delta-like ligand and was evaluated in the Dellphi-300 trial against small cell lung cancer (SCLC) with poor prognosis. Asymptomatic patients with stable brain metastasis were enrolled. Safety was the primary end point. ICANS was similar to patients with or without brain metastasis (any grade 10.5% (four of 38) vs. 12.3% (14 of 114)), resolving within 4 and 9 days, respectively. Continuing patients on tarlatinib had grade 1 or 2 cytopenia or asthenia, with one patient having a TRAE (neutropenia). ORR was 25% (95% CI 18.3 to 32.7) with four CRs and 34 PRs. Median DOR was 11.2 months (95% CI 6.6 t0 22.3). Also, 17 patients had a median DOR of 14.9 months (95% CI 14.2 to 61.7), who received 10 mg tarlatanib once every 2 weeks, with a median OS of 20.3 months (95% CI 5.1–NE); 25 patients (15.1%) had sustained disease control, defined as greater than 52 weeks on time on treatment. Of these SCLC patients, 23 (95.8%) had detectable DLL3 expression. Intracranial disease control occurred in 87.5% (14 of 16). Greater than 30% CNS tumor shrinkage was observed in 10 of 16 patients (62.5%). Because no new safety signals occurred, the authors concluded in the DeLLphi-300 trial that tarlatanib demonstrated unprecedented survival [25].

7.6.1 *Amivantamab*

Leighi et al. performed an analysis on patients with advanced refractory EGFR-mutant NSCLC comparing subcutaneous versus intravenous administration amivantamab (Fig. 7.6). "EGFR-mutated advanced NSCLC who progressed after osimertinib and platinum-based chemotherapy were randomly assigned 1:1 to

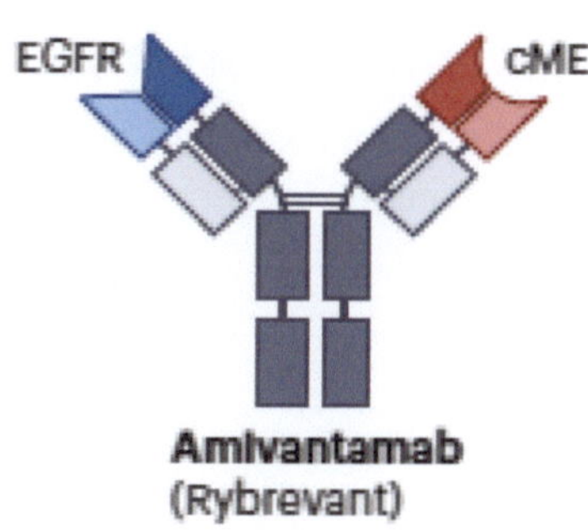

Fig. 7.6 Amivantamab. (Adapted from Klein)

receive subcutaneous or intravenous amivantamab, both combined with [TKI-CNS] penetrant lazertinib" in primary results from the phase III PALOMA-3 trial. The authors posited that a subcutaneous formulation "could improve tolerability and reduce administration time while maintaining efficacy." The PAPILLON trial established the use of this bispecific antibody as first-line treatment with chemotherapy, whereas the phase I CHRYSALIS established it as monotherapy. The phase III MARIPOSA trial showed the superior PFS of this combination over that of osimertinib. The phase I PALOMA was a study that evaluated the subcutaneous formulation of amivantamab. Endpoints included coprimary pharmacokinetic outcomes and disease assessments through imaging and safety. ORR and PFS were key secondary outcomes.

7.6.1.1 Key Results

Pharmacokinetic Profiles

Mean C_{trough} Cycle 2 Day 1 subcutaneous (SC) 365 ug/mL; intravenous 314 ug/mL
Mean C_{trough} Cycle 4 Day 1 subcutaneous 224 ug/mL; intravenous 162 ug/mL
Geometric mean ratio: Cycle 2 Day 1 subcutaneous to intravenous 1.15
Cycle 4 Day 1 subcutaneous to intravenous 1.43

Efficacy

ORR (CR or PR): 30% (95% CI 24 to 37) in the subcutaneous group; 33% (95% CI 26 to 39) in the IV group

SD: 45% in the SC group
38% in the IV group
DCR: 75% (95% CI 69 to 81) in subcutaneous group
71% (95% CI 64 to 77) in IV group

PFS 6.1 months (95% CI 4.3 to 8.1) versus 4.3 months (95% CI 4.1 to 5.7) with OS significantly longer

Safety

Most events were grade 1. The most common grade 3 event was dermatitis.
Serious AEs: 29% and 30% for subcutaneous and intravenous, respectively

The phase III MARIPOSA study was also the first to show the impact of prophylactic anticoagulation against venous thromboembolism (VTE) risk for the combination therapy, which is higher in lung cancer with molecular driver alterations and those receiving the combination. The study recommended this lower

VTE rate. The authors concluded that SC amivantamab–lazertinib demonstrated noninferior pharmacokinetics and ORR with a potential greater durability of response and better PFS and OS when compared with IV administration with reduced venous thromboembolic events in the SC formulation. Shorter treatment times that led to better patient convenience were also observed from SC administration when compared with IV administration, and SC administration may become a treatment option [26].

Zenocutuzumab (MCLA-128) is a BsAb targeting HER2 and human EGFR 3 (HER3 and ERBB3) signaling in NRG1 fusion+/ER+ breast cancer that induces sustained tumor regression after progression on a CDK4/6 inhibitor (unreported targeted agent). NRG1 stands for neurelulin-1 gene and encodes a membrane-bound glycoprotein. The chimeric NRG1 fusions have been detected in 0.04–0.7% of breast cancer cases. The mechanism of action of NRG1-mediated HER2/HER3 signaling is described next.

Uncontrolled tumor growth occurs when a free NRG1 and an NRG1 fusion ligand bind to HER3, leading to the docking-site transphosphorylation of the p85 subunit of the PI-3 kinase of the HER3 cytoplasmic domain through the HER2 kinase resulting in HER2:HER3 activation. Targeted agents that inhibit signaling at different points in the pathway are shown. A BsAb, zenocutuzumab, by docking itself on the HER2 arm via the anti-HER2 arm, optimally positions itself on the anti-HER3 arm, blocking the interaction of ligand/receptor and inhibiting HER2:HER3 dimerization and downstream signaling, as illustrated in Fig. 7.7.

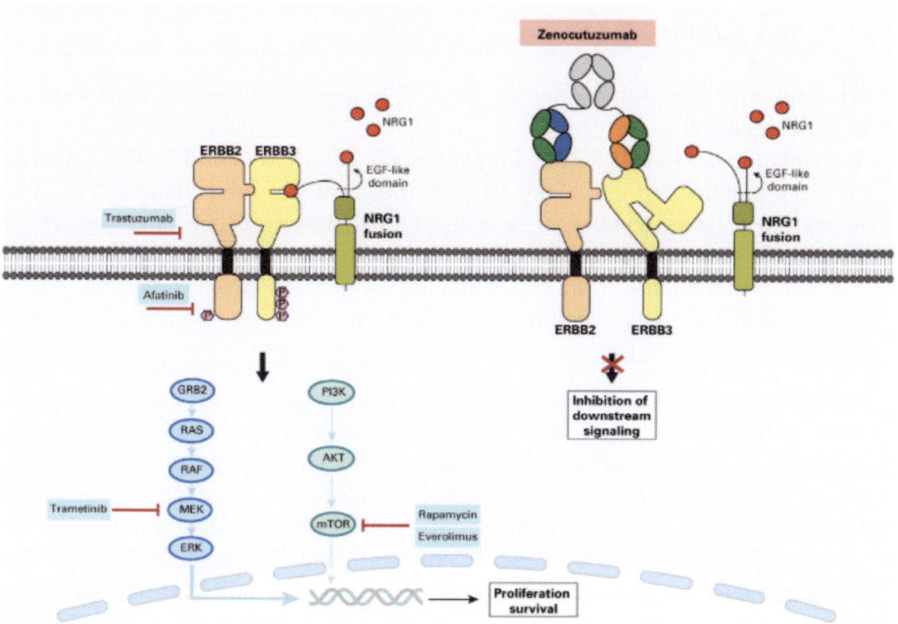

Fig. 7.7 Zenocutuzumab. (Adapted from Fontana et al. [27])

MCLA-128 is a bispecific antibody that consists of a humanized full-length IgG1 antibody that leads to ADCC activity, which, along with its ability to dock on the abundantly expressed HER2 protein that blocks ligand binding to HER3 and prevents HER2-HER3 dimerization, is responsible for its dual anticancer mechanism. In one patient, an Oncofocus (that targets 505 genes) companion diagnostic test "identified an SLC3A2-NRG1 gene fusion between exon 5 of the SLC3A2 gene and exon 6 of NRG1, at the locus position of chr11:62649538—chr8:32585467," and a PR was reported. No other data were reported [27].

Two bispecific immune cell engagers were evaluated in a phase 3 MARIPOSA trial with lazertinib for EGFR-mutated advanced NSCLC with no prior treatment and a first in human (FIH) study also targeting EGFR on solid tumors. Regarding the first study, the combination of amivantanab (an EGFR-MET BsAb with an optimized Fc domain) and lazertinib (a CNS-penetrant third-generation TKI that has shown positive clinical outcomes in EGFR-mutated and T790M mutated malignancies) as a treatment was first evaluated in the phase 1 CHRYSALIS trial. MARIPOSA is an international trial that randomized patients with an EGFR mutation in a 2:2:1 fashion, evaluating the treatment with the third-generation agent osimtertinib. The scientific rationale of MARIPOSA was that downstream resistance to osimeritinib was leading to a lack of response, and the study authors hypothesized that this could be mitigated with amivantanab–lazertinib treatment. PFS as assessed through an independent central review was the primary endpoint, with OS and response rates serving as secondary endpoints.

7.6.1.2 Key Results

- Amivantamab (n = 42), osimertinib (n = 429), and lazertinib (n = 216) were the therapeutic agents.
- The amivantamab and lazertinib immunotherapy duo had an mPFS of 23.7 months (vs. 16.6 months; HR 0.70; 95% CI 0.58–0.85); 86% of the patients (95% CI 83 to 89) and achieved an ORR in the amivantamab–lazertinib cohort vs. 85% (95% CI 81 to 88) in the osimertinib arm.
- The amivantamab–lazertinib group and the osimertinib group had different confirmed response values: confirmed response n = 336 vs. confirmed response n = 314.

Adverse events included venous thromboembolism (37% in the combination arm and 9% in the control group), with grade 1 and 2 side effects being the most common. Dose reduction occurred in 249 patients (54%) as a result of adverse events, and the authors note that discontinuations of any trial agent were due to paronychia and infusion-related reactions, being the most common AEs, and that the HR for death was 0.80 in terms of OS and was not significant. The authors conclude that PFS was found to be superior in the amivantamab and lazertinib treatment combination in comparison with osimertinib for EGFR-mutated advanced NSCLC in the first-line setting [28].

In a dose-escalation FIH phase 1 study, the investigational tetravalent bispecific innate cell engager AFM24 was evaluated in EGFR-positive tumors, primarily NSCLC and CRC (MSI-high and MSS) patients (n = 35), as reported by El-Khoueiry et al. in *Clinical Cancer Research.* The primary endpoints were safety, tolerability, and pharmacokinetics. The most common adverse events were infusion-related reactions and GI events such as nausea and pyrexia. In this study, 77.1% of patients experienced IRRs, with 34.3% experiencing grade 1, 37.1% grade 2, and 5.7% grade 3. Nausea was reported by 25.7% of patients; dermatologic acne was seen in 22.9% of patients, with one grade 3 event. One grade 3 and grade 4 event of lymphocytopenia was seen, and reported in 8.6% of patients. This agent was found to have a unique mechanism of action in not targeting EGFR signaling pathways that characterize many small molecule inhibitors, but the mutated EGFR that activates innate and adaptive immune system, given that both NK and CD3 T cells were observed to be activated in vitro and from an analysis of tumor biopsies. Tumor regression was determined. The recommended phase 2 dosage was 480 mg. EGFR expression was maintained throughout treatment, and those at higher doses (greater than 160 mg) showed increased CD3+ T-cell infiltration, accompanied by an increase in "CD56dim NK and CD8 T cell-specific markers genes and cytotoxicity associated genes," as shown through gene expression profiling. Thus, NK and T-cell functions were confirmed to be augmented in tumors with AFM24 treatment, providing proof-of-concept evidence for evaluating the agent in combination with other immunotherapies, such as immune checkpoint inhibitors. The study authors included that the "tolerable safety profile and promising correlative biomarker data, whereby AFM24 demonstrated activation of the innate and adaptive immune systems in paired tumor biopsies, highlighting a unique mechanism of action" [29].

Riha-Paul et al. conducted a multicenter, open-label, dose-escalation FIH phase I study of the bispecific antibody molecule cinrebafusp alfa that targets HER2 on advanced solid tumors while leading to stimulatory 4-1BB agonism on innate and adaptive immune cells, including NK cells and T cells on heavily pretreated patients that were HER2+ that progressed on these prior regimens. Generated from the fusion of the trastuzumab with the "anticalin protein specific for 4-1BB using a silenced IgG4 isotype to avoid Fc-mediated immune cell engagement," in preclinical models, the compound showed promise for generating antitumor activity. The primary endpoints were safety and tolerability, along with the determination of clinical activity and pharmacokinetics and pharmacodynamics and with the assessment of immunogenicity and the presence of biomarkers. Dosing was intravenous administration "over 2 hours at dose levels ranging from 0.0005 to 18 mg/kg."

7.6.1.3 Key Results

Drug discontinuation due to grade 3 pleural effusion on day 28 at the 12 mg/kg dose arm in one patient with breast cancer and one DLT were reported. However, no MTD was identified for the treatment of cinrebafusp alfa up to 18 mg/kg doses.

- TRAEs were shown in 44 patients, or 56.4% of them (grade 3 TRAE: 11, or 14.1%; grade 4 TRAE: one patient (1.3%); no grade 5 TRAEs reported as due to the drug).
- IRR were the most frequent at 21.8%, with fatigue at 14.1% ($n = 11$) and nausea at 11.5% ($n = 9$). Most were less than grade 2, with four patients (5.1%) experiencing grade ≥ 3 IRRs and one patient (1.3%) experiencing grade 3 fatigue.

Five patients (12.5%) displayed antitumor activity, with one CR and four PRs. Also, 16 patients (40%) showed a confirmed SD with a DCR of 52.5%, and antitumor activity was shown in waterfall plots, where the greatest change and percentage change from baseline was seen at the 18 mg/kg t2W dosing in CRC, with an dose-dependent increase in T-cell activation and localized increase in T cells observed in the assessment of paired tumor biopsies. The study investigators also reported that to "achieve optimal 4-1BB pathway engagement and immune cell activation," a minimal dose of 8 mg/kg was required. The study investigators concluded that in a heavily pretreated HER2 positive patient population, tumor-agnostic 4-1BB treatment is tolerated and shows antitumor activity, and they added that thanks to "its bispecific design, cinrebafusp alfa enhances immune cell activation while avoiding the hepatotoxicity associated with conventional 4-1BB antibodies" [30].

7.7 Investigational Agents and Studies

Bispecific antibodies in clinical trials include pertosemtamb (MCLA-158), which binds the cancer stem cell surface receptor EGFR and LGR5 for advanced HNSCC. Izalontamab (SI-B001) targets both HER3 and EGFR and is under evaluation for locally advanced and metastatic epithelial tumors. Dual checkpoint inhibitors reduce undesired side effects and simultaneously target two different checkpoint proteins while increasing the efficacy and probability of resistance, providing complementary immune stimulating signals, and improving selectivity for T cells that express checkpoint proteins. According to Klein et al., the development of BsAbs include exploratory work for checkpoint inhibition that targets the HER-family of RTKs on the tumor cell surface, and when combined with anti-PD1/PD-L1 signaling "as a second functionality" to target the ICI to tumor cells, it results in increased specificity and activity toward EGFR tumor cells by directing the PD-L1 binding agent to these tumor cells. Cadonilimab is a bispecific antibody that has a mechanism of action that increases targeted binding to PD-1 and CTLA-4 as a result of its tetravalency, which in addition to Fc mutations that abolish Fc gamma receptors (FcγR) engagement has a favorable therapeutic index. In a phase I/Ib study, cadolinilimb had both antitumor activity and a relatively small number of irAEs and is approved in China for metastatic cervical cancer progressing on chemotherapy. MEDI5752 also binds CTLA-4 and PD-1, has displayed PD-1-mediated targeting, and is "preferentially saturated CTLA4 on PD1+ T cells, and caused rapid internalization and degradation of PD-1." PD-L1 and TGFβ BsAb targets are in development, including the BsAb-like antibody fusion protein bintrafusp alfa that has the mechanism of action of activating both the innate and adaptive immune systems, leading to tumor growth and metastasis—as opposed to individual targeting of PD-L1 and TGF-β, which is trapped by an extracellular domain (ECD) of human TGF-β receptor II82. Retlirafusp alfa (SHR-1701) also targets PDL1 and TGF-β and is undergoing evaluation in phase III studies in patients with cervical cancer and gastric or GE junction cancer; YM101a TGF-β × PDL1 BsAb is also undergoing development in preclinical studies. As Klein et al. explain, the combinatorial approaches counteract both the inhibitory TGF-β and PD1/PDL1 pathways simultaneously showing evidence of greater in vivo antitumor activity when compared with individual binding alone; however, clinical proof of concept has not been shown [32].

Roy et al. reported on an investigational agent, AGR2, that leads to angiogenesis and fibroblast invasion while promoting VEGF activity and the migration of fibroblasts and inducing wound healing, mediated by the adhesion domain of the molecule. Higher expression of AGR2 (located in the ER and contributing to protein folding also present in the plasma membrane), EXC, and cytoplasm is linked to lung cancer progression and has been observed in other cancers. A T-cell-engaging BsAb targets both AGR2 and PD1, redirecting cytotoxic T cells to treat AGR2-overexpressing solid tumors. Many solid tumors, including lung adenocarcinoma, are rich in AGR2, thus leading the investigators to conduct a preclinical study on the potential and synergistic effects of a bispecific antibody with the simultaneous targeting of PD-1 and AGR2 while binding tumor cells and immune cells together. According to the authors, the putative mechanism of action is that when the agent engages cytotoxic T cells to target tumor cells, activated T cells release perforin, inducing membrane perforation in the target T-cell membrane, binding both targets while cross-linking them to damage membrane integrity and cytotoxicity, and this represents a superior approach to monoclonal antibodies. The T-cell activation and expression of caspase 3, granzyme B, and perforin are also enhanced "in a contact-dependent manner" in a culture of AGR2-overexpressing tumor cells, further enhancing in vivo the colocalization of both PD1 and AGR2 in the AGR2-rich tumor site. In AGR2XPD-1-treated mice, tumor growth was significantly reduced when compared to control groups, and tumor formation was also significantly inhibited. High levels of T-cell activation were also observed; also, when compared to the control group and monoclonal antibody-treated group, a greater attachment to and a greater infiltration of CD8 + cytotoxic T cells into the TME were observed. The BsAb was also shown to inhibit AGR2 angiogenesis. A T-cell-induced damaged membrane led to the higher expression of perforin and upregulation in the AGR2xPD1 BsAb–treated group. The engagement and infiltration of activated CD8 T cells and the redirecting of immune cells to the tumor site occurred as a result of multiple mechanisms in AGR2 overexpressing TME as well as blocking paracrine signaling in the inhibition of AGR2 cellular functions. Significantly, the inhibition of PD1/PDL2 cross-talk takes place as a result of PDL1 overexpression, as induced by AGR2. As the study authors concluded that the AGR2xPD1 BsAb serves as a potential candidate for AGR2 overexpressing solid tumors by inducing the suppression of AGR2 and mediating cytotoxic T-cell activity, promoting T-cell activation and enhancing the action of cytolytic proteins [33].

A phase II trial on immune checkpoint–based bispecific antibodies with a lenvatinib TKI was conducted on advanced HCC and served as the first exploratory study of its kind that evaluated a TKI with a bispecific antibody. The agent, the bispecific antibody KN046 directed at PD-L1 and CTLA-4, was shown in an open-label study to have an ORR of over 40% (45.5% (95% CI 31.97–59.45)) and an mPFS of 11.0 months (95% CI 8.21–15.24), indicating "promising efficacy as first-line treatment for advanced unresectable or metastatic HCC," but it necessitated management for grade ≥ 3 TRAEs, present in 47.3% of patients. Other key results included a DCR of 89.1% (95% CI 77.75–95.89). TRAEs occurred in 100% of patients, with 23.6% experiencing irAE; treatment discontinuation was observed in five patients (9.1%), and TRAEs leading to death due to interstitial lung disease occurred in one patient.

The most common TRAEs occurring in > 30% of patients were as follows:

- Decreased platelet count (26 (47.3%))
- Fatigue (22 (40.0%))
- Hypertension (22 (40.0%))
- Proteinuria (21 (38.2%))
- Elevated blood bilirubin (19 (34.5%))
- Elevated aspartate transaminase (18 (32.7%))

The most common grade ≥ 3 TRAEs (> 2%) were as follows:

- Hypertension (7 (12.7%))
- Elevated blood pressure (5 (9.1%))
- Decreased platelet count (3 (5.5%))
- Fatigue (2 (3.6%))
- Elevated aspartate aminotransferase (2 (3.6%))
- Weight loss (2 (3.6%))
- Hyponatremia (2 (3.6%))

The most common grade ≥ 3 TEAEs (> 5%) were as follows:

- Hypertension (7 (12.7%))
- Elevated blood pressure (5 (9.1%))
- Decreased platelet count (3 (5.5%))
- Hyponatremia (3 (5.5%))

According to biomarker analysis, frequently mutated genes were TP53 (59.1%), TERT (47.7%), and LRP1B (27.3%), with Wnt and SWI/SNF pathways being the most commonly mutated pathways. Additionally, copy number variations (CNVs) such as CCND1 and FGF19 were more frequent in patients with stable disease and disease progression (nonresponders) than in patients with CR + PR (responders). No difference in TMB was observed between responders and nonresponders, and ctDNA status was that achieving ctDNA clearance was closely associated with efficacy and with worse prognosis. When KN046 was combined with lenvatinib, promising efficacy was shown as a first-line treatment for advanced unresectable or metastatic HCC, becoming a potential treatment option and substantiating support for conducting a phase III trial [34].

References

1. Hays P. Clinical development and therapeutic applications of bispecific antibodies. In: Hays P, editor. Cancer immunotherapies. Cham: Springer Nature; 2022.
2. Epperly R, Gottschalk S, Velasquez MP. Biology and clinical evaluation of T/NK cell engagers. In: Ghobadi A, DiPersio JF, editors. Gene and cellular immunotherapy for cancer. Cham: Springer Nature; 2022. p. 329–43.
3. Mateos MV, Chari A, Usmani SZ, Goldschmidt H, Weisel K, Qi K, et al. Comparative efficacy of Teclistamab versus physician's choice of therapy in the long-term follow-up of APOLLO, POLLUX, CASTOR, and EQUULEUS clinical trials in patients with triple-class exposed relapsed or refractory multiple myeloma. Clin Lymphoma Myeloma Leuk. 2023;23(5):385–93.
4. van de Donk, Niels et al.. MM-163 Long-Term Follow-Up From MajesTEC-1 of Teclistamab, a B-Cell Maturation Antigen (BCMA) × CD3 Bispecific Antibody, in Patients With Relapsed/Refractory Multiple Myeloma (RRMM). Clinical Lymphoma, Myeloma and Leukemia, Volume 23, S477 - S478.
5. Kang C. Teclistamab: first approval. Drugs. 2022;82(16):1613–9.
6. Lesokhin AM, Tomasson MH, Arnulf B, Bahlis NJ, Miles Prince H, Niesvizky R, et al. Elranatamab in relapsed or refractory multiple myeloma: phase 2 MagnetisMM-3 trial results. Nat Med. 2023;29(9):2259–67.
7. Grosicki S, Crafoord J, Koh Y, White D, Mellqvist U-H, Leip E et al. MagnetisMM-5: An open-label, multicenter, randomized phase 3 study of elranatamab as monotherapy and in combination with daratumumab in patients with relapsed/refractory multiple myeloma. Abstract. American Society for Clinical Oncology. 2022.
8. FDA grants accelerated approval to elranatamab-bcmm for multiple myeloma; 2023. Accessed March 2025. https://www.fda.gov/drugs/resources-information-approved-drugs/fda-grants-accelerated-approval-elranatamab-bcmm-multiple-myeloma.
9. Lee HC, Bumma N, Richter J, Zonder JA, Hoffman JE et al. Indirect Comparison of Linvoseltamab vs Teclistamab for theTreatment of Triple-Class Exposed Relapsed/Refractory Multiple Myeloma. Clinical Lymphoma, Myeloma and Leukemia. 2025 preprint.
10. Chari A, Minnema MC, Berdeja JG, Oriol A, van de Donk N, Rodriguez-Otero P, et al. Talquetamab, a T-cell-redirecting GPRC5D bispecific antibody for multiple myeloma. N Engl J Med. 2022;387(24):2232–44.
11. Ye JC, Biran N, Nair S, Lin X, Qi K, et al. Talquetamab Versus Real-World Physician's Choice Treatment: Comparative Effectiveness in Patients With Triple-Class Exposed Relapsed/Refractory Multiple Myeloma. Clinical Lymphoma, Myeloma and Leukemia. 2024, Vol. 25, No. 2, 124–134.
12. Cohen YC, Magen H, Gatt M, Sebag M, Kim K, Min CK, et al. Talquetamab plus Teclistamab in relapsed or refractory multiple myeloma. N Engl J Med. 2025;392(2):138–49.
13. Hutchings M, Morschhauser F, Iacoboni G, Carlo-Stella C, Offner FC, Sureda A, et al. Glofitamab, a novel, bivalent CD20-targeting T-cell-engaging bispecific antibody, induces durable complete remissions in relapsed or refractory B-Cell Lymphoma: a phase I trial. J Clin Oncol. 2021;39(18):1959–70.
14. Dickinson MJ, Carlo-Stella C, Morschhauser F, Bachy E, Corradini P, Iacoboni G, et al. Glofitamab for relapsed or refractory diffuse large B-Cell Lymphoma. N Engl J Med. 2022;387(24):2220–31.

15. FDA grants accelerated approval to glofitamab-gxbm for selected relapsed or refractory large B-cell lymphomas; 2023. Accessed March 2025. https://www.fda.gov/drugs/drug-approvals-and-databases/fda-grants-accelerated-approval-glofitamab-gxbm-selected-relapsed-or-refractory-large-b-cell.
16. van der Horst HJ, de Jonge AV, Hiemstra IH, Gelderloos AT, Berry D, Hijmering NJ, et al. Epcoritamab induces potent anti-tumor activity against malignant B-cells from patients with DLBCL, FL and MCL, irrespective of prior CD20 monoclonal antibody treatment. Blood Cancer J. 2021;11(2):38.
17. Hutchings M, Mous R, Clausen MR, Johnson P, Linton KM, Chamuleau MED. Dose escalation of subcutaneous epcoritamab in patients with relapsed or refractory B-cell non-Hodgkin lymphoma: an open-label, phase 1/2 study. Lancet. 2021;398:1157.
18. Thieblemont C, Phillips T, Ghesquieres H, Cheah CY, Clausen MR, Cunningham D, et al. Epcoritamab, a novel, subcutaneous CD3xCD20 bispecific T-cell-engaging antibody, in relapsed or refractory large B-cell lymphoma: dose expansion in a phase I/II trial. J Clin Oncol. 2023;41(12):2238–47.
19. FDA grants accelerated approval to epcoritamab-bysp for relapsed or refractory follicular lymphoma; 2024. Accessed March 2025. https://www.fda.gov/drugs/resources-information-approved-drugs/fda-grants-accelerated-approval-epcoritamab-bysp-relapsed-or-refractory-follicular-lymphoma#:~:text=On%20June%2026%2C%202024%2C%20the,more%20lines%20of%20systemic%20therapy.
20. FDA D.I.S.C.O. Burst Edition: FDA approval of Lunsumio (mosunetuzumab-axgb) for adult patients with relapsed or refractory follicular lymphoma after two or more lines of systemic therapy; 2022. Accessed March 2025. https://www.fda.gov/drugs/resources-information-approved-drugs/fda-disco-burst-edition-fda-approval-lunsumio-mosunetuzumab-axgb-adult-patients-relapsed-or#:~:text=On%20December%2022%2C%202022%2C%20the,more%20lines%20of%20systemic%20therapy.
21. Matasar M, Bartlett NL, Shadman M, Budde LE, Flinn I, Gregory GP, et al. Mosunetuzumab safety profile in patients with relapsed/refractory B-cell Non-Hodgkin lymphoma: clinical management experience from a pivotal phase I/II trial. Clin Lymphoma Myeloma Leuk. 2024;24(4):240–53.
22. Budde EL, Sehn LH, Matasar M, Schuster SJ, Assouline S. Mosunetuzumab monotherapy is an effective and well-tolerated treatment option for patients with relapsed/refractory (R/R) follicular lymphoma (FL) who have received 2prior lines of therapy: pivotal results from a phase I/II study. CLML. 2022;22:S387.
23. Kim TM, Taszner M, Novelli S, Cho SG, Villasboas JC, Merli M, et al. Safety and efficacy of odronextamab in patients with relapsed or refractory follicular lymphoma. Ann Oncol. 2024;35(11):1039–47.
24. Zeng X, Zhang H, Guo J, Yang D, Zhu Y, Liu N, et al. A novel bispecific T-cell engager using the ligand-target csGRP78 against acute myeloid leukemia. Cell Mol Life Sci. 2024;81(1):371.
25. Dowlati A, Abbas A, Chan T, Henick B, Wang X, Doshi P, et al. Immune checkpoint blockade outcome in small-cell lung cancer and its relationship with retinoblastoma mutation status and function. JCO Precis Oncol. 2022;6:e2200257.
26. Leighl NB, Akamatsu H, Lim SM, Cheng Y, Minchom AR, Marmarelis ME, et al. Subcutaneous versus intravenous Amivantamab, both in combination with Lazertinib, in refractory epidermal growth factor receptor-mutated non-small cell lung cancer: primary results from the phase III PALOMA-3 study. J Clin Oncol. 2024;42(30):3593–605.
27. Fontana E, Torga G, Fostea R, Cleator S, Wasserman E, Murat A, et al. Sustained tumor regression with Zenocutuzumab, a bispecific antibody targeting human epidermal growth factor receptor 2/human epidermal growth factor receptor 3 signaling, in NRG1 fusion-positive, estrogen receptor-positive breast cancer after progression on a cyclin-dependent kinase 4/6 inhibitor. JCO Precis Oncol. 2022;6:e2100446.
28. Cho BC, Lu S, Felip E, Spira AI, Girard N, Lee JS, et al. Amivantamab plus Lazertinib in previously untreated EGFR-mutated advanced NSCLC. N Engl J Med. 2024;391(16):1486–98.

29. El-Khoueiry A, Saavedra O, Thomas J, Livings C, Garralda E, Hintzen G, et al. First-in-human phase I study of a CD16A bispecific innate cell engager, AFM24, targeting EGFR-expressing solid tumors. Clin Cancer Res. 2025;31(7):1257–67.
30. Piha-Paul S, Olwill SA, Hamilton E, Tolcher A, Pohlmann P, Liu SV, et al. A first-in-human study of Cinrebafusp Alfa, a HER2/4-1BB bispecific molecule, in patients with HER2-positive advanced solid malignancies. Clin Cancer Res. 2025;31(2):288–98.
31. Pan D, Richter J. Management of Toxicities Associated with BCMA, GPRC5D, and FcRH5-targeting bispecific antibodies in multiple myeloma. Curr Hematol Malig Rep. 2024;19(6):237–45.
32. Klein C, Brinkmann U, Reichert JM, Kontermann RE. The present and future of bispecific antibodies for cancer therapy. Nat Rev Drug Discov. 2024;23(4):301–19.
33. Roy D, He Y, Wang Y, Xu P, Jin B, Xiao H, et al. Bispecific antibody simultaneously targeting AGR2 and PD1 mediates cytotoxic T-cell-induced antitumor response in AGR2-dependent manner and inhibits AGR2-induced PDL1 upregulation. Sci Rep. 2025;15(1):6015.
34. Xu D, Wang H, Bao Q, Jin K, Liu M, Liu W, et al. The anti-PD-L1/CTLA-4 bispecific antibody KN046 plus lenvatinib in advanced unresectable or metastatic hepatocellular carcinoma: a phase II trial. Nat Commun. 2025;16(1):1443.

Chapter 8
Antibody Drug Conjugates

Antibody drug conjugates (ADCs) constitute a specific type of targeted therapy and are considered breakthroughs in their drug design by being combinations of monoclonal antibodies and chemotherapy's cytotoxic potential that would enable "drug delivery to targeted cells." One of the major advancements in ADCs is the development and approval of the anti-HER2 ADC trastuzumab deruxtecan that incorporates the monoclonal antibody trastuzumab and a topoisomerase inhibitor for HER2 low breast cancer. Incidences of interstitial disease and resistance mechanisms have been observed. Two reviews by Chen and Zeng and Coleman et al. were conducted on ADCs for lung cancer, which were referred to as "pioneering the way" with "revolutionary potential" at the "dawn of a new era" and as "agents of precision oncology." HER2, HER3, TROP2, CEACAM, and MET1 targeted ADCs are described in terms of target antigens and antibodies, linkers, and payloads for lung cancer with a discussion of the general mechanisms of action for ADCs, mechanisms of resistance, combination therapies, and toxicities [1, 2].

ADCs are composed of a monoclonal antibody directed to a target antigen on tumor cells, a cytotoxic payload, and a cleavable linker conjugating the two components. The properties of an effective ADC include having a cytotoxic payload that can survive circulation and be released intracellularly under specific conditions and a target expressed on malignant cells as opposed to normal cells. The three main examples of linkers are those that cleave in acidic environments (acidic), the reductive environment induced by reducing agents such as glutathione (disulfide linkers), and enzyme-labile linkers cleaved by enzymatic activity [3]. Three classes of toxins make up current ADCs: topoisomerase I inhibitors (SN38/Dxd/exatecan), DNA-damaging agents (including DNA-alkylators, such as duocarmycin (DUBA)/pyrrolobenzodiazepines), and microtubule toxins (e.g., monomethyl auristatin E and F (MMAE/MMAF)). They are widely based on two payload classes: DNA-interactive damaging agents (calicheamicin, DXd, PBD, and SN38) and tubulin inhibitors (DM1, DM4, MMAE, and MMAF), which disrupt microtubule formation. The

P. Hays, *Personalized Medicine in Oncology*,
https://doi.org/10.1007/978-3-032-14437-9_8

purpose of ADCs in cancer is to minimize drug exposure in healthy tissue and improve the therapeutic index of cytotoxic agents [4].

Due to differential target antigen expression on normal tissue versus tumor tissue, the complexities of intracellular trafficking in endosomes that modulate ADC activity, poor drug antibody ratios, poor linker chemistry, and inefficiency in cytotoxic payload, ADCs, once thought of as "magic bullets," have had their clinical success limited. However, several very effective ones have been developed, such as brentuximab vedotin for Hodgkin lymphoma in combination with chemotherapy, polatuzumab vedotin-piiq for diffuse large B-cell lymphoma (DLBCL), enfortumab vedotin for urothelial carcinoma (UC), trastuzumab deruxtecan for HER2+breast cancer, and sacituzumab govitecan for metastatic triple-negative breast cancer (TNBC). ADCs are representative of precision medicine in oncology and are the goal of the paradigm in targeted therapeutic drug development in the oncology of "developing therapeutic compounds that selectively and potently inhibit cancerous tissue while sparing normal tissue" [5] (Fig. 8.1).

Drugs approved by the US Food and Drug Administration (as of 2024) include the following:

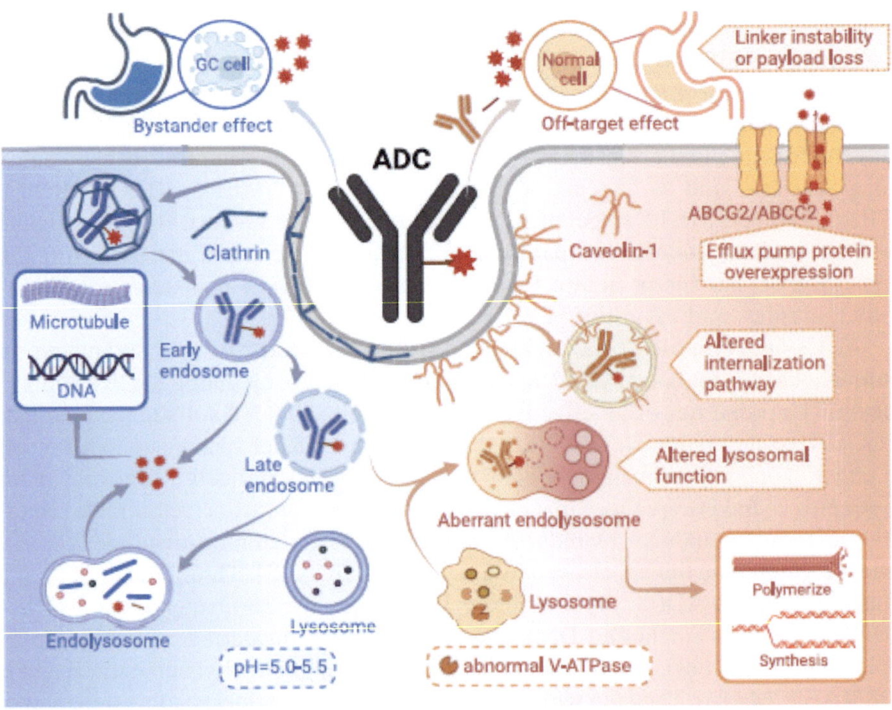

Fig. 8.1 How antibody conjugates work. (Adapted from Hao et al. [6])

- Brentuximab vedotin, composed of a monoclonal antibody targeting the CD20 antigen and conjugated to microtubule disrupting agent monomethyl auristatin, which serves as the payload, is for chronic Hodgkin's lymphoma (cHL).
- Trastuzumab emtansine (T-DM1), composed of the monoclonal antibody trastuzumab targeting HER2 conjugated to the microtubule inhibitor payload emtansine, for breast cancer.
- Belantamab mafodotin, composed of a monoclonal antibody targeting B-cell maturation antigen and conjugated to the cytotoxic payload monomethyl auristatin F (MMAF), a microtubule disrupting agent, is for multiple myeloma (MM).
- Gemtuzumab oxogamicin targets the CD33 receptor on myeloid cells and is approved for acute myeloid leukemia (AML).
- Inotuzumab ozogamicin targets the CD22 receptor on the B-cell precursor leukemic cells and is approved for acute lymphoblastic leukemia (ALL).

8.1 Components of ADCs: Design and Construction (Figs. 8.2 and 8.3)

The components of ADCs—a target antigen, an antibody, a linker, and a payload—are frequently described in the literature. The antigen serves as the target for the ADC, enabling direct binding and identification and thus communication while reducing off-target toxicity because the antigen is tumor bearing but absent from normal cells. Tumor-specific antigens are expressed as glycoproteins, extracellular matrix proteins, and cell-surface proteins. An effective target is nonsecreted such that its circulation is minimal and ADCs are not bound beyond tumor sites, leading to the cytotoxic payload unloading onto tumor cells and to intracellular transfer. On the tumor cell surface where the target antigen is, the circulating antibody can attach effectively, with internalization properties to lead to efficient ADC entry into the cell while enhancing cytotoxic potency. Many of the antigen targets, such as ERBB2 (HER2) and TROP2, are expressed more than 100 times on tumor cells versus healthy noncancer tissue, presenting a wider therapeutic window and decreasing systemic toxicities, hematologic targets, BCMA, CD30, and CD22 on multiple myeloma, acute myeloid leukemia, and lymphomas.

Antibody selection for ADCs must be balanced between the efficient infiltration of tumor tissues and maintaining specificity and must have increased in vivo half-lives to adequately assist in linking the target antigen to the ADC. Monoclonal antibodies serve as the primary element in ADC design. Produced by plasma cells, they are composed of glycoproteins that specifically attach to an antigen. The ideal antibody binds to a target antigen and has limited immunogenicity while maintaining proficient internalization. Higher affinity speeds up the internationalization of the antigen–antibody complex; however, this can impede tumor penetration. Larger antibodies face internationalization issues, whereas smaller ones, lacking the Fc

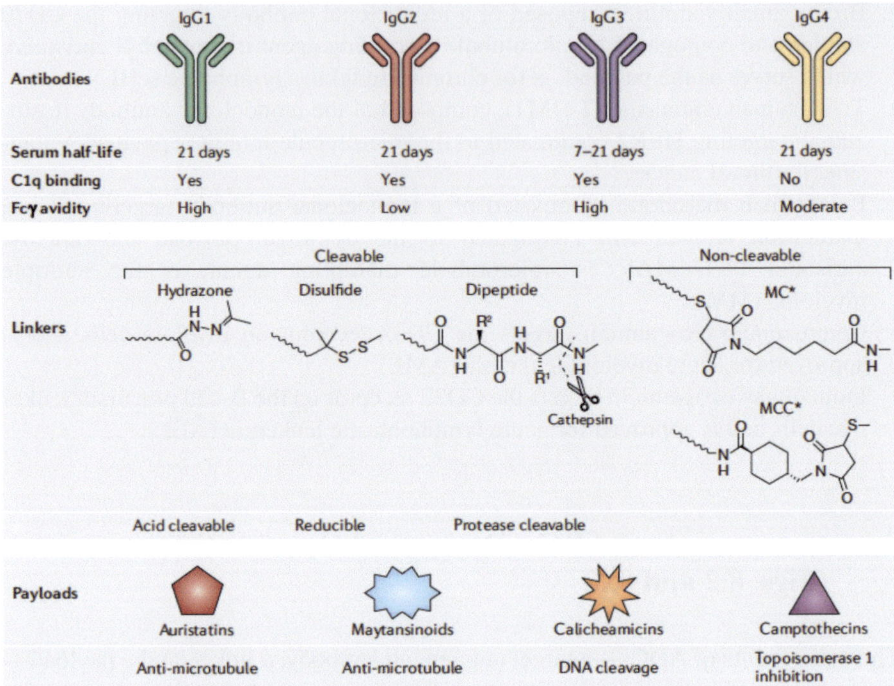

Fig. 8.2 The components of ADCs. (Adapted from Dumontet [7])

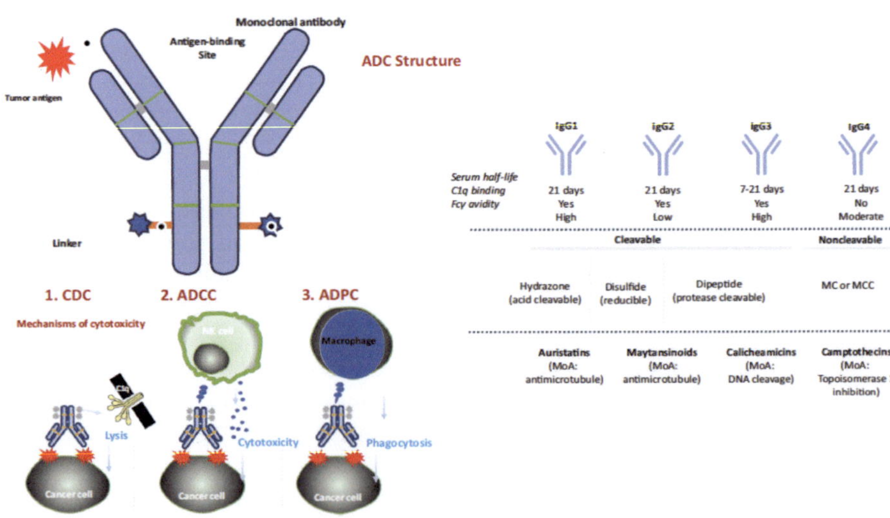

Fig. 8.3 The structure and components of ADCs. (Adapted from Coleman [2])

construct, have shorter half-lives in vivo. Different Fcy regions on immune effector cells have distinct affinities for each IgG subclass, with a majority of ADCs developed on the basis of IgG1 architecture, optimally combining solubility, binding affinity, and long serum half-life for Fcy receptors and greater complement fixation. IgG1 serves as a scaffold for ADCs due to its hinge structure, but IgG2- and IgG4-based ADCs lessen nontarget tissue aggregation. Different immunogenic responses result from the distinct antibody isotypes with an indirect mAb cytotoxic mechanism, including complement-dependent cell-mediated cellular toxicity, antibody-dependent cytotoxicity, and complement-dependent cellular toxicity. Different epitopes also have varying rates of internalization, whereas miniaturized antibodies maintain specificity and high affinity and also make traveling into the vasculature of solid tumors, which is more challenging for ADCs, easier.

Payloads are part of the ADC with cytotoxic properties and with intracellular targets such as tubulin and nucleic acids. They ideally have a low molecular weight and high solubility with functional groups such as potent inhibitors of tubulin and agents of DNA. They fall under the categories of auristatins (antimicrotubules affect microtubule structure: MMAE and MMAF), maytansinoids (antimicrotubules affect microtubule structure: ravtansine), calichaemicins (DNA cleavage: firmly attach to minor DNA grooves, leading to breaks in double-stranded DNA and cellular death), and camptothecins (topoisomerase 1 inhibition leading to apoptosis), all of which induce G2/M arrest and thus apoptosis by inhibiting microtubule polymerization. Their activity is limited by low cellular internalization, restricted tumor antigen expression, limited permeability into tumor tissue, and degradation while circulating. When potent, they have remarkably cytotoxic activity with tumor cell elimination with IC50 in nanomolar and picomolar concentration ranges and would cause severe toxicity if given systemically. Immunomodulatory agents such as immune-stimulating antibody conjugates that constitute noncytotoxic payloads that activate myeloid APCs are also emerging. They have a different mechanism of action that activates toll-like receptors, causing a signaling pathway cascade that activates NF-KappaB, which causes the secretion of chemokines and cytokines and activates lymphocytes. The drug-to-antibody (DAR) ratio is defined by the average number of payload moieties that are attached to each mAb, which ranges between two and eight, with high DARs being more potent with faster clearance and with in vitro activity directly correlating with DAR. The payload must also have the property of being stable in the acidic lysosomal environment, with the ability even after degradation to retain cytotoxicity.

The fourth main constituent of an ADC is the linker, which connects the antibody to the cytotoxic drug via covalent bonds for targeted delivery, impacting DAR, therapeutic index, pharmacokinetic (PK) and pharmacodynamic (PD) characteristics of the drug, and payload release and playing a significant role in the stability, efficacy, and safety of an ADC. They come in two classes: cleavable (disulfide, acid labile, protease cleavable) and noncleavable. Cleavable linkers have the property of maintaining stability while circulating and undergoing cleavage within the acidic lysosomal intracellular milieu with elevated glutathione. Other studies have categorized linkers into chemical or disulfide and hydrazone bonds, on one hand, and enzyme linkers or peptide and glucuronide bonds (including those used in polatuzumab vedotin, enfortumab vedotin, Sacituzumab govitecan, and trastuzumab deruxtecan (T-DXd), brentuximab vedotin), on the other. The amino acids phenylalanine–lysine (Phe-Lys), valine–citrulline (Val-Cit), and valine–alanine (Val-Ala) dipeptide linkers are employed in the construction of the linker, relying on the lysosomal protease Cathepsin B, overexpressed in tumor cells that can recognize and cleave specific peptide sequences such as Phe-Lys and Val-Cit, leading to the release of the connected cytotoxic payload by exerting its protease activity, such as the large payload doxorubicin.

Hydrozone, being pH sensitive, maintains stability in systemic circulation and releases the payload when exposed to the acidic environment of the lysozyme; an example of an ADC utilizing a hydrazone linker is gemtuzumab ozogamicin. Acid labile linkers are sensitive to external pH and the acidic environment of lysosomes and endosomes; protease cleavable linkers are specific to lysosomal proteases; and disulfide linkers are sensitive to glutathione reduction and rely on the high concentration of glutathione reducing molecule in the cytoplasm to release the payload. The variation in reduction potential that occurs when ADCs, having reducible linkers, enter cancer cells leads to payload release. Examples of ADCs utilizing reducible disulfide linkers are indatuximab ravtansine and mirvetuximab soravtansine. Payload release occurs in a precise and guided way through tumor-associated factors that distinguish between tumor cells and other cells when circulating systemically. Recent cleavable linkers (e.g., enfortumab vedotin, sacituzumab govitecan, and trastuzumab deruxtecan (T-DXd)) are stable when systemically circulated, in contrast to noncleavable linkers (e.g., ado-trastuzumab emtansine (TDM1)). Hydrazone linkers are more labile than other cleavable linkers and undergo hydrolysis at physiological pH and thus has more off-target toxicities.

Noncleavable linkers release their payload after internationalizing and after the breakdown of the mAb component in the lysosome and have high stability. An example would be TDM1, which is thioether based and links the anti-HER2 mAB with mertansine (DM1). This cleavage mechanism enhances systemic circulation prior to the active drug release of DM2 but after Ab degradation. Noncleavable linkers often result in the retention of the charged amino acids within the payload, affecting cell permeability.

Stability is crucial for linkers because their chemical stability is necessary to avoid off-target toxicity and for the effective release of the payload at the targeted site. The complete lysosomal enzymatic degradation of the antibody must take place to detach the linker, also leading to higher potency, decreased extracellular payload release, decreased off-target toxicity, and a high therapeutic index. However, stable linkers have limitations in that they have lower release efficacy and are unable to induce bystander effects (explained later), and PK/PD analysis and toxicity profiles must be assessed before utilizing the noncleavable linker technology [1, 2, 7].

8.2 The Development of Antibody Drug Conjugates

First-generation ADCs were viewed as improvements over initial constructions combining immunoglobulins with chemotherapeutic drugs with a noncleavable linker. However, they lacked superiority over free cytotoxic drugs, and later, first-generation drugs led to improved safety, achieved by stronger cytotoxic drugs that received market approval, examples being inotuzumab ozogamicin and gemtuzumab Ozogamicin. However, these were later removed due to excessive liver toxicity, in addition to shorter half-life, linker instability, and lower potency, and further advancements were needed. Three Food and Drug Administration (FDA)-approved ADCs, namely inotuzumab ozogamicin, ado-trastuzumab emtansine, and brentuximab vedotin, followed, with better cytotoxic payloads, with better linkers, and featuring the more careful selection of mABs (IgG1 subtype) to increase tumor cell specificity and decrease cross-reactivity with normal cells. They serve as more-potent molecules when compared with first-generation ADCs, with better chemistry manufacturing and controls (CMC) characteristic and linkers modified for increased stability and more uniformity in DAR distribution. More-cytotoxic payloads, such as mytansinoids and auristatins are used, with better binding ability and better water solubility. However, they face diminished therapeutic windows due to off-target toxicity and quick clearance. ADCs such as enfortumab vedotin (EV), Pola-V, and T-DXd are examples of third-generation ADCs. Site-specific conjugation is key to the production of successful ADCs, leading to lower off-target toxicity and higher PK effectiveness, due to a process of site-specific linkage utilized to generate ADCs with DARs of 2 or 4; their more powerful payloads; and their having entire humanized antibodies with less immunogenicity. Certain investigations are also being conducted to make ADCs more stable in circulation, to make them more easily internalizable by tumor cells, and to use Fabs as substitutes for full mAb in various forms of ADCs and the use of PEGylation linkers, with an increase in the therapeutic index [8].

8.3 ADCs' Mechanism of Action (Figs. 8.4 and 8.5)

ADCs trigger genome/cellular death by aiming at cancer cells. They achieve drug delivery selectively to cancer cells and lessen off-targeted toxicities through a multifaceted mechanism: antibody to target antigens, followed by internationalization and payload release within cells. According to Chen, the canonical mechanism of action involves distinct steps of specific binding to the target within systemic circulation, with ADCs selectively binding to the target antigen on the tumor cell surface; the internalization binding of ADCs triggers a process of receptor-mediated

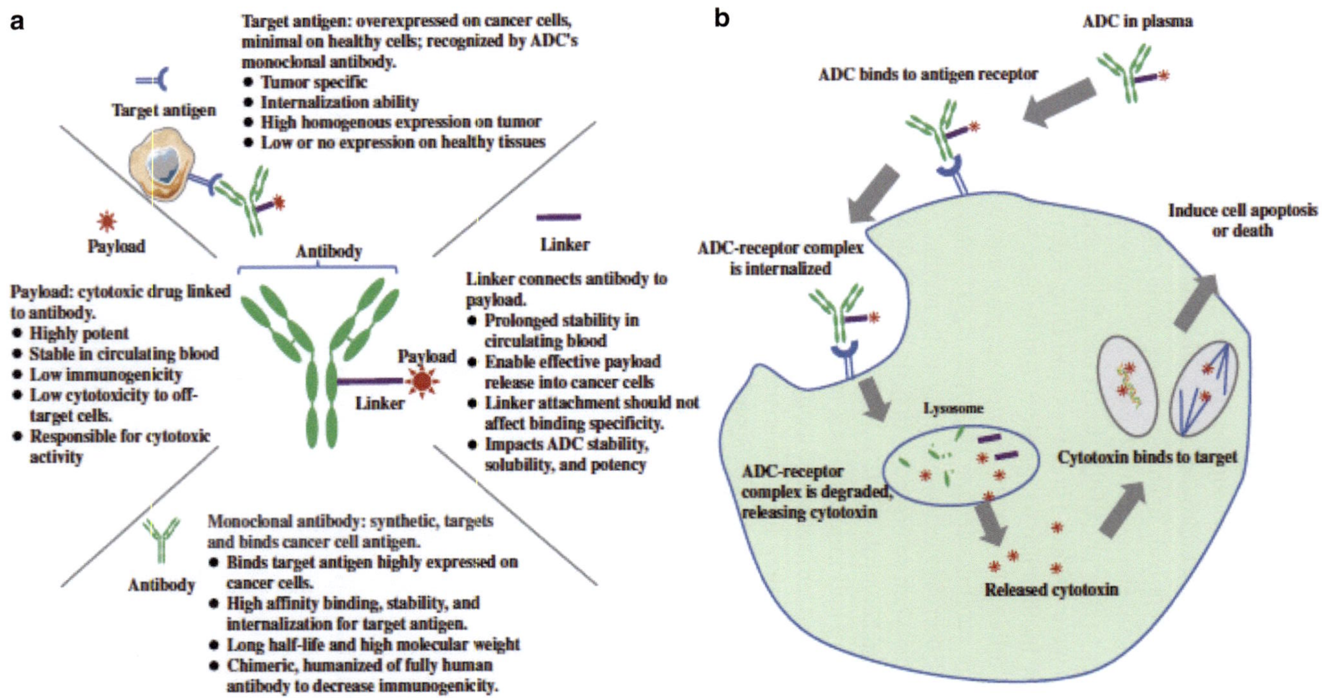

Fig. 8.4 ADCs' mechanism of action. (Adapted from Chen [1])

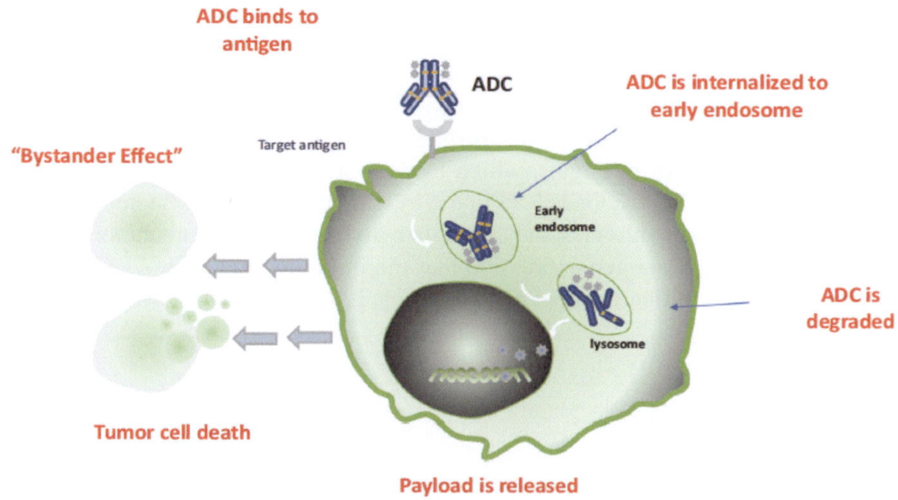

Fig. 8.5 Another depiction of ADCs' mechanism of action. (Adapted from Coleman [2])

endocytosis that promotes tumor cell internalization for ADC uptake; a complex intracellular trafficking process of transporting to lysosomes for metabolism and linker cleavage takes place where the linker molecule is chemically or enzymatically cleaved and the drug is finally released, at which point the cytotoxic drug is liberated from the antibody within lysosomes. At that point, the cytotoxic effect is exerted; the cytotoxic drug has various mechanisms to exert its toxicity, including the inhibition of DNA synthesis, microtubule formation disruption, inducing apoptosis, and interfering with pathways involved in cellular signaling. Coleman offers a more complicated picture of the way that ADCs act as "agents of precision medicine" or "biological homing missiles," specifically targeting tumor cells and inducing cellular death, allowing for increased drug delivery. After the antibody on the ADC binds to the target antigen on the tumor cell, the ADC is then internalized by the cancerous cell. After lysosomal fusion, the cytotoxic agent is released. The bystander effect can further enhance the ADC efficacy, which is when a free drug in circulation is released and unintentionally kills adjacent cancer cells that do not express the target cell antigen on its cell surface when the ADC crosses the cell membrane of the target tumor after internationalization and degradation, thereby enhancing ADC efficacy. This can also be enhanced by the linker effect, with the conjugation to the lysine residue, as an example, leading to an attenuated bystander effect, "as charged residues" promote drug persistence within the tumor cell target. This picture is further complicated by an ADC's activity as a prodrug in vivo, where each ADC has distinct half-lives and differing peak times. ADCs are usually in circulation as naked Ab, intact conjugate, and free payload owing to incomplete conjugation. Inefficient tumor penetration is also common, with tumor payload being released before engaging with the antigen–antibody complex. However, the active antibody component may dampen downstream signaling by engaging with immune effector cells before payload is ever released. ADC activity may be affected by the degree of target internalization and turnover and constitute an important contributor, because after engaging with an antigen, most ADC internalization occurs via endocytosis, with targets being bound. Lysosomes possess a proteolytic or redox environment and once inside ADCs release their payload to diffuse into cytoplasm, acting on substrates from targets, which leads to genome/cell death. This review notes that hydrophobic payloads lead to the bystander effect, because being able to diffuse through cell membranes, they result in cytotoxicity toward neighboring cells irrespective of target antigen expression that might be important for ADC efficacy with heterogenous antibody target expression [1, 2, 7] (Table 8.1).

8.4 Clinical Studies

The antitrophoblast cell-surface antigen-2 (TROP2) in its humanized version forms part of the antibody drug conjugate. Datopotamab deruxtecan (Dato-DXd) is linked to the potent topoisomerase I inhibitor payload via a cleavable linker. Dato-DXd was evaluated in the TROPION-PanTumor01 phase I dose-escalation/dose-expansion trial for safety, tolerability, antitumor activity, and pharmacokinetics solid tumors with prior therapy, including HR+/HER2- breast cancer and TNBC. Out of

Table 8.1 FDA-approved antibody conjugated antibodies [9]

Drug name	Targets	Conjugated agents	Indications in hemato-oncology
Antibody drug conjugates			
BelantamabMafodotin	BCMA	Monomethyl auristatin F	MM
BrentuximabVedotin	CD30	Monomethyl auristatin E	HL, sALCL, or other CD30-positive PTCL, CTCL
GenturumabOzogamicin	CD33	Calicheamicin	AML
InotuzumabOrogamicin	CD22	Calicheamicin	ALL
LoncastuximabTesirine	CD19	Tesirine	FL
PolatuzumabVedotin	CD79b	Monomethyl auristatin E	DLBCL
Immunotoxins			
Denileukin-Diftitox	CD25	Diphtheria toxin	CTCL
MoxetumomabPasudotox	CD22	PE38	HCL
Tagraxofusp	CD123	Diphtheria toxin	BPDCN
Radio immunotherapeutic			
IbritumomabTiuxetan	CD20	90 yttrium (β-radiation)	FL

ALL acute lymphoblastic leukemia, *AML* acute myeloid leukemia, *BPDCN* blastic plasmacytoid dendritic cell neoplasm, *CTCL* cutaneous T-cell lymphoma, *DLBCL* diffuse large B-cell lymphoma, *FL* follicular lymphoma, *HL* Hodgkin lymphoma, *HCL* hairy cell leukemia, *MM* multiple myeloma, *PTCL* peripheral T-cell lymphoma, *sALCL* systemic anaplastic large cell lymphoma the 85 patients enrolled (HR+/HER2– BC = 41 and TNBC = 44), ORR through blinded independent central review (BICR) was 26.8% (95% CI 14.2 to 42.9) and 31.8% (95% CI 18.6 to 47.6) with median DOR not evaluable and 16.8 months for breast cancer (BC) and TNBC, respectively. Median progression-free survival (mPFS) was 8.3 months and 4.4 months for BC and TNBC, respectively. Furthermore, 100% of BC and 41.5% of TNBC patients experienced all-cause treatment-emergent adverse events (TEAEs). The study investigators concluded that Dato-DXd showed potential clinical response and a tolerable safety profile [10].

Following this study, a preclinical analysis was conducted to assess antitumor activity and determine biomarkers for datopotamab deruxtecan in breast cancer in patient-derived breast cancer xenograft models. The authors reiterated that Dato-DXd is a humanized anti-TROP2 igG1 mAb linked to a topoisomerase I inhibitor payload, and they sought to determine the importance of TROP2 expression and determinants of response. Their experimental design involved showing the effects of TROP2 expression on Dato-DXd activity in vitro and in vivo in breast cancer patient–derived xenograft-derived cell lines. Their results included that a 10 mg/kg dosing of Dato-DXd led to objective response (OR). In 36% of models, the prolongation of event free survival (EFS) was statistically significant in eight models (73%), compared to fewer events for the IgG-DXd at the same dosing levels, with higher levels of TROP2 mRNA and protein in Dato-DXd-sensitive models. Overexpression conferred the antitumor activity of Dato-DXd in vitro and in vivo. Activity in breast cancer models was shown by Dato-DXd mediated by TROP2-dependent and -independent antitumor activity. The authors additionally demonstrated that the membrane expression of TROP2 was highly correlated with matched patient derived xenograft models (PDXs) in patient tumors. Four models (36.4%) had a PR when treated with the ADC, with all five models having high TROP2 expression, demonstrating antitumor activity and tumor regression in these models, with low TROP2 expression showing variable antitumor activity.

According to the results, two of "the BCXs that regressed with 10 mg/kg Dato-DXd (BCX.022 and BCX.024) also had tumor regression with 10 mg/kg IgG-DXd. However, at equivalent 1 mg/kg doses of Dato-DXd and IgG-DXd, Dato-DXd had greater activity in these models. Four models had greater sensitivity to 10 mg/kg Dato-DXd compared with the equivalent dose of IgG-DXd." After the stratification of BCXs into responders and nonresponders, the investigators showed that the responders had significantly more TROP2 expression, as shown through immunohistochemistry (IHC), where RNA-seq showed that RNA expression was also higher, with Dato-DXd significantly increasing the percentage of apoptotic cells in these TROP2-overexpressing cell lines versus controls. Dato-DXd induced DNA damage markers pCHK1, pCHK2, γH2AX, and pKAP1, showing increased expression in Dato-DXd responsive models, which ranged from a modest to a high increase in levels. In one experiment, Dato-DXd was combined with olaparib, and the combination (1mg/kg Dato-DXd) led to significantly greater durable response and better antitumor activity (data not shown). The study authors conclude that TROP2 expression was associated with Dato-DXd response with variable sensitivity to IgG-DXd and was associated with payload for subsequent membrane binding and internationalization, confirming the importance of TROP2 expression for Dato-DXd activity [11].

Three clinical trials reported in *JCO* illustrated positive outcomes from evaluating ADCs with or without ICIs in metastatic and advanced urothelial cancer. Sheng et al. conducted a combined analysis of two phase II clinical trials to evaluate the efficacy and safety of disitamib vedotin, a novel humanized anti-HER2 antibody conjugated with MMAE in HER2 positive local advanced or metastatic UC patients refractory to the standard of care. Patients received 2 mg/kg intravenous (IV) infusion once every 2 weeks. ORR was the primary endpoint, and progression-free survival (PFS), overall survival (OS), and safety were assessed. ORR was 50.5 (95% CI 40.6 to 60.3), PFS was 5.9 months (95% CI 4.3 to 7.2), and OS was 14.2 months (95% CI 9.7 to 18.8); 58 patients (54.2%) experienced grade 3 treatment-related adverse events (TRAEs), including neutropenia and peripheral neuropathy. Waterfall plots indicted an 82.2% change in tumor size shrinkage, and swimmer plots demonstrated positive patient responses from the start of treatment [12].

Milowsky reported on outcomes on patients with advanced UC receiving the antibody drug conjugate enfortumab vedotin (EV) with and without pembrolizumab who were ineligible for cisplatin in a phase Ib/II trial. Quality of life (QOL) and functioning symptoms were evaluated by using EORTCQLQ-C30. Monotherapy and dual therapy were administered in a 1:1 ratio: Of 149 patients, 65 were EV + P and 63 were EV mono. Improvements in pain, emotional functioning, and insomnia were assessed at week 24, and clinically meaningful improvements in pain were observed after EV + P at weeks 12 and 24 (−14.41 and 14.99) for EV mono. QOL remained stable, with insomnia (−14.46) and constipation (−10.09) at week 24. The authors concluded for cisplatin ineligible patients that improvement in or the preservation of QOL functioning and symptoms was seen in both treatment arms [13].

Enfortumab vedotin (EV) is an anti-NECTIN4 ADC approved for patients with metastatic urothelial carcinoma (mUC) ; however, its benefit for the NECTIN4+population is not well characterized, because clinical benefit is seen in a small subset. Located on 3q23.3 and 1q2.3, it represents frequent copy number variations (CNVs). Furthermore, 108 patients were evaluated, and CNVs were correlated with membranous NECTIN4 protein expression, EV treatment responses, and durable outcomes. The Cancer Genome Atlas (TCGA) data were also queried, eliciting 10,712 patients across 32 cancer types for NECTIN4 CNVs. In muscle-invasive bladder cancer, NECTIN4 amplifications are frequent genomic events that represent stable genomic alteration and indicate progression. NECTIN4 amplification was associated with objective response to EV (96% vs. 27 of 28) compared with 32% (24 of 74) in the nonamplified subgroup adjusted for age and sex, with a 92% reduction in the risk of death. TCGA analysis indicated that NECTIN4+amplification occurred in other cancers (5–10% of breast and lung cancer). The amplification of NECTIN4+is seen as predictive of long-term EV responses in terms of genomic events [14].

The efficacy and safety results of sacituzumab govitecan (SG) in metastatic TNBC were reported in the ASCENT trial conducted by Bardia et al. SG ($n = 235$) was compared to chemotherapy ($n = 233$) as a single agent prespecified by the investigator (54% eribulin, 20% vinorelbine, 13% capecitabine, and 12% gemcitabine). Consistent with investigator assessments, mPFS according to blinded central independent review (BCIR) was 5.6 months (95% CI 4.3 to 6.3) versus 1.7 months (95% CI 1.5 to 2.6) for SG and chemotherapy, respectively (HR, 0.41; 95% CI 0.32 to 0.52), which was consistent with investigator assessments (5.5 months vs1.7 months) (HR, 0.35; 95% CI 0.28 to 0.44). Median OS was 12.1 months (95% CI 10.7 to 14) versus 6.7 months (95% CI 5.8 to 7.7) for SG versus chemotherapy, respectively (HR 0.48; 95% CI 0.38 to 0.59). Neutropenia (63% vs. 43%), diarrhea (59% vs. 12%), nausea (57% vs. 26%), alopecia (46% vs. 16%), fatigue (45% vs. 30%), and anemia (34% vs. 24%) were the most common TRAEs. Grade 3 or higher events of neutropenia, leukopenia, and anemia were reported: 51% vs. 33%, 10% vs. 5%, and 8% vs. 5%, respectively.

Other Key Results

Serious TRAEs occurred in 39 patients (15%) and 19 patients (8%) when treated with SG and chemotherapy respectively, leading to dose reductions in each arm from AEs of similar frequency (22% vs. 26%).

The investigators concluded that the utilization of SG benefited all clinical subgroups, including those receiving PD-1 and PD-L1 inhibitors as prior treatment. The odds ratio (OR) was higher when compared to chemotherapy (35% vs. 5%); improvements in PFS and OS were also seen as in a full trial of patients with or without brain metastasis [15].

SG in combination with pembrolizumab was assessed in patients with mUC that progressed after platinum-based chemotherapy in the TROPHY-U-01 trial, specifically cohort 3. Pembrolizumab is the standard of care for this patient population but meets with a 21% response. SG received accelerated FDA approval for mUC patients receiving a platinum-based chemotherapy and an immune checkpoint inhibitor (ICI). The open label, multicohort phase II study evaluated patients who were ICI naive and metastatic in the adjuvant setting. Patients received 10 mg/kg of SG once on days 1 and 8 and 200 mg of pembrolizumab on day 1 of 21-day cycles. ORR per a central review was the primary endpoint. PFS, DOR, and clinical benefit rate were also reported. With a median follow-up, key results include the following:

- ORR of 41% (95% CI 26.3 to 57.9)
- CRR of 20%
- Clinical benefit rate (CBR) of 46% (95% CI 30.7 to 62.6)
- Median DOR of 11.1 months (95% CU 4.8 to not estimable (NE))
- PFS of 5.3 months (95% CI 3.4 to 10.2)
- OS of 12.7 months (range, 10.7 to NE)
- Grade 3 TRAEs of 61%, including neutropenia (37%) leukopenia (20%), and diarrhea (20%) (most common)

The authors concluded that SG + ICI demonstrated a high response rate with a favorable safety profile, with no new safety signals in the mUC population who progressed after platinum-based chemotherapy.

Sacituzumab govitecan was also evaluated in comparison to docetaxel for previously treated metastatic and advanced non–small cell lung cancer (NSCLC). The open label, randomized phase III EVOKE-01 study enrolled patients assigned in a 1:1 ratio to receive SG (n = 299) in a 10 mg/kg intravenous infusion or docetaxel (n = 304) 75 mg/m^2 in 21-day cycles. OS served as the primary endpoint, and key secondary endpoints were PFS, ORR, and safety. OS was 11.1 versus 9.8 months in the SG and docetaxel arm, respectively (HR 0.84; 95% CI 0.68 to 1.04). Median PFS was 4.1 months versus 3.9 months (HR 0.9; 95% CI 0.77 to 1.11). Consistent across histologies was an mNSCLC nonresponse to prior anti-PD-L1-containing regimens: a 3.5-month mOS increase and an HR of 0.75 (95% CI 0.58 to 0.97). TRAE discontinuations were 6.8% versus 14.2%, respectively. TRAEs leading to death were 1.4% versus 1.0%, respectively. The study authors concluded that OS was numerically improved in SG versus docetaxel [16].

Telisotuzumab vedotin (Teliso-V) is an ADC that is c-Met directed with a monomethyl auristatin E cytotoxic payload was evaluated in the phase II LUMINOSITY trial for c-Met protein overexpressing wild-type EGFR NSCLC with prior treatment. C-Met overexpression was defined as greater than 25% tumor cells with 3+staining.

The dosing of Teliso-V was 1.9 mg/kg every 2 weeks, and ORR served as the primary endpoint. Of the 172 patients enrolled, those in stages I and II received Teliso-V. ORR was 28.6% (95% CI 21.7 to 36.2).

- C-Met high: 34.6% (95% CI 24.2 to 46.2)
- C-Met intermediate: 22.9% (95% CI 14.4 to 33.4)
- Median DOR: 8.3 months
  - C-Met high: 9.0 (95% CI 4.2 to 13.0)
  - C-Met intermediate: 7.2 (95% CI 5.3 to 11.5)
- Median OS: 14.5 months (95% CI 9.9 to 16.6)
  - C-Met high: 14.6 (95% CI 9.2 to 25.6)
  - C-Met intermediate: 14.2 (95% CI 9.6 to 16.6)
- Median PFS: 5.7 months (95% CI 4.6 to 6.0)
  - C-Met high: 5.5 (95% CI 4.1 to 8.3)
  - C-Met intermediate: 6.0 (95% CI 4.5 to 8.1)

AEs included peripheral sensory neuropathy of grade 3 or greater (30%), peripheral edema (16%), and fatigue (14%). The authors concluded that in c-Met overexpressing wild-type EGFR NSCLC, Teliso-V was associated with durable responses and with manageable AEs in comparison to docetaxel in this cohort [17].

Among biliary tract cancers (BTCs), which encompass a range of tumors, including cholangiocarcinomas and gallbladder cancer, only 10–40% are considered resectable. T-DXd demonstrated efficacy in HER2-expressing solid tumors. In a single-arm, multicenter phase II trial, the antibody drug conjugate demonstrated efficacy in patients refractory to a gemcitabine treatment regimen. In total, 32 patients who received 5.4 mg/kg dosing with a confirmed ORR of 36.4% (90% CI

19.6 to 56.1) were enrolled. Stratified according to HER2 expression, as revealed through IHC analysis, patients exhibited different response rates, showing durable response and more tumor shrinkage in high-HER2-expressing patients. Median PFS in the HER2-postive and HER2-low was 5.1 and 3.5 months, respectively, which was considered clinically meaningful with no treatment after third-line intensive therapy; manageable adverse events observed included grade 3 or higher hematologic toxicities, such as anemia and neutropenia [18].

SG was further evaluated in the TROPICS-3 trial, a phase II basket study in patients with solid tumors NSCLC, head and neck squamous cell carcinoma (HNSCC), and squamous cell carcinoma. ORR was the primary endpoint, and clinical benefit rate (CBR), DoR, PFS, CR, PR, and SD served as the secondary endpoints. Checkpoint inhibitors dostarlimab and pembrolizumab were evaluated in the phase III RUBY trial on recurrent endometrial carcinoma (EC) patients with mismatch repair (MMR)–proficient disease. SG has a humanized anti-TROP2 antigen, and mAB combination is linked to irinotecan and is marked by the high specificity of the antigen and a high DAR (7.6:1), with efficient payload release in Trop-2-expressing cancer cells in the tumor microenvironment (TME) as well as having a bystander effect enhancing its antitumor effect in adjacent cells not expressing Trop-2. SG has also shown antitumor activity against mTNBC in a dose expansion stage followed a proof-of-concept stage. In TROPICS-3, eight patients (20%) were microsatellite instability (MSI) high (MSI-H); 17% had a serous type histology; and 49% had endometroid histology. Median DOR was 8.8 months (95% CI 2.8 months to NE). Median PFS was 4.8 months (95% CI 2.8 to NE). Trop-2 expression was observed in 92% of tumor samples. No correlation was observed from baseline between the best change in tumor volume against tumor Trop-2 score. SD, PD, and PR showed "a similar range of tumor Trop-2 expression." Low and high Trop-2 expression both experienced PD, suggesting limited correlation between Trop-2 expression and SG efficacy. The three most common TEAEs were diarrhea ($n = 23$, or 56%), nausea ($n = 22$, or 54%), and fatigue ($n = 21$, or 51%). Grade 2 TEAEs included "neutropenia ($n = 13$, or 32%), diarrhea ($n = 8$, or 20%), febrile neutropenia ($n = 7$, or 17%), anemia ($n = 6$, or 15%), hypokalemia ($n = 6$, or 15%) and decreased neutrophil count ($n = 5$, or 12%)." Spider plots revealed tumor response over time [19].

Yao et al. [20] performed a trial on the safety, efficacy, and pharmacokinetics of SHR-A1811—an investigational anti-HER2 monoclonal antibody—combined with a topoisomerase inhibitor. Patients' tumors expressed HER2, had refractory advanced or metastatic solid tumors, and received intravenous doses of 1.0 to 8.0 mg/kg once every 3 weeks. The primary endpoints included dose-limiting toxicity, safety, and recommended dosing for the phase II trial. The solid tumors in 464 patients included HER2+breast cancer ($n = 90$) , HER2 low breast cancer ($n = 209$), BTC ($n = 23$), UC ($n = 23$), colorectal cancer (CRC) ($n = 14$), and gynecological cancer (GC) ($n = 10$), and these patients were selected for a dose-escalation stage, a pharmacokinetics stage, and an indication expansion stage. Dosing ranges included the following:

- Dose-escalation stage: 1.0 mg/kg ($n = 6$), 2.0 mg/kg ($n = 6$), 3.2 mg/kg ($n = 6$), 4.8 mg/kg ($n = 6$), 6.4 mg/kg ($n = 8$), and 8.0 mg/kg ($n = 3$)
- Pharmacokinetics expansion stage: 4.8 mg/kg ($n = 28$), 5.6 mg/kg ($n = 25$), 6.4 mg/kg ($n = 27$), and 8.0 mg/kg ($n = 16$)
- Indication expansion stage: 4.8 mg/kg ($n = 98$) and 6.4 mg/kg ($n = 78$)

Assessments in tumor response were performed every 6 weeks for the first 24 weeks. CT and MRI were used to measure tumor responses. Regarding the safety profile, AEs were observed in 300 or 97.7% of 307 patients.

The decreased neutrophil count was 204 (66.4%); anemia was in 198 patients (64.5%) and nausea in 188 (61.2%). Also, 87 patients (60.9%) experienced grade 3 or higher adverse events. Serious adverse events were reported in 70 (22.8%) with 40 (13.0%) considered treatment-related. The authors of this phase 1 first-in-human (FIH) umbrella trial concluded that SHR-A1811 offers "promising antitumor activity and a manageable safety profile." As "an ADC," it is considered an active agent in HER2 expressing cancers, for which clinical trials will be used to determine "different toxicity profiles."

8.5 Further Clinical Studies

8.5.1 Trastumuzumab Deruxitcan

A recent study evaluated the genomic profiles of HER-2 positive advanced gastric cancer tumors in a real-world study to predict sensitivity to trastumuzumab deruxtican and determine the impact of genomic alterations. Notably, 20% of advanced GC patients are HER2+. A retrospective study with real-world clinical data and comprehensive genomic profilling (CGP) performed through next-generation sequencing (NGS) was conducted to show that although the most frequently altered genes were TP53 (82%), ERBB2(80%), and CCNE1 (36%), CCNE1 amplification and alterations in cell-cycle genes were predictive of shorter PFS when T-DXd treatment was compared with non-T-DXd treatment (mPFS, 131 days versus 189 days; HR 1.90 (95% CI 1.02 to 3.53)). PFS was significantly higher in patients with ERBB2 amplification than in those without (41% in ERBB2-amplified tumors vs. 11% in ERBB2-nonamplified tumors).

Key Results

In this study, 1450 gastric and gastroesophageal junction (G/GEJ) cancers were analyzed, demonstrating CCNE1/ERBB2 coamplification at a rate of 41% versus 11% CCNE1 amplification in ERBB2-nonamplified tumors. Here, 3.7% of G/GEJ cancers and 8.8% of HER2+tumors treated with T-DXd had ERBB2-activating mutations, with mutated tumors having decreased PFS when compared to nonmutating tumors (mPFS 105 versus 180 days). Additionally, 28 patients experienced PR (25%), and 40 patients experienced SD (35%). Median PFS was 169 days (95%

CI 131 to 194), and further genomic analysis was conducted in high TMB samples (18%). S310F/Y, V842I, and R678Q were the most frequent mutations in the extracellular domain (ECD), kinase domain, and juxtamembrane domain, respectively. The study authors also surmised that because cyclin E1 overexpression via cell-cycle dysregulation leads to chromosomal instability, different carcinogenic mechanisms may be involved in CCNE1/ERBB2 coamplification in G/GEJ tumors when compared to other solid tumors and that tumor-agnostic drug development may be conducted for this mutation, leading to the conclusion that CCNE1 amplification may lead to T-Dxd drug resistance [21].

8.5.2 Enfortumab Vedotin and Pembrolizumab/Trastuzuamb Deruxtecan and TKI

Two original investigations reported in *JAMA Oncology* evaluated ADC combination therapy and the optimal sequencing of agents after a tyrosine kinase inhibitor. A systematic review and meta-analysis conducted by Yajima et al. had the objective of determining EV and pembrolizumab combination approaches in metastatic urothelial carcinoma. Frenel et al. analyzed the complexity in the optimal sequencing of the ADC trastuzumab deruxtecan followed by the TKI tucatinib in patients with ERBB2-positive (formerly HER2) metastatic breast cancer (mBC). In total, 101 mBC patients with prior trastuzumab deruxtecan treatment were followed up with to determine the clinical outcomes of tucatinib in combination with trastuzumab and capecitabine (TTC) treatment. The primary endpoints included PFS, OS, and ORR. The median number of prior treatments of exposure was four at TTC treatment initiation, with 82 patients (81.2%) having prior trastuzumab plus pertuzumab and 94 (93.1%) having prior trastuzumab emtansine exposure. Lastly, 18 patients (17.8%) had stopped ADC treatment due to drug toxicity. For 86 patients (85.1%), TTC was the immediate treatment (Table 8.2).

The rationale behind the design of the study was shown to be clinical evidence of resistance to trastuzumab deruxtecan, which is now considered a first-line therapy choice for mBC patients without active brain metastasis because it outperforms chemotherapy. Few studies have posited mechanistic hypotheses accounting for this resistance, and "only 15% of patients in the DESTINY-Breast03 trial had received a previous TKI, while no patients enrolled in the HER2CLIMB clinical trial had received prior [T-DXd]." The authors concluded that "the present study found a meaningful intracranial DCR of 62.5% based on the RECIST guideline, version 1.1, with an ORR of 18.8%, a median PFS of 4.7 (95% CI 3.0–7.3) months, and a median TTNT of 5.6 (95% CI 4.4–NR) months in patients with active brain metastases at TTC initiation" [24].

Metastatic urothelial carcinoma typically presents with poor prognosis, and treatment options remain limited to chemotherapy regimens such as docetaxel. The ADC enfortumab vedotin targeted to nectin-4 on pooled analysis showed clinically meaningful results over chemotherapy as monotherapy and in combination with

Table 8.2 Clinical Outcomes for mBC patients with prior TDxt followed-up with tucatinib and TTC treatment.

TTC (trastuzumab and capecitabine)	mPFS (median progression free survival)	mOS (median overall survival)	Median TTNT (time to new treatment)	Best ORR (objective response rate)	DCR (disease control rate)	Intracranial ORR
	4.7 (95% CI 3.9–5.6)	13.4 (95% CI 11.1–NR)			64%	
Immediately after initial exposure	5.0 (95% CI 4.2–6.0)	13.4 (95% CI 11.9–NR)	5.5 (95% CI 4.8–7.2)			
After ADC toxicity-related discontinuation	7.3 (95% CI 3.0–NR)			32.6%		
Brain metastasis	4.7 (95% CI 3.0–7.3)	12.4 (95% CI 8.3–NR)	5.6 (95% CI 4.4–NR)			
Brain metastasis documented at site of progression			5.2 (95% CI 4.5–7.0)			20.0%

pembrolizumab, and Yajima et al. provided a comprehensive analysis of the safety and clinical efficacy of the ADC in combination with ICI and as monotherapy with a novel putative mechanism of action to overcome resistance. Pooled DCRs and pooled ORRs were associated with heterogeneity (79% (95% CI 74%–83%) (pooled DCR, moderate heterogeneity); (53% (95% CI 45%–61%), high heterogeneity). The pooled 1-year survival rate had high heterogeneity, at 67% (95% CI 56%–76%). All grade AEs reported a pooled incidence of 94% (95% CI 90%–96%); high-grade AEs reported a pooled incidence of 55% (95% CI 47%–62%).

Network meta-analysis allowed for the evaluation of three key randomized controlled trials (RCTs) in terms of comparative effectiveness and safety, which showed higher disease control rates and higher response rates when compared with chemotherapy:

- DCR
  - For EV plus pembrolizumab, OR 2.13 (95% CI 1.13–4.01)
  - For enfortumab monotherapy, OR 1.87 (95% CI 1.00–3.51)
- ORR
  - For EV plus pembrolizumab, OR 3.47 (95% CI 1.49–8.09)
  - For EV monotherapy and chemotherapy, statistical significance not reached and OR 2.29 (95% CI 0.97–5.42)

In terms of hematologic toxicities, anemia was less frequent in the combination arm when compared with chemotherapy (OR, 0.20; 95% CI 0.05–0.84); however, EV plus pembro led to higher frequencies of peripheral neuropathy when compared with chemotherapy (OR, 6.13; 95% CI 1.97–19.10). The study authors concluded that the dual treatment achieved historical benchmarks for mUC, with a DCR of 86% and an ORR of 68%, representing a great leap forward in disease management. EV monotherapy when compared with chemotherapy at later settings was also associated with higher response rates and a favorable safety profile in this meta-analysis of 11 studies [25].

8.5.3 *Polatuzumab Vedotin*

Polatuzumab vedotin (PV) belongs to the class of ADCs that target the CD79b antigen on B cells and delivers the microtubule inhibitor MMAE to cells after binding to the B-cell receptor on both normal B cells and B-cell malignancies, DLBCL being an example. Polatuzumab vedotin showed promise as monotherapy for DLBCL and the combination of PV with bendamustine and rituximab (BR), or Pola-BR, yielded encouraging ORRs (13–56%) for R/R DLBCL despite having a low CR rate (0–15%). One of the first studies reporting on the Pola-BR in comparison with polatuzumab vedotin with bendamustine and obinutuzumab (Pola-BG) as well as in comparison with BR alone was evaluated in a single-arm cohort conducted by Sehn et al. [26] in a phase Ib/II trial enrolling a randomly assigned single cohort consisting of R/R DLBCL patients ineligible for transplantation, published in *JCO* in 2019. The (Independent Review Committee) (IRC) assessment of Pola-BR versus BR was evaluated in the phase II portion at the end of treatment. PFS, DFS, and OR were also presented in Kaplan–Meier curves.

Key Results

The Pola-BG CR rate and mOS were 29.6% and 10.8 months. In total, 80 patients in the Pola-BR arm had a significantly higher CR (40.0% vs. 17.5%), PFS (median, 9.5 vs. 3.7 months; HR, 0.36, 95% CI 0.21 to 0.63), and OS (median, 12.4 vs. 4.7 months; HR, 0.42; 95% CI 0.24 to 0.75), as assessed through IRC at a median follow-up of 22.3 months. Grade 3–4 events included neutropenia (46.2 vs. 33.3%), anemia (28.2% v 17.9%), thrombocytopenia (41% vs. 23.1%), and grade 3–4 serious infections (23.1% vs. 20.5) in each cohort, respectively, with peripheral neuropathy resolving (43.6%). The CR rate was 50%, with remission in all three patients at a median follow-up of 37.6 months (DOR 28.9 to 38.2 months). One nonresponder remained alive after receiving subsequent therapy, and two died as a result of disease progression. In the combined phase of the Pola-BG arm, the CR rate was 29.6%, mPFS was 6.3 months, and mOS was 10.8 months, respectively. Four patients reported durable responses lasting at least 20 months (20.7–22.5 months) without requiring additional treatment. Two patients proceeded to autologous and allogeneic stem cell transplantation (SCT). Eight patients remained alive, 17 died due to progressive disease (120) and AEs (five), and two discontinued due to one physician decision and an AE. PFS and OS were significantly increased with Pola-BR versus BR at a 22.3-month median follow-up. Peripheral neuropathy (PN) led to Polatuzumab vedotin (PV) dose reduction in two patients, with PN resolving. Fatal AEs were reported in nine Pola-BR patients, and 11 patients died due to infection (four BR and four Pola-BR), occurring after PD.

Significantly, levels of CD79b expression did not correlate with clinical outcome, including PFS and OS, in all subgroups, including refractory and heavily pretreated patients. The study authors concluded that "Pola-BR represents a novel, effective therapeutic regimen to address the unmet need of patients with transplantation-ineligible R/R DLBCL".

Pola-BR was also evaluated in patients with R/R FL, the most common indolent form of NHL (iNHL); however, the results determined that the regimen conferred no clinical benefit in a similarly designed study: A phase Ib safety analysis of Pola-BR and Pola-BG was followed by phase II randomization to investigate Pola-BR versus BR and phase II expansion to investigate Pola-BG. IRC-assessed safety and tolerability served as the primary endpoints in phase IB, and secondary endpoints included end of treatment (EOT) and the best objective response. Biomarker analysis of CD79b expression, investigator-assessed DoR, PFS, EFS, and OS were exploratory secondary endpoints.

Key Results

Randomized group

- Pola-BR arm
  - Median investigator-assessed DOR: 16.4 months
  - Median PFS: 18.5 months (95% CI 15.9–30.4)

- BR arm
  - Median IV-assessed DOR: 18.1 months (95% CI 12.5–35.0)

Dose-expansion phase

- Pola-BR arm
  - Median PFS not reached

SAEs were reported in 61.4% (27/440) in the Pola-BR arm and 29.3% (12/41) in the BR arm, which were mostly infections. PN was seen in 43.2% (19/44) in the Pola-BR group and 26.8% (11/41) in the Pola-BR group. EC, AML, CRC, and HL were reported as secondary malignancies (9.8%;4/41) in the Pola-BR group, and basal cell carcinoma, gastrointestinal (GI) adenocarcinoma (each $n = 2$), prostate cancer (PC), rectal cancer, and squamous cell carcinoma of the skin in 4% (1/26) (each $n = 1$) in the BR group and one endometrial adenocarcinoma in the Pola-BG group were reported.

The study authors surmised that the lack of ostensible clinical benefit when combining Pola-V with bendamustine and adding an anti-CD20 agent may be related to the considerable activity of bendamusine in FL patients; however, in "this analysis, safety results were found to be consistent with the known safety profiles of polatuzumab vedotin, bendamustine, obinutuzumab, and rituximab." The study authors concluded that the addition of PV to BR was not superior to BR/BG alone and that no differences were observed between BR and Pola-BR, with the latter regimen being associated with a greater incidence of SAEs and cytopenia, leading to the conclusion that adding Pola to BR does not lead to any clinical benefit for R/R FL [27].

The combination of the off-the-shelf, CD20xCD3 T-cell-engaging bispecific antibody mosunetuzumab and polatuzumab vedotin (mosun-pola or mos-PV) administered in an outpatient setting was evaluated for R/R aggressive LBCL. Mosunetuzumab is associated with a favorable safety profile in R/R DLBCL patients. Durable responses were observed, and treatment-related adverse events consistent with other studies were shown with incidences of CRS and Immune Effector Cell–Associated Neurotoxicity Syndrome (ICANS), typically associated with bispecific T-cell engager treatment. This phase 1b part was a dose-escalation study for finding recommended phase 2 dosing, which was followed by a phase 2 dose-expansion cohort to determine efficacy. IRC-assessed best ORR served as the primary endpoint. According to the study, mosunetuzumab had an RP2D determined to be 1/2/60/30 mg, with 1.8 mg/kg of polatuzumab vedotin in six patients. Moreover, 98 R/R LBCL patients enrolled in phase 2 were treated according to the 1/2/60/30 mg of mosunetuzumab dose schedule in combination with 1.8 mg/kg of polatuzumab vedotin. The Best ORR according to IRC assessment was 59.2% (95% CI 48.8–69.0). Per investigator assessment, the best ORR was 63.3% (95% CI 52.9–72.8), and the best CR was 51.0% (95% CI 40.7–61.3). The IRC and investigator concordance assessment of DoR was 82%. Median PFS values of 16.5 months (95% CI 5.6–23.4) with one previous treatment and 11.4 months (95% CI 5.7–18.7) with two or more treatments were shown. Patients with high-risk pathology or

Table 8.3 Safety results between the overall population and the dose-expansion cohort

	Fatigue	Neutropenia	Diarrhea	Pyrexia
Common AEs	46.7%	35.0%	30.8%	20%
Grade 3/4 AEs	6.7%	25%		
Grade 3/4 TRAEs (38.3%)		25%		
Grade 5 TRAEs: PD 5; COVID-19 pneumonia one patient (0.8%)				
Mos-PV discontinuation: 12; 8TR; grade 3 pneumonitis (*n* = 1), grade 3 cellulitis (*n* = 1), grade 4 encephalopathy (*n* = 1), PN (grade 1 and 2): 2				
CRS: Occurred in 20 of 120 patients (16.7%) Grade 1 CRS: 10% (*n* = 12); Grade 2 CRS: 4.2% (n = 5); Grade 3: 2.5% (*n* = 3)				
(ICANS) Immune Effector Cell–Associated Neurotoxicity Syndrome: *n* = 6; 5 in the dose-expansion cohort. AEs; Adverse Events, TRAEs Treatment Related Adverse Events; PD Progressive Disease, (Mos-PV) mosunetuzumab and polatuzumab vedotin; Cytokine Release Syndrome (CRS) Grade 1 events: Lethargy, syncope, confusion, mental status change (*n* = 1 each)				

clinical disease course showed durable responses with the administration of mosun-pola.

At RP2D, the safety results were similar between the overall population and the dose-expansion cohort (Table 8.3).

According to the authors, the phase 1b/2 dose-escalation/dose-expansion study showed that mosun-pola had durable responses and a favorable safety profile in R/R DLBCL. RP2D was established as 1/2/60/30 mg in combination with PV, with no MTD reached. The report also pointed out that the step-up dosing of mosunetuzumab in combination with PV reduced tumor burden to mitigate the number of CRS events occurring, which was limited to Grade 1 and occurred only in 16.7% of patients, with no grade 4 events and grade 3 events in 2.5% of patients—which was lower than mosunetuzumab monotherapy, similar to other BsAbs, and in contrast to CAR T-cell therapy. ICANS events were also limited to grade 1 events at a 5% incidence. The study investigators concluded that the ADC-directed bispecific antibody targeted agent against "two biologically relevant B-cell targets" induced durable responses in R/R LBCL patients, as demonstrated in the phase 1b/2 study using a mosun-pola combination regimen [28].

8.5.4 EGFR-Based Antibody Drug Conjugates

Two anti-EGFR-based antibody drug conjugates were evaluated in both in vitro studies and preclinical models, for TNBC and GBM. Jain et al. evaluated two investigational ADC agents in preclinical glioblastoma models that were delivered through convection-enhanced delivery (CED) for direct infusion. The study found that this "enhanced delivery" led to pronounced survival benefits in PDX models (three EGFRviii-amplified GBM PDXs, namely GBM6, GBM39, and GBM108, and an EGFR-nonamplified GBM10). PDX was accompanied by neurotoxicity as a result of linker stability, however. These two agents with similarity in having auristatin toxins, namely losatuxizumabm vedotin (ABBV-221) and depatuxizumab mafodotin (Depatux-M), are EGFR-targeting ADCs that have an auristatin toxin cell-impermeant MMAF and a cell-permeant MMAE, respectively. The CED infusion of MMAF is linked to an ADC in a noncleavable fashion at much greater concentrations than a similar ADC with a cleavable linker and a cell-permeable MMAE.

ABBV-221 led to in vitro bystander cytotoxicity.

Key Results

- GBM39 was found to be exceptionally sensitive to free toxins, with all four cell lines being highly sensitive in the subnanomolar range. EGFR-targeted antibodies conjugated to MMAE or MMAF were also evaluated, and infusions led to significantly reduced BLI signal in GBM6 and GBM39 models versus AB095 and AB095 models.
- "CED infusions of ABBV-221 (66 μg/mouse) and Depatux-M (60 μg/mouse) significantly extended the survival of all three PDX models.
  - GBM39 (median: 195 and > 300 days).
  - GBM6 (median: 125 and 140 days).
  - GBM108 (median: > 300 and 219 days, compared with AB095 (120 μg/mouse) control (medians: 20, 49 and 36 days, respectively))."

The negative charge of MMAF prevents the released toxin from entering cells, despite both ADCs releasing similar toxins (Cys-mc-MMAF or MMAE) in the brain TME after CED infusion in nontumor-harboring models. As the study authors conclude, in GBM PDX models, the intracranial administration of Depatux-M and ABBV-221 showed remarkable efficacy in EGFRviii-amplified GBM models, with the latter having neurotoxicity that may be mitigated by improving linker stability with the brain TME in the context of bystander effects from microtubules, neurotoxins, and cell penetrance [29].

Cheung et al. constructed an ADC that targeted EGFR with a CDK inhibitor in an elegant preclinical study evaluating this investigational agent against TNBC in a set of experiments designed to target EGFR on TNBC cells with a payload designed to elicit cytotoxicity through intereference with cell-cycle regulation, leading to tumor cell cytotoxicity. Cetuximab was the selected EGFR inhibitor for the generation of a cetuximab-SNS-032 ADC conjugated via a thiol-maleimide reaction, and the ADC was found to restrict EGFR-expressing cancer cell growth both in vitro and in xenograft models.

Toxicity was also limited in that non-EGFR normal breast cancers went mainly unaffected. Although cetuximab has not shown clinical efficacy in TNBC, due to intrinsic and acquired resistance and tumor heterogeneity, and although CDK4/6 inhibitors have limited activity in decreasing TNBC cell growth, a targeted approach combining the CDK2/cyclin E driving G1/S-phase transition dysregulation with the

EGFR expression of TNBC in an ADC was the scientific rationale for the study. EGFR would be directly attacked, and cell-cycle dysregulation would result from CDK inhibition. Also, scRNA single-cell sequencing and spatial transcriptomic analyses confirmed EGFR expression and cyclin A, cyclin E, and CDK2 levels in the breast cancer cells. As Cheung et al. explain, in basal-like BCs/TNBCs, even though CDK4/6 are upregulated, they are accompanied by cyclin D, CDK7/cyclin H, and CDK9/ cyclin T downregulation, which leads to the development of an ADC on the basis of cetuximab combined with a CDK inhibitor. This ADC is constructed by conjugating SNS-032, a selective inhibitor of CDK2/7/9, over CDK4/6 to cetuximab through a maleimide linker, with an antibody-bearing vehicle with specific delivery to tumor cells. The significant finding is that the expression of EGFR is necessary for this EGFR-specific ADC therapy.

Some of the key results are that levels of EGFR are higher in TNBC and both non-TNBC with the basal-like PAM50 molecular subtype and that key "cell cycle regulators CDK4/6/cyclin D (G1-phase), CDK2/cyclin E (G1/S-phase transition), and CDK2/cyclin A (S-phase) … are activated sequentially." CDK7/cyclin H and CDK9/cyclin T have RNA pol II activity, and CDK7 leads to the active phosphorylation of the CDK2/cyclin E complex for G1/S-phase progression. In ADC-treated mice, tumor growth delay was measured, and when compared with vehicle, cetuximab, and SNS-032 in cetuximab-resistant MDA-MB-468 xenografts, the delay was even more significant due to the molar fraction (1.65%) of the SNS-032 dose measurement of free uncoupled inhibitor treatment. The authors also note that two ADC doses of 10 mg/kg were given to animals, whereupon tumors demonstrated significantly inhibited tumor growth.

The study investigators conclude that in cancer cells that are EGFR-mutated; and when ADC was compared to cetuximab alone, cell-cycle arrest was induced, and cytotoxic activity was produced, with payload release and bystander cytotoxicity against neighboring EGFR-low cells in heterogenous TMEs. Cetuximab-SNS-032 ADC led to restricted cell viability and growth and cell-cycle inhibition, with a bystander effect in EGFR-low cells despite the low molar fraction of the inhibitor dose for cetuximab antitumor effects from orthotopic in vivo TNBC xenograft growth. "This ADC strategy could potentially be considered for further research to treat EGFR-expressing patients with limited treatment options and unfavorable prognoses" [30].

8.5.5 ADC Targets for NSCLC

ADC targets for NSCLC include HER2 T-DM1, T-DXd TROP2, Dato-D, SG, HER3, patritumab deruxtecan, Mesenchymal-Epithelial Transition factor (MET) Teliso-V, CEACAM, and tusamitamab ravtansine. HER2 targets include gene amplification, gene mutation, and elevated protein levels. HER2's signaling pathway is characterized by prolonged activation and the ability to form heterodimers with other membranes of the HER2 family, where ADCs targeting this family cause effective cytotoxic activity. Ado-trastuzumab emtansine, an HER2 mAB, is connected to tubulin polymerization inhibitor DM1, linked by a noncleavable maleimidyl 4-(N-maleimidomethyl) cyclohexane-1-carboxylate linker. In a phase 1 trial, ten patients achieved a PR (ORR 55.6%), mPFS was 11.3 months, a median DOR of 10.7 months was achieved, and an ORR of 72.7% (n = 8) in patients with HER2- mutant NSCLC was demonstrated (exon 20: n = 6). In phase 2 trials, the agents have shown limited-to-moderate efficacy, with PFS rates ranging from 2 months (n = 18) to 5 months (including 2.8 months). Corresponding ORRs are 44% and 38.1%, with a DCR of 52.4%. One trial with a cohort of 49 patients had an ORR not reached in HER2 IHC 2 overexpression and a 20% ORR in HER2 IHC3+groups, with an mPFS of 2.6 versus 2.7 months and an OS of 12.2 months versus 15.3 months. In NSCLC patient populations, T-DXd has shown greater cytotoxic potency and, antitumor activity when compared to tyrosine kinase inhibitors, and a bystander effect as a result of its DAR. Composed of an anti-HER2 IgG1 mAb connected to a topoisomerase inhibitor via a cleavable peptide linker, HER2 NSCLC showed substantial efficacy in a phase 1 trial, with an ORR of 72.7% and an mPFS of 11.3 months. The DESTINY-Lung01 also showed the efficacy of this ADC, with a 55% confirmed ORR, an mPFS of 8.2 months, and an mOS of 17.8 months, with responses in both HER2 mutant and nonexpressing cases. "At doses of 5.4 mg/kg and 6.4 mg/kg, T-DXd exhibited response rates of 53.8% and 42.9%, respectively." Dato-DXd employs a TROP2 mAb linked via a tetrapeptide linker with a topoisomerase payload in the TROPION, which was also effective in NSCLC patients exhibiting an mPFS of 6.9 months and an mOS of 11.4 months. In the phase III trial, when compared to docetaxel in advanced non-small cell lung cancer (aNSCLC), a confirmed ORR of 26.4% versus was 12.8% was shown, with an mDOR of 7.1 versus 5.6 months. In a patient population with prior immunotherapy and platinum-based chemotherapy, ORRs ranged from 21% to 25% at 4 mg/kg (23%), 6 mg/kg (21%), and 8 mg/kg (25%), with "one confirmed CR at 6 mg/kg, 32 PRs in 20 patients, 8 PRs in 29 patients at 4.0 mg/kg, 4 PRs in 20 patients at 6.0 mg/kg, and 20 PRs in 76 patients at 8.0 mg/kg. In NSCLC (n = 34), ORR was 35% (95% CI 19.7–53.5) and median DOR was 9.5 months (95% CI 3.3–NE)." SG had "encouraging therapeutic effectiveness," with moderate responses rates of 16.7% and an mOS of 7.3 months in a median response duration of 6 months, and nine patients achieved PR. In a pretreated population of three prior therapies in mNSCLC, an ORR of 19% was achieved, with an mDOR of 6 months, an mPFS of 5.2 months, and an mOS extending to 9.5 months. In the phase I/II IMMU-132-01 basket trial, Trop2 expression patients were treated with 8–18 mg/kg on a tumor-agnostic basis, and "in the NSCLC cohort, 54 patients received 8, 10, or 12 mg/kg; ORR was 16.7% (7.9–29.3), there were 9 PRs (16.7%), 22 SDs (40.7%). mDOR was 6.0 months (2.5–21.0), mPFS was 4.4 months, and mOS was 7.3 months. 10 mg/kg dose was selected for further development in dose-expansion studies."

Patritumab deruxtecan is an HER3-directed ADC composed of IgG mAB patritumab conjugated to an MAAA-1181 topoisomerase inhibitor payload linked with a tetrapeptide-based cleavable linker, and it has shown activity in EGFR-mutant NSCLC, with ORRs and mPFS reported as 39% and 8.2 months, respectively, in a phase I trial. In non-EGFR tumors receiving prior chemotherapy, a confirmed ORR of 28% was achieved, with 13 PRs and 22 SDs and a nmPFS of 5.4 months at a median DOR of 5.7 months. In a dose-expansion/dose-escalation study, at an HER3-DXd dose of 5.6 mg/kg, the safety and activity data confirmed evidence of preliminary antitumor activity in heavily pretreated aEGFR-mutated NSCLC patients. Telisotuzumab vedotin is composed of ABT-700 mAb directed to c-Met via MMAE, which is linked via a cleavable valine–citrulline. In a phase 1 trial, the mDoR was reported as 4.8 months, whereas the mPFS was reported as 5.7 months. Also evaluated in the LUMINOSITY trial, the monotherapy regimen elicited a 36.5% ORR in aNSCLC with prior treatment without EGFR and elevated c-Met expression. At moderate c-Met levels, a 52.2% ORR was reported. The strategic implementation of the CEACAM5-targeting ADCs is based on its expression in many tumors, including colorectal and lung cancer. A member of the carcinoembryonic antigen family, it is a glycoprotein that is prominently displayed on the cell surface. Tusamitamab ravtansine targets CEACAM5 and has a humanized mAB with a cytotoxic maytansinoid payload that was found to be a well-tolerated and potent agent in preclinical models, leading to dose-dependent cell death in CEACAM5 cell lines. In a phase 1 trial, an ORR of 7.1% and two confirmed PRs were yielded. Additionally, 13 PRs and 27 SDs resulted in a high CEACAM5 expression subgroup. The CARMEN-LC05 phase II study investigated the efficacy and safety of tusamitamab ravtansine with pembrolizumab ± chemotherapy in patients with CEACAM5-positive nonsquamous NSCLC, with a DCR and ORR of 88% and 40%, respectively. Reported common adverse events with each of these agents included fatigue, nausea, and neutropenia [1, 2].

8.6 Investigational Agents

8.6.1 SGN-B6A (Preclinical and Phase 1 Study)

SGNB6A is constructed with an integrin beta-6 targeting antibody that delivers an MMAE cytotoxic payload to cancer cells. The proof of concept of the target was determined through multiple investigations, which validated the overexpression of integrin beta-6 on advanced solid tumors, including CRC, NSCLC, and gastric cancer. The molecule was also found to play a role in metastasis in that it promotes epithelial mesenchymal transition (EMT), which allows cancer cells to invade adjoining healthy tissues. In a preclinical study conducted by Lyon et al., SGN-B6A was found to exhibit cytotoxicity and have a good tolerability profile, "capable of inhibiting tumor growth or regressing tumor volume in multiple integrin beta-6-positive carcinoma models." TCGA confirmed the expression of integrin beta-6 (ITGB6) in cancer tissues. Pancreatic cancer, lung cancer, esophageal cancer, HNSCC, and bladder carcinoma showed high levels of integrin beta-6 expression.

Key results include the observation of the antigen-dependent cytotoxic activity of SGNB6A in all subcutaneous xenograft 21 PDX models (10 adenocarcinoma and 11 squamous cell carcinoma, according to histology) among varied EC50 values that include tumor growth delay in the least responsive models and tumor volume reductions and tumor eradication in up to 25% of the more responsive models, as shown at the best response as a percentage change from baseline. Although dose-dependent antitumor activity was observed, variability existed in the durability and depth of response, including 3 mg/kg SGN-B6A response that led to durable tumor regression at day 40, with 2/8 mice remaining at complete tumor regression by the end of the study. Responses were across both pretreated and treatment-naive models, which were the best responding. No life-threatening toxicities were observed. The study authors concluded that in this PDX study of various histologies of NSCLC as recapitulated in tumor xenograft models, 12 of 21 had tumor reductions induced, with nine models having a reduction greater than 30% in both squamous cell and adenocarcinomas across varied integrin beta-6 expression assessed through IHC [5].

In a dose-escalation/dose-expansion study, SGNB6A was evaluated for safety, PK, and antitumor activity in patients with advanced NSCLC, HNSCC, and EC solid tumors. In total, 148 patients were enrolled (Part A = 88; Part B = 60). Grade 3 TEAEs (most common: neutropenia, 8.1%) were observed in 50.7% of patients out of a total of 88.5% (most common fatigue, 35.1%), and 37.2% were serious; 6.1% of patients discontinued therapy (due to peripheral neuropathy and pneumonia, 1.4% each), and three patients died due to TEAEs; however, none were treatment related. The study authors conclude that the agent had a favorable safety profile with antitumor activity (data not shown) in this heavily pretreated population. A randomized phase 3 study evaluating SGN-B6A is underway [31].

8.6.2 M9410

An investigational agent, M9140, an anti-CEACAM5 antibody drug conjugate (ADC) with an exatecan cytotoxic payload that showed antitumor activity, potency, and the bystander effect (the property of the cytotoxic payloads of ADCs that confers antitumor activity in cells with low antigen expression due to the improved permeability of the ADC) in a preclinical model was evaluated in a FIH phase 1 trial against mCRC malignancies. CEACAM5 is expressed on the tumor cells of advanced solid malignancies such as mCRC, and exacetan releases the topoisolsomerase inhibitor TOP1. The two components are conjugated by a ß-glucuronide linker that has stable circulation. Furthermore, 40 patients mCRC patients from the United States, Europe, and Japan were enrolled and evaluated for safety and pharmacokinetic profiles. According to the abstract presented at ASCO2024 by Kopetz et al., the "primary objectives of Part 1A were to determine the maximum tolerated dose (MTD) and/or recommended dose(s) for expansion (RDE)."

Key Results

Four out of 10 patients experienced PR, (2.4 mg/kg); 17 (42.5%) experienced SD; and PD was confirmed in six patients (15%), with a 100-day response. The MTD was 2.8 mg/kg, and recommended dose expansion took place at 2.8 mg/kg, shown through PD analysis. At 3.2 mg/kg, hematologic events were most common, and at

2.8 mg/kg, patients experienced grade 5 sepsis. Grade 3 TEAEs were thrombocytopenia and anemia in 11 (27.5%) each, with neutropenia in 16 patients (40%). White blood cell (WBC) count was decreased in 10 patients (25%). No ocular toxicity or interstitial lung disease (ILD) were reported. As the abstract concludes, M9410 had promising activity in heavily pretreated CRC, with a predictable safety profile, and even more significantly, no ILD or ocular toxicities were reported, leading to further evaluation in the CRC patient population in the dose-expansion part of the study [22].

8.6.3 20D9h3-DUBA

A preclinical study on in vitro, ex vivo, and PDX cells targeting the FLT-3 mutation in AML described the construction of an investigational ADC utilizing a DNA-damaging agent and a microtubule inhibitor as cytotoxic payloads. The specific monoclonal antibody targeted quiescent leukemic stem cells and the characterization of a monoclonal antibody. FLT3, or Fms-like tyrosine kinase, has high expression on AML cells and leukemic stem cells and correspondingly low expression on healthy stem cells. Because a DNA-damaging agent exhibits a more quiescent phenotype, the study authors hypothesized that a cytotoxic payload containing this type of agent would elicit greater in vitro cytotoxicity and have greater potency than microtubule disrupting agents and would spare healthy leukemic stem cells.

A humanized FLT3-directed antibody (20D9h3) was generated and conjugated to DUBA, a DNA alkylating agent.

Key Results

An EC50 of 11.0–11.4 ng/mL for VL120D9h1-20D9h4 was observed for monoclonal antibodies versus 29.3–111.6 for all other mAbs, with the rapid internalization of 20D9h3 in FLT3 expressing cells and presence in the intracellular domain after 1 hour that is dependent on the FLT3 surface expression level. IC50 for DUBA was the most efficient at 50%: between 0.58 and 21.25 nM. Even though it had a lower DAR, 20D9h3-DUBA and 20D9h3-MMAF had similar cytotoxicity in FLT3-positive MOLM-13, MOLM-13, MV4–11, and OCI-AML3 cells.

The ADC constructed, namely 20D9h3-DUBA, had a mechanism of action leading to G1/S arrest, which arrested MV4–11 cells with no induced bystander effect. FLT3-negative HL-60 cells were spared in the presence of the ADC. At 0.3 µg/mL, 20D9h3-DUBA eradicated CFCs AML-388 and AML-393: "AML-388 LTC-IC-derived CFC (LTC-IC-CFC) to 0% ± 0% (0.3 µg/mL) and 86.1% ± 1.4% (0.025 µg/mL) of untreated control, respectively, and AML-393 LTC-IC-CFC to 2.8% ± 0.6%."

As the authors further note, 1 µg/mL of 20D9h3-DUBA impaired cytotoxicity only in healthy progenitor CFCs when compared to untreated controls. As the investigators conclude about the analysis of the DNA-alkylator payload, DUBA payload when conjugated to the FLT-3-directed antibody 20D9h3 led to the cytotoxicity of quiescent LSCs and nonproliferating cells. The ATR-CHK1 DNA damage repair pathway is activated by the 20D9h3-DUBA ADC with superior cytotoxicity toward leukemic cells and PDX cells when compared to 20D9h3-MMAF, irrespective of the lower DAR of 4.8 versus 8 [23].

8.6.4 CLDN6-23-ADC

A novel ADC evaluated in xenograft and in vitro models in a preclinical study was identified: CLDN6–23-ADC in the treatment of CLDN6-positive solid tumors. Claudin-6 has a high expression level in solid tumors such as ovarian cancer (OC), with no expression in healthy tissues, making it an ideal target. A CLDN6-targeting ADC was "generated from a fully humanized anti-CLDN6 antibody conjugated to MMAE, resulting in a potential therapeutic ADC." The investigators found robust tumor regression in CLDN6 + xenograft models, and the inhibition of the tumors led to markedly enhanced survival after treatment, with IHC assessment demonstrating elevated levels of CLDN6 in 29% of ovarian epithelial cells. Claudin-6 belongs to a family of membrane proteins that consist of 27 distinct proteins that are characterized by two extracellular loops and four transmembrane domains, which due to its location in tight junctions between epithelial cells may play a role in barrier functions and some signaling pathways (YAP-1-snail1 axis and CLDN6 signaling). Implicated in the initiation, progression, and metastasis of cancers, with aberrant expression in ovary, stomach, lung, and cervix, it is largely restricted to malignant tissues. Also, mRNA analysis of TCGA identified antigens as suitable targets, and the CLDN6 gene showed variegated expression across 30 histologic subtypes. Efficacy was observed in CLDN6-xenograft models, which demonstrated optimal CLDN6 binding on membranes of positive cell lines, which led to significant tumor inhibition. Support for the development of a CLDN6-targeting ADC and conjugation potential to a cytotoxic payload was shown through the internalization and colocalization of LAMP1 and the intracellular trafficking of CLDN6 to the lysosome with the mAb. CLDN6–23-ADC exhibited significant antitumor activity in xenografts expressing CLDN6. Treatment resulted in tumor growth when compared to treatment with an unconjugated antibody, and significant and sustained growth inhibition, tumor regression, and overall robust decreased tumor size was observed when compared with IgG control, which was assessed continually beyond the 21-day treatment period and sustained for 189, 166, or 123 days. The ADC also showed retained selective binding to CLDN6 versus CLDN3, 4, and 9, with a similar degree of internalization when compared to the CLDN6–23-mAb. After validation for a selective and sensitive antibody targeting CLDN6 + cells, including ovarian epithelial cell cancer expressing the protein at 29% levels, healthy tissues were shown to not express detectable levels of CLDN6, suggesting a "wide therapeutic window for clinical studies of an anti-CLDN6 therapeutic." As the study authors conclude, the investigational ADC is a potential therapy for CLDN6 ovarian and endometrial cancers, with CLDN6 positivity determined through IHC tumor-agnostic analysis. Based on preclinical efficacy results, a FIH trial was initiated to determine safety, tolerability, and antitumor activity for advanced cancer patients with endometrial and ovarian cancer solid tumors [5].

8.6.5 SEZ6 Conjugated to ABBV-011

A FIH phase I study of an ADC targeting seizure-related homolog protein 6 (SEZ6) conjugated to calicheamicin ABBV-011 in R/R NSCLC patients was conducted to determine the MTD, safety profiles, and initial ORRs. Initial outcomes were reported in *Clinical Cancer Research*. The dose-escalation phase involved 0.3–2 mg/kg IV of ABBV-011 once every 3 weeks and expansion. Patients displayed SEZ6-positive tumors according to IHC (> 25% of tumor cells) and were preselected for expansion. Tolerability and safety, along with antitumor activity, were evaluated. The patient population was a heavily pretreated one (32%, 41%, and 26% received one, two, and more than three prior therapies, respectively). The MTD was not reached. Fatigue (50%), nausea (42%), and thrombocytopenia (41%) were reported, with hepatic TEAEs of increased AAT (22%), gamma-glutamyltransferase (21%), and hyperbilirubinemia (17%). The ORR was 19% (19/98). In the dose-expansion cohort (n = 40, 1 mg/kg), ORR was 25% and mPFS was 3.5 months (95% CI 1.5–4.2). This study constituted an effort to find options for extensive-stage small-cell lung cancer (SCLC) that has poor prognosis and a 5-year survival rate of 6.8%, with standard treatment being chemoradiotherapy, which is associated with an mPFS of 13.5 to 15.4 months and a 5-year PFS of 25%, with most patients experiencing relapse. Second-line treatment has less benefit, and a high unmet need exists.

SCLC is also an attractive target possessing a high level of SEZ6 expression given that ABBV-011 has a DAR of 2. A dose-escalation phase study was conducted to evaluate doses at 0.3, 0.6, 1.2, 1.6, and 2.0 mg/kg every 3 weeks, on day 1 of each 21-day cycle or at 0.5 mg/kg on days 1 and 8 of each 21-day cycle.

SEZ6 expression was correlated with efficacy in xenograft models with greater than 25% tumor cells. In terms of the safety profile, no MTD was identified, and 2 mg/kg every 3 weeks was selected for the expansion phase during the dose-limiting toxicities (DLT) evaluation period. Delayed-onset hepatotoxicity occurred in 5/14 patients (36%), with Gamma-glutamyl transferase (GGT) increase. Bilirubin increases led to a reduction in the expansion phase (1.6 mg/kg and 1.2 mg/kg). Continued findings of hepatotoxicity led to additional dose reductions. TEAEs included nausea (42%), fatigue (50%), and thrombocytopenia (41%). Grade 3 TEAEs were in 63 patients (64%), with fatigue and thrombocytopenia at 9% each and increased GGT and pneumonia at 7%, the most frequent AEs. ORR rates were 19% for the 0.6 mg/kg dose or greater and 25% for the 1 mg/kg dose-expansion cohort. For patients with one or two prior lines of therapy, ORR was 25% and 27% for patients with chemotherapy-free intervals of less than and greater than 90 days, respectively.

8.6.6 *MRG003*

MRG003, an anti-EGFR ADC, was evaluated in a nonrandomized phase I clinical study for humanized IgG1 mAB with anti-EGFR conjugated with MMAE via a valine–citrulline linker. The study was divided into a phase 1a/1b dose-escalation/dose-expansion trial, featuring the recruitment of EGFR-positive patients with refractory advanced colorectal cancer (CRC), squamous cell carcinoma of the head and neck (SCCHN), and nasopharyngeal cancer (NPC) in phase 1b. An IV dose of 0.1 to 2.5 mg/kg of MRG003 was administered every 3 weeks in phase 1a. Dose-limiting toxic effects in phase Ia and ORR in phase Ib served as the primary endpoints, with safety, tolerability, and immunogenicity also assessed. The results included 19 patients (31%) reporting grade 3 events, including hyponatremia (8%), leukocytopenia (7%), neutropenia (5%), increased AAT levels, and febrile neutropenia. Moreover, 5% of patients achieved PR, and five (23%) achieved stable disease; 13 patients had PD. In phase Ib, 8 patients (21%) achieved confirmed PR and 12 (31%) achieved SD. ORRs were 40%, 44%, and 0% for SCCHN, NPC, and CRC, respectively. Increased AATs were reported in 39% of patients. ORR and DCR were 4.5% (1/22 patients) and 27.3% (6/22 patients), with the EGFR subgroup having ORRs of 11% and 66.7%, respectively. At the data cutoff date, "mPFS was 2.8 months (95% CI 1.2–4.1 months) and the PFS of SCCHN, NPC, and CRC was 2.8 (95% CI 0.6–6.8) months, 4.0 (95% CI 1.2–not reached) months, and 1.2 (95% CI 0.5–2.8) months, respectively." Only the SCCHN cohort reached the mOS at 11.8 (95% CI 3.4–11.8) months. The study authors concluded that MRG003 at a dose of 2.5 mg/kg was tolerable for advanced and metastatic solid tumors but that the optimal dosing scheme and the benefit–risk ratio require further investigation; however, its antitumor activity in EGFR-expressing SCCHN and NPC tumors is encouraging with the initiating of phase 2 studies in this patient population. In this nonrandomized clinical trial, the authors concluded that the results were encouraging of the antitumor activity of MRG003 in EGFR-advanced SCCHN and NPC and was found tolerable in most patients with advanced and metastatic solid tumors when administered at a dose of 2.5 mg/kg, "but the optimal dosing scheme, as well as the risk and benefit ratio of MRG003, requires further investigation, and phase 2 studies in patients with advanced SCCHN and NPC have been initiated" [35].

- 1 mg/kg dose-expansion cohort ($n = 40$): 3.5 months (95% CI 1.5–4.2)
- One prior line of therapy: 5.4 months (95% CI 1.4–8.3)
- Two or more prior lines of therapy: 2.7 months (95% CI 1.4–4.1)

At 1 mg/kg every 3 weeks, an ORR of 25% was shown in R/R SCLC patients in this FIH study evaluating ABBV-001 with no on-targeted ocular toxicities or neurotoxicities reported, nor hepatotoxicity, such as a class effect of calicheamicin-based ADC (GGT and bilirubin increases). RP2D will be confirmed once the results of the 0.8 mg/kg dose cohort are available [33].

ADC targets were identified in the histologic subtypes (neuroendocrine and non-endocrine types) of small-cell lung cancer, which typically have little response to chemotherapy and poor prognosis and which also have less response to bispecific antibodies and targeted therapies.

The study investigators conducted an investigation into expression levels for genetic marker–based ADC targetability, clinical characteristics, and tumor heterogeneity with variation in temporal expression assessed. Four targets were identified: SEZ6 had the highest expression in SCLC, followed by CD276, DLL3, and TACTSD2. Spatial sequencing identified extensive heterogeneity within these targets among SCLC cell lines; SEZ6, DLL3, and CD276 expression remained unchanged, whereas TACSTD2 decreased significantly. Some of the findings were in the ASCL1 subtype DLL3, and in neuroendocrine subtypes, CD276 had a high expression. When compared to primary tumors, TACSTD2 had lower and attenuated levels in brain metastases and the lymph nodes. The study underscored the determination of precise targeting in the selection of ADCs for targeting SCLC [34].

8.7 Mechanisms of Resistance

Abelman et al. discuss the resistance that has emerged with the use of ADC mBC and reported on the incidence of TOP1 mutations emerging in this setting. In characterizing this mutation, they compared patients with mBC not receiving treatment and in TCGA. Plasma-based genotyping identified TOP1 mutations (S57C, R364H, W401C, and G359E) in 4/31 patients (12.9%) at disease progression ADC compared with 3/420 (0.7%) in non-ADC-treated patients. Cross-resistance resulted from sequential treatment (455 days for the first ADC and 52 days for the second ADC), and the novel TOP1 mutant proteins showed resistance to ADC payloads SN38 and deruxtecan, diminished covalent DNA binding, and reduced enzymatic activity. The authors note that TROP2 and HER2 are poor predictors of response to ADC and that no other clinically actionable markers were identified prior to their study; their discovery of TOP1 mutations provides "direct evidence" that they confer TOP1 inhibitor resistance by disrupting TOP1 function. The quantitation of the emergence of TOP1 mutations in temporal fashion was assessed through mutation specific assay and ddPCR analysis of isolated DNA from both tissue samples and blood samples for determining the prevalence of each mutation in the context of the sequential treatment. Serial DNA specimens revealed the emergence of the increased frequency of mutations in TOP1 that were consistent at the start of ADC therapy. The decline in MAF in other tumor mutations suggested that TOP1 mutations conferred the growth of resistant subclones. The increase in the TOP1 MAF was correlated with a lack of therapeutic response. Resistance to the TOP1 inhibitor was associated with statistically significant decreased DNA damage. The authors also suggest that because the mutations could be detected through plasma analysis, a clinical decision-making strategy could result. The study authors conclude that in mBC receiving ADCs with TOP1 inhibitor payloads, TOP1 mutations are rare, but patients still experience disease progression and resistance. The mutations are cross-resistant ones that emerge with the sequential administration of existing ADCs with detectable TOP1 inhibitor payloads, which establishes that these mutations in clinical diagnostics may be necessary for the optimal and rational sequencing of the future development of ADCs for overcoming TOP1-associated clinical resistance [32].

ADC is often characterized by limited efficacy when used clinically, arising from PD profiles featuring the insufficient tumor penetration of the mAb-payload complex. Tumor progression often results from the development of therapy resistance due to diminished payload concentrations as a result of defective antibody/antigen internalization. Modifications in apoptosis signaling are also implicated in resistance mechanisms. Combination strategies, discussed below, are being employed to attenuate resistance mechanisms. Kumari et al. expound on the major challenges in ADC resistance that are the result of the interface of complicated factors. Alterations in cancer antigen are preventing the interaction of mAb with tumor cells, mutations in targets binding payload, antigen downregulation, pathway alterations in payload transfer through tumor membranes, and apoptotic dysregulation brought on by, for example, BCL-2 alterations in signaling pathways. Making modifications to the dual drug-delivery system is considered a plausible solution through the use heterofunctional linkers that offer multidrug loading and site specificity—for example, N-aryl-maleimide as a linker for the attachment of two drugs. Also being proposed is a new model of action using a new drug composed of short DNA and RNA fragments, both being able to interact with the immune system and affecting tumor growth at the transcriptional and translational levels. The diversity of target antigens is also increasing with the development of folate receptor alpha, tissue factors, HER3, c-Met, mesothelin, and CEACAM5. In silico techniques utilizing RNA-sequencing and protein expression are comprising computational techniques to help in the discovery of potential targets for ADC development, with research showing that GD2 ADCs may be useful in the future for the treatment of tumors expressing GD2. ADCs are being optimized to trigger adaptive immunity that helps immune therapies to overcome resistance, with understandings of synergistic mechanisms of action and risk assessment ongoing [1, 8].

8.8 Toxicity

Much of the literature on the toxicities of ADCs has focused on unbound conjugates existing free in circulation for systemic damage and contributing to off-target toxicities, which is attenuated by cleavable linkers that promote the delivery of unconjugated cytotoxic agents into systemic circulation, with T-DXd and SG administration leading to significant increases of unconjugated payloads in the bloodstream. In terms of specific side effects, Chen et al. describe those associated with the administration of ADC in lung cancer such as alopecia, neutropenia, and GI AEs and interstitial lung disease, ocular toxicities, and skin disease, warranting attentive monitoring and strategic implementation to mitigate these AEs. Ocular manifestations are the most varied, with lacrimation and blurred vision that necessitates management though palliative therapy and eye examinations. ADCs in breast cancer lead to cardiotoxicity, left ventricular disease (LVD), QT prolongation, myocardial infarction (MI), arrhythmias, and heart failure. Trastuzumab-based ADCs are associated with left ventricular dysfunction and drug-related cardiotoxicity, and routine echocardiography is recommended. Chen et al. note that these toxicities are due to off-target effects attributed to the untimely liberation of ADC payload within circulation or the TME of the ADC binding to nonmalignant cells expressing the target antigen. Another mechanism may be that ADC delivers the cytotoxic payload directly to HER2-expressing cardiomyocytes, with the interruption of the ERBB-neuregulin signaling axis as a mediator of cardiotoxicity. Interstitial disease and pneumonitis may result from high binding affinity for TROP2, HER3, and HER2 to tumor cells, leading to increased exposure of payload to normal tissue, increasing the potential for dose-dependent and direct toxicity, which triggers tissue damage as a result of local inflammation.

Other toxicities are enfortumab vedotin, associated in 40% of patients with dysgeusia, which is related to nectin4 expression in salivary glands. MMAE is associated with anemia, peripheral neuropathy, and neutropenia. The properties of the cytotoxic payload also lead to certain toxicities, with MMAF and DM4 being associated with ocular toxicity and DM1 being associated with thrombocytopenia and hepatotoxicity. "Also, subtle chemical changes in linker and payload structure can manifest clinically. MMAF when released retains a charge and therefore accumulate intracellularly in corneal epithelia, whereas the more hydrophobic MMAE payload delivered via a cleavable linker can diffuse out of corneal epithelial cells." The latter mechanisms may explain why nearly all ADCs, especially those that deliver DM4 and DM1, are associated with ocular toxicities. There are also examples of one ADC causing different toxicities depending on the tumor type. At the same dose, glembatumumab vedotin, a gpNMB-targeted ADC-carrying MMAE, led to severe rash in melanoma (30%) and breast cancer (4%). With a complicated set of factors at play, the safety profiles of ADCs are difficult to predict, requiring close patient monitoring, careful dose selection, and "diligent AE reporting and attribution in clinical trials, with needed preclinical and translational studies of the ADC toxicity mechanism clearly warranted" [1, 7].

8.9 Combination Strategies

The combined application of ICIs and ADCs has become a "research hotspot," with demonstrated efficacy in solid tumors resistant to treatment and refractory in several studies. Lv et al. have written an excellent description of the process of immunogenic cell death, which forms the basis of the mechanism of action of these combined potent agents. ICD is related to the release of tumor associated antigens (TAAs) and Damage-Associated Molecular Patterns (DAMPs), which leads HSP70 and HSP90 to contribute to the phagocytosis of dying cells and the release of ATP and cytokines. Tumor cells engaging in these processes of aberrant DAMP release pathways, such as autophagy, are unresponsive to stimuli and trigger ICD. Increasing DAMP and its consequent recognition leads to dendritic cell processing, the presentation of MHC II molecules, and the activation of both CD4+and CD8+T cells, which is synergized by the activity of anti-CTLA4 and anti-PD-L1 therapies. Preclinical antitumor activity has been shown in MC38 tumors, with complete tumor rejection shown to be more effective than ADCs and ICIs alone. This synergy is shown to be enhanced by the ADC capacity to generate memory T cells, as supported by the in vivo findings of D'Amico and Iwata, in which fully cured mice responsive to T-DXd were reinoculated with cancer cells, remained in remission, and grew rapidly when introduced to control mice. In a phase Ib trial, 45 HER-2 BC-positive patients who were treated with T-DXd in combination with nivolumab had an ORR of 65.6% and an mPFS of 7 months. Metastatic UC patients who were also HER2+had an ORR of 36.7%, an mPFS of 6.9 months, and an mOS of 11 months when receiving the combination. The trial authors evaluated the antitumor effects of "[p]embrolizumab in combination with T-DXd in HER-2e and HER-2m NSCLC patients. The latest interim analysis showed that patients in both cohorts demonstrated significant antitumor activity (ORR: 54.5% vs 66.7%; mPFS: 15.1 vs 11.3 mo)." Trop-2 targets such as SG have been combined with pembrolizumab and have shown superiority over monotherapy, with an mPFS of 11.1 versus 6.7 months (prolonged by 4.4 months) and an mOS of 18.5 months versus 12.5 months (prolonged by 6 months). In the BEGONIA trial, Dato-DXd showed activity in TNBC in combination with durvalumab, with an ORR of 79% (6/62) and 43 PRs, and durable antitumor activity was shown when combined with pembrolizumab for NSCLC in patients in any PD-L1 expression state. Nectin-4 ADC targets, such as enfortumab vedotin, approved for mUC, has been shown in a phase III trial to have demonstrated efficacy in treatment-naive patients, with an mPFS of 12.5 months, demonstrating significantly higher performance than that of chemotherapy (mOS 31.5 months vs. 6.3 months; ORR 67.7% vs. 44.4%), with a reduced risk of disease progression of 55% and risk of death reduced by 53%. In the phase II EV-202, the confirmed ORR of EV monotherapy in head and neck cancer (HNC) was 23.9%, showing good antitumor activity with potential for therapy with pembrolizumab [36].

Villacampa et al. performed systematic reviews and meta-analyses in a safety and efficacy analysis on the combination treatments of ADC and ICIs and compared them with monotherapy. As Villacampa et al. note, limited information is available on the safety profiles of ADC-ICI combination treatment. They identified 16 clinical trials evaluating the dual therapy on a total cohort of 1133 patients and found that 55.3% of patients developed grade 3 or greater AEs, of which 30% led to treatment discontinuation and 3% led to death. When compared to ADC as a single agent, T-DXd plus ICI had a greater rate of pneumonitis and interstitial lung disease (15% vs. 11.5%), highlighting the need for monitoring. The study overall aimed to estimate the incidence of TEAEs and determine whether the combination increases their prevalence. Advanced tumors included UC ($n = 6$), OC ($n = 1$), cervical cancer ($n = 1$) and NSCLC (n-10. The ADCs included enfortumab vedotin ($n = 3$), trastuzumab emtansine ($n = 3$), SG ($n = 5$), and tisotumab vedotin ($n = 1$). The ICIs were pembrolizimab (n = 9), atezolizumab (n = 3), nivolumab (n = 2), durvalumab (n = 1), and ipilumumab and nivolumab (n = 1). Common AEs were peripheral neuropathy (52.3%), rash and pruritis (50.3% and 38%, respectively) for enfortumab vedotin (n = 561); fatigue (40.6%) and pyrexia (30.2%) for T-DM1 (n = 192); nausea (70%), fatigue (52.2%), and vomiting (44.1%) for T-DXd (n = 140); neutropenia (57.4%), diarrhea (51.9%), and nausea (50%) for SG (n = 121); and diarrhea (54.4%), alopecia (45.6%), and nausea (45.6%) for tisotumab vedotin (n = 68). The percentage of grade 3 anemia was 20.6%. When compared with monotherapy, the percentage of grade 3 or greater was higher with the combination at 55.3% compared to ADC or ICI alone, which were at 49% and 29.5%, respectively). The combination led to increases in mild GI events, but no serious GI AEs. The combination also increased the risk of increased Alanine Aminotransferase (ALT) and Aspartate Aminotransferase (AST) by 5% when compared to ADC alone and by 10% when compared to ICI alone. When T-DXd is combined with ICI, the increase in ILD/pneumonitis rose to 3.5% when compared to monotherapy and 10.2% when compared to single-agent ICI (15.0% vs. 11.5% and 4.8%, respectively). When comparing SG alone and in combination, no significant differences in the incidence of neutropenia were observed. EV in combination led to a higher incidence of grade ≥ 3 rash than when used as monotherapy or with ICI alone (16.2%, 10.4%, and 0.2%, respectively), and the authors note that, overall, "the 3.0% rate of treatment-related deaths observed with the combination therapy was numerically higher than that reported in most trials involving ADC monotherapy." In their meta-analysis, the ADC-ICI combination therapy resulted in a similar rate of grade 3 AEs when compared to traditional ADC therapy and associated side effects, with the rise in the potential synergistic effects increasing toxicities. They surmised that the increasing incidence of ILD/pneumonitis and diarrhea resulted from an overlapping mechanism as opposed to a synergistic effect, with better therapy in cervical cancer as opposed to TNBC, where SG monotherapy was shown to be superior [37].

8.10 Next-Generation ADCs

Numerous strategies for enhancing the efficacy of ADCs utilize the capacity of ADCs to either target different epitopes in the design and construction of biparatopic ADCs or different antigens, as in the case of bispecific ADCs. One example is the targeting of two anti-HER2 antibodies while binding to two epitopes, leading to the formation of receptor-antibody clusters, endocytosis, and lysosomal trafficking, such as in MED14276, a tetravalent HER2 targeting ADC with an single chain variable fragment (scFv) from trastuzumab fused with another anti-HER2 IgG1 antibody, and zanidatamab zovodotin (ZW49), which has a "heterodimerized Fc region fused with an scFv targeting HER2 CED4 and Fab targeting ECD2 of the same protein, conjugated to an auristatin payload." The biparatopic ADCs through the receptor clustering of HER2 displayed faster internalization and lysosomal trafficking. MED14276 had preclinical activity in mouse xenograft models in HER2 breast cancer lines but did not demonstrate clinical activity in BC, with a low ORR (9.4%, three of 32). ZW49, unlike the tetravalent MED14276, is bivalent, and in a phase II study, it was shown to have an RP2D of 2.5 mg/kg every 3 weeks. Among 29 evaluable patients, ZW49 achieved in multiple HER2+advanced cancers an ORR of 28% and a DCR of 72%, with only 9% of patients experiencing TRAEs. REGN5093-M114 is a biparatopic ADC designed to target two epitopes on MET linked with a maytansine derivative payload, which is being evaluated clinically with NSCLC. Bispecific ADCs targeting both EGFR and MET are also being developed and tested preclinically and clinically, such as AZD9592, equipped with a topoisomerase I inhibitor payload that showed promising antitumor activity as both monotherapy and in combination with osimertinib in EGFR-mutant NSCLC. M1231 is a "MUC1-EGFR-targeted bispecific ADC constructed from a heterodimeric antibody with an anti-MUC1 scFv and an anti-EGFR Fab domain" linked with a valine–citrulline linker to a hemiasterlin payload with antimicrotubule activity, and M1231 was evaluated in a phase I dose-escalation study assessing safety, PK, and preliminary efficacy activity. Other bispecific ADCs have been constructed on the basis of the ability of receptors to undergo rapid lysosomal trafficking after endocytosis, such as the prolactin receptor and amyloid precursor-like protein, which constitutes an improvement in intracellular processing and payload release kinase and efficient trafficking to lysosomes and recycling back to the cell surface. Both PRLR and APLP2 targeting ADCs showed improved trafficking and enhanced in vitro potency, but the HER2-APLP2 did not have improved preclinical activity in breast cancer models. Immunostimulatory antibody conjugates (ISACs) are bound to tumor-specific antigens and internalized into APCs, leading to the intracellular release of tumor-associated peptides and conjugated PRRs, such as TLRs and Stimulator of Interferon Genes (STING). When these mediators synergistically trigger the release of proinflammatory cytokines from immune cells, they are attracted to the tumor site, and antigen presentation is enhanced, leading to a robust and specific antitumor immune response. The hydrophobic nature of the PRR can lead to a bystander effect with delivery of agonists to APCs after internalization into tumor cells following intracellular diffusion. Examples are "BDC-1001, a HER2-targeted ISAC with a TLR7/8 agonist payload; TAC-001, a CD22-targeted ISAC with a chemically modified CpG TLR9 agonist payload; [and] XMT-2056, a HER2-targeted ISAC with a dimeric amidobenzimidazole (diABZI) STING agonist payload."

Preclinical evaluation has demonstrated the potential advantages of ISACs over conventional ADCs, where ISACs mediate antitumor response through the release of damage-associated molecular patterns. One commercialized ISAC is pertuzumab zuvotolimod, with a TLR8 agonist conjugated to pertuzumab via a cleavable linker, evaluated as monotherapy and in combination with pembrolizumab and cemiplimab in a phase I study and with other HER2 targeted therapies in a phase I/II study, but it was curtailed by the lack of range among doses being administered with pembrolizumab. NJH395, which is composed of a TLR7 agonist conjugated with a HER2 antibody via a noncleavable linker, was being evaluated in a phase I trial but was discontinued due to insufficient efficacy and prevalent toxicity. BDC-1001, a HER2-targeted ISAC based on trastuzumab equipped with a TLR7/8 agonist via a noncleavable linker, is currently being tested in a phase I/II trial as monotherapy and in combination with nivolumab and pertuzumab. One anti-PD-L1 ISAC demonstrated robust antitumor immune response through TLR7/8 activation, showing the substantial suppression of tumor growth in syngeneic models with an efficient payload release and a potent activation of tumor-associated macrophages. Both bispecific ADCs and ISACs form a class of promising new immunotherapies with encouraging initial clinical trial results, both as monotherapies and in combination with TKIs and anti-PD-1/PD-L1 agents [38].

References

1. Chen X, Zeng C. Pioneering the way: the revolutionary potential of antibody-drug conjugates in NSCLC. Curr Treat Options in Oncol. 2024;25(4):556–84.
2. Coleman N, Yap TA, Heymach JV, Meric-Bernstam F, Le X. Antibody-drug conjugates in lung cancer: dawn of a new era? NPJ Precis Oncol. 2023;7(1):5.
3. Jackson DY. Development of Antibody-Drug conjugates. Bioprocessing, Bioengineering and Process Chemistry in the Biopharmaceutical Industry. 2024. p. 345–79.
4. Lyon RP, Jonas M, Frantz C, Trueblood ES, Yumul R, Westendorf L, et al. SGN-B6A: a new vedotin antibody-drug conjugate directed to integrin beta-6 for multiple carcinoma indications. Mol Cancer Ther. 2023;22(12):1444–53.
5. McDermott MSJ, O'Brien NA, Hoffstrom B, Gong K, Lu M, Zhang J, et al. Preclinical efficacy of the antibody-drug conjugate CLDN6-23-ADC for the treatment of CLDN6-positive solid tumors. Clin Cancer Res. 2023;29(11):2131–43.
6. Walko CM and West H. Antibody Drug Conjugates for Cancer Treatment.JAMA Oncology Patient Page. 2019.
7. Dumontet C, Reichert JM, Senter PD, Lambert JM, Beck A. Antibody-drug conjugates come of age in oncology. Nat Rev Drug Discov. 2023;22(8):641–61.
8. Kumari S, Raj S, Babu MA, Bhatti GK, Bhatti JS. Antibody-drug conjugates in cancer therapy: innovations, challenges, and future directions. Arch Pharm Res. 2024;47(1):40–65.
9. Schmidts, I., Haferlach, T., Hoermann, G. (2022). Precision Medicine in Therapy of Non-solid Cancer. In: Cascorbi, I., Schwab, M. (eds) Precision Medicine. Handbook of Experimental Pharmacology, vol 280. Springer, Cham.
10. Bardia A, Krop IE, Kogawa T, Juric D, Tolcher AW, Hamilton EP, et al. Datopotamab deruxtecan in advanced or metastatic HR+/HER2- and triple-negative breast cancer: results from the phase I TROPION-PanTumor01 study. J Clin Oncol. 2024;42(19):2281–94.
11. Meric-Bernstam F, Yuca E, Evans KW, Zhao M, Maejima T, Karibe T, et al. Antitumor activity and biomarker analysis for TROP2 antibody-drug conjugate Datopotamab Deruxtecan in patient-derived breast cancer xenograft models. Clin Cancer Res. 2025;31(3):573–87.
12. Sheng X, Wang L, He Z, Shi Y, Luo H, Han W, et al. Efficacy and safety of Disitamab Vedotin in patients with human epidermal growth factor receptor 2-positive locally advanced or metastatic urothelial carcinoma: a combined analysis of two phase II clinical trials. J Clin Oncol. 2024;42(12):1391–402.
13. Milowsky MI, O'Donnell PH, Hoimes CJ, Petrylak DP, Flaig TW, Moon HH, et al. Patient-reported outcomes in patients with advanced urothelial cancer who are ineligible for cisplatin and treated with first-line Enfortumab Vedotin alone or with pembrolizumab. J Clin Oncol. 2024;42(12):1403–14.
14. Klumper N, Tran NK, Zschabitz S, Hahn O, Buttner T, Roghmann F, et al. NECTIN4 amplification is frequent in solid tumors and predicts Enfortumab Vedotin response in metastatic urothelial cancer. J Clin Oncol. 2024;42(20):2446–55.

15. Bardia A, Hurvitz SA, Tolaney SM, Loirat D, Punie K, Oliveira M, et al. Sacituzumab Govitecan in metastatic triple-negative breast cancer. N Engl J Med. 2021;384(16):1529–41.
16. Paz-Ares LG, Juan-Vidal O, Mountzios GS, Felip E, Reinmuth N, de Marinis F, et al. Sacituzumab Govitecan versus docetaxel for previously treated advanced or metastatic non-small cell lung cancer: the randomized, open-label phase III EVOKE-01 study. J Clin Oncol. 2024;42(24):2860–72.
17. Camidge DR, Bar J, Horinouchi H, Goldman J, Moiseenko F, Filippova E, et al. Telisotuzumab Vedotin monotherapy in patients with previously treated c-met protein-overexpressing advanced nonsquamous EGFR-wildtype non-small cell lung cancer in the phase II LUMINOSITY trial. J Clin Oncol. 2024;42(25):3000–11.
18. Ohba A, Morizane C, Kawamoto Y, Komatsu Y, Ueno M, Kobayashi S, et al. Trastuzumab deruxtecan in human epidermal growth factor receptor 2-expressing biliary tract cancer (HERB; NCCH1805): a multicenter, single-arm, phase II trial. J Clin Oncol. 2024;42(27):3207–17.
19. Santin AD, Corr BR, Spira A, Willmott L, Butrynski J, Tse KY, et al. Efficacy and safety of Sacituzumab Govitecan in patients with advanced solid tumors (TROPiCS-03): analysis in patients with advanced endometrial cancer. J Clin Oncol. 2024;42(29):3421–9.
20. Yao H, Yan M, Tong Z, Wu X, Ryu MH, Park JJ, et al. Safety, Efficacy, and Pharmacokinetics of SHR-A1811, a Human Epidermal Growth Factor Receptor 2-Directed Antibody-Drug Conjugate, in Human Epidermal Growth Factor Receptor 2-Expressing or Mutated Advanced Solid Tumors: A Global Phase I Trial. J Clin Oncol. 2024;42(29):3453–65.
21. Yamaguchi K, Ito M, Isobe T, Koreishi S, Taguchi R, Uehara K, et al. Impact of genomic alterations on efficacy of Trastuzumab Deruxtecan against human epidermal growth factor receptor-2-positive advanced gastric cancer. JCO Precis Oncol. 2024;8:e2300681.
22. Kopetz S, Boni V, Kato K, Raghav KRP, Pallis P et al. First-in-human trial of M9140, an anti-CEACAM5 antibody drug conjugate (ADC) with exatecan payload, in patients (pts) with metastatic colorectal cancer (mCRC). Meeting Abstract: 2024 ASCO Annual Meeting I.
23. Able M, Kasper MA, Vick B, Schwach J, Gao X, Schmitt S, et al. Effective eradication of acute myeloid leukemia stem cells with FLT3-directed antibody-drug conjugates. Leukemia. 2025;39(3):632–42.
24. Frenel JS, Zeghondy J, Guerin-Charbonnel C, Mailliez A, Volant E, Poumeaud F, et al. Tucatinib combination treatment after Trastuzumab-deruxtecan in patients with ERBB2-positive metastatic breast cancer. JAMA Netw Open. 2024;7(4):e244435.
25. Yajima S, Hirose K, Masuda H. Enfortumab Vedotin with or without pembrolizumab in metastatic urothelial carcinoma: a systematic review and meta-analysis. JAMA Netw Open. 2025;8(3):e250250.
26. Sehn LH, Herrera AF, Flowers CR, Kamdar MK, McMillan A, Hertzberg M, et al. Polatuzumab Vedotin in Relapsed or Refractory Diffuse Large B-Cell Lymphoma. J Clin Oncol. 2020;38(2):155–65.
27. Flowers CR, Matasar MJ, Herrera AF, Hertzberg M, Assouline S, Demeter J, et al. Polatuzumab vedotin plus bendamustine and rituximab or obinutuzumab in relapsed/refractory follicular lymphoma: a phase Ib/II study. Haematologica. 2024;109(4):1194–205.
28. Budde LE, Olszewski AJ, Assouline S, Lossos IS, Diefenbach C, Kamdar M, et al. Mosunetuzumab with polatuzumab vedotin in relapsed or refractory aggressive large B cell lymphoma: a phase 1b/2 trial. Nat Med. 2024;30(1):229–39.
29. Jain S, Griffith JI, Porath KA, Rathi S, Le J, Pasa TI, et al. Bystander effects, pharmacokinetics, and linker-payload stability of EGFR-targeting antibody-drug conjugates Losatuxizumab Vedotin and Depatux-M in glioblastoma models. Clin Cancer Res. 2024;30(15):3287–97.
30. Cheung A, Chenoweth AM, Johansson A, Laddach R, Guppy N, Trendell J, et al. Anti-EGFR antibody-drug conjugate carrying an inhibitor targeting CDK restricts triple-negative breast cancer growth. Clin Cancer Res. 2024;30(15):3298–315.
31. Hollebecque A, Lopez JS, Piha-Paul SA, Dowlati A, Patnaik A et al. SGN-B6A, an integrin beta-6 (ITGB6)-targeted antibody-drug conjugate (ADC), in patientswith advanced solid

tumors: Updated results from a phase 1 study (SGNB6A-001). Meeting Abstract. American Society of Clinical Oncology. 2023
32. Abelman RO, Wu B, Barnes H, Medford A, Norden B, Putur A, et al. TOP1 mutations and cross-resistance to antibody-drug conjugates in patients with metastatic breast cancer. Clin Cancer Res. 2025;31(10):1966–74.
33. Morgensztern D, Ready N, Johnson ML, Dowlati A, Choudhury N, Carbone DP, et al. A phase I first-in-human study of ABBV-011, a seizure-related homolog protein 6-targeting antibody-drug conjugate, in patients with small cell lung cancer. Clin Cancer Res. 2024;30(22):5042–52.
34. Ajay A, Wang H, Rezvani A, Savari O, Grubb BJ, McColl KS, et al. Assessment of targets of antibody drug conjugates in SCLC. NPJ Precis Oncol. 2025;9(1):1.
35. Qiu MZ, Zhang Y, Guo Y, Guo W, Nian W, Liao W, et al. Evaluation of safety of treatment with anti-epidermal growth factor receptor antibody drug conjugate MRG003 in patients with advanced solid tumors: a phase 1 nonrandomized clinical trial. JAMA Oncol. 2022;8(7):1042–6.
36. Lv Y, Cui X, Li T, Liu C, Wang A, Wang T, et al. Mechanism of action and future perspectives of ADCs in combination with immune checkpoint inhibitors for solid tumors. Clin Exp Med. 2025;25(1):139.
37. Villacampa G, Cresta Morgado P, Carita L, Navarro V, Pascual T, Dienstmann R. Safety and efficacy of antibody-drug conjugates plus immunotherapy in solid tumours: a systematic review and meta-analysis. Cancer Treat Rev. 2024;131:102847.
38. Tsuchikama K, Anami Y, Ha SYY, Yamazaki CM. Exploring the next generation of antibody-drug conjugates. Nat Rev Clin Oncol. 2024;21(3):203–23.

Chapter 9
Chimeric Antigen Receptor T-Cell Therapy

Chimeric antigen receptor (CAR) T-cell therapy is one of the most studied and prominently evaluated cancer immunotherapies. With proven clinical efficacy in hematologic malignancies such as B-cell acute lymphoblastic leukemia (ALL) and mantle cell lymphoma (MCL), they are in use for cancers with poor prognosis and have robust outcomes (tisagenlecleucel (tisa cel) and axi cel). They are effective for a number of reasons, one being that they are MHC independent and can activate T cells even with reduced human leukocyte antigen (HLA) expression. CAR designs include those in first-, second-, third-, and fourth-generation categories, with improving efficacy and safety profiles. New combination therapies are being designed for less toxicity, including CAR macrophage combinations [1].

9.1 CAR T-Cell Therapy (Figs. 9.1 and 9.2)

P. Hays, *Personalized Medicine in Oncology*,
https://doi.org/10.1007/978-3-032-14437-9_9

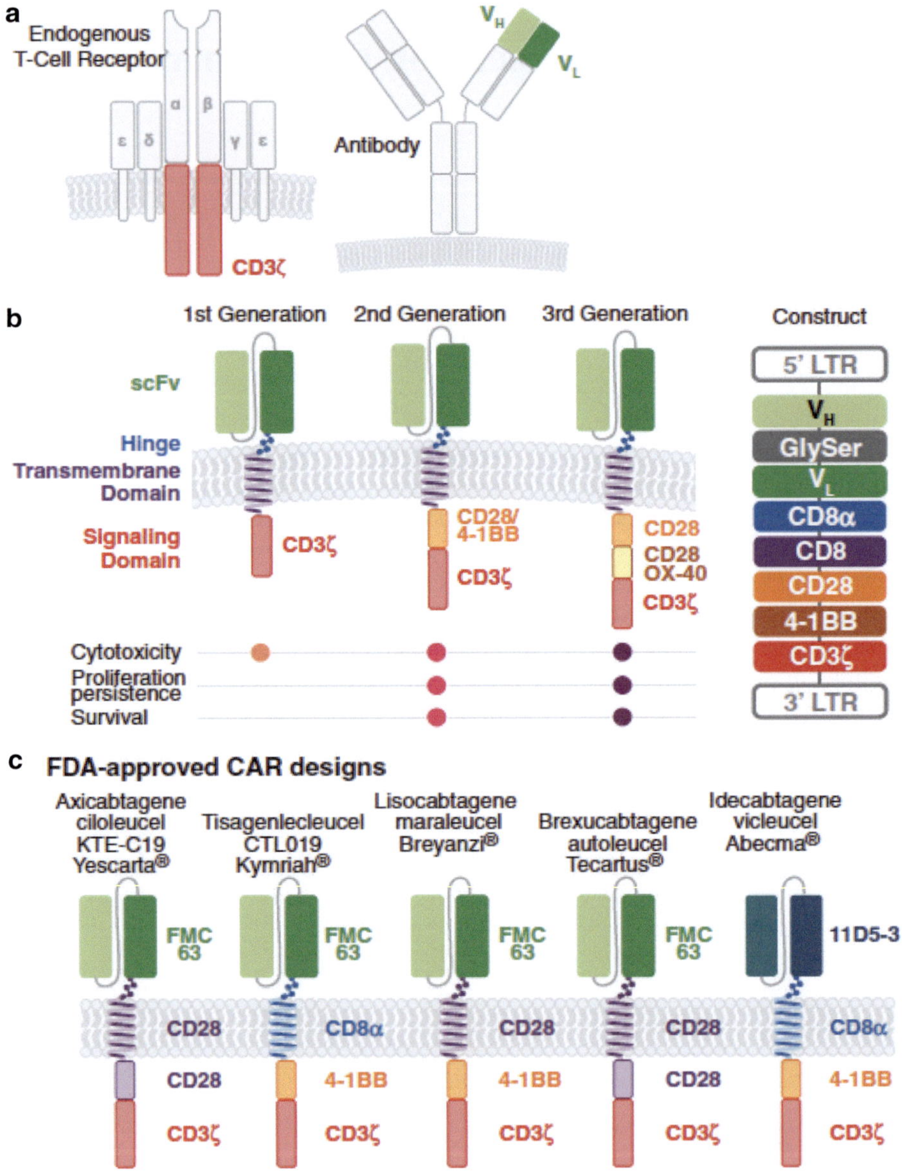

Fig. 9.1 The biology of CAR T cells [1]

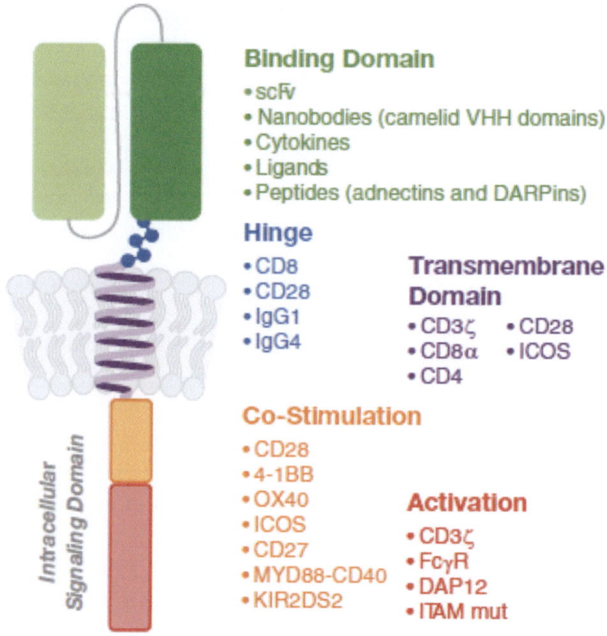

Fig. 9.2 The design of CAR T cells [1]

9.2 CAR T-Cell Combinations

Natural killer (NK) cells form 5–15% of peripheral blood leukocytes and express CD56 rather than CD3 and T-cell receptors. They are key mediators of ADCC and can effect tumor cell killing independent of antigen-specific T-cell receptors while also secreting chemokines and cytokines and activating T cells. With these characteristics, they constitute an ideal choice for combination treatments with CAR T cells, having better toxicity profiles as well by not being associated with graft-vs-host disease (GvHD).

9.3 CAR T-Cell Therapies Approved for Lymphomas and Myeloid Malignancies (Table 9.1)

This chapter discusses CAR T-cell therapies and their challenges in treating hematologic malignancies and solid tumors, which given tumor escape, tumor heterogeneity, diminished capacity to proliferate, and an immunosuppressive TME pose a number of issues for the effectivity of this T-cell-based treatment. A review of the clinical and robust outcomes for CAR T-cell therapy for urological cancers describes the evolution of first-, second-, third-, and fourth-generation CAR T-cell therapy constructs, with each generation overcoming the cytotoxic challenges faced by the previous generation. The optimization and enhancement of CAR T cells result from

Table 9.1 CAR T cells approved by the US Federal Drug Administration (FDA)

Drug name	Target	Costimulatory receptor	Indications in hemato-oncology
Axicaltagene Ciloleucel	CD19	CD28	Large B-cell lymphoma
Brexucabtagene Autoleucel	CD19	CD28	Mantle cell lymphoma, acute lymphoblastic leukemia
Tisagenlecleucel	CD19	4-1BB	Acute lymphoblastic leukemia, diffuse large B-cell lymphoma, follicular lymphoma
Lisocabtagene Maraleucel	CD20	4-1BB	Large B-cell lymphoma
Ciltacabtagene Autoleucel	BCMA	4-1BB	Multiple myeloma
Idecabtagene Vicleucel	BCMA	4-1BB	Multiple myeloma

increasing their capability to proliferate and kill malignant cells through the inclusion of costimulatory molecules located intracellularly in the receptor. First-generation CAR T cells consisted of a relatively uncomplicated design when compared to second or third generation CAR T cells, with a CD3ζ as the costimulatory domain located intracellularly but with no costimulatory signal for the activation of the CAR T cell. In second-generation CAR T cells, the costimulatory domain CD28 and 4-1BB domains were introduced with significantly improved immune activation and durability, possessing distinct antitumor characteristics, with CD28 T-cell activation leading to strong mortality and 4-1BB leading to T-cell activation that has greater persistence with antitumor abilities. Third-generation CARs display increased persistence and better-balanced tumor killing with CD27, OX40, and ICOS costimulatory domains and an elevated CD8:CD4 ratio, leading to decreased exhaustion. However, they also have impaired mitochondrial function and lead to T-cell exhaustion. This led to the development of fourth-generation CAR T cells that coexpressed IL-7, IL-12, and IL-18, the proinflammatory cytokines, to positively regulate T cells. With their inducible domain and receptor activation, they have improved ability for cytokine expression and CAR T-cell persistence with antitumor activity. IL-12 has a significant role in activating T cells and modulating the immune and vascular TME while also recruiting cancer cells to attach cancer cells unrecognizable by CAR T cells [2].

9.3.1 Axicabtagene Ciloleucel

Axicabtagene ciloleucel (axi cel), investigated in the ZUMA-1 study ($n = 108$), is a CD19-directed CD3ζ/CD28-costimulated CAR approved for relapsed/refractory (R/R) large B cell lymphoma (LBCL) and follicular lymphoma (FL) after two or more lines of therapy without T-cell selection taking place during the manufacturing process while also possessing a gamma-retrovirus vector and being administered to patients after lymphodepletion [1]. Axi cel was approved by the FDA for use in third-line, second-line, and high-risk LBCL patients. In ZUMA-1, out of 101 patients enrolled, the objective response rate (ORR) was 82% (95% CI 73–89), with a 54% response rate. Duration of response (DOR) was reported as 11.1 months (95% CI 3.9–nonestimable). However, 93% experience cytokine release syndrome (CRS), 13% being grade 3 or higher, and 64% experience immune effector cell–associated neurotoxicity syndrome (ICANS), 28% being grade 3. The 5-year overall survival (OS) rate was 42.6% (95% CI 32.8–51.9). For second-line LBCL, ZUMA-7 demonstrated event free survival (EFS) improvement in the axi cel arm versus chemoimmunotherapy—i.e., standard of care (SOC)—8.3 months vs. 3.0 months, HR 0.398) in second-line LBCL. In high-risk LBCL (with adverse molecular alterations such as MYC, BCL2, and BCL6), the single-arm, multicenter phase 2 ZUMA-12 trial showed that axi cel in these patients has high-risk profiles after patients received chemoimmunotherapy and after demonstrating positron emission tomography (PET) positivity. Of the 37 patients, ORR was reported as 89% (95% CI 75–97), and the complete response (CR) rate was reported as 78% (95% CI 62–90). With a 16-month median follow-up, 71% had a CR, exhibiting that the therapy was durable in response. The high performance of axi cel in this trial motivated a phase 3 study, ZUMA-12, also comparing first-line axi cel to the SOC in high-risk patients. The FDA and EMA approved axi cel in 2017 in R/R LBCL patients as third-line therapy or as subsequent lines of therapy [3].

Locke et al. conducted a trial reported in *Blood* in 2024 evaluating axi cel vs. SOC in second-line-setting LBCL, measuring clinical outcomes through a new prognostic measure of tumor burden and metabolic tumor volume, as determined through fluorodeoxyglucose (FDG)–positron emission tomography (PET)–computed tomography (CT), or FDG-PET-CT, which could serve as a promising prognostic indicator of LBCL, as shown through an analysis in the phase 3 ZUMA-7 trial. R/R LBCL patients after 12 months after receiving chemoimmunotherapy (CIT) were administered axi cel ($n = 175$) or SOC (CIT followed by CT and autologous stem-cell transplant (ASCT); $n = 165$). EFS served as the primary endpoint, in the time from randomization to disease progression. Low MTV corresponded to higher EFS, whereas high MTV corresponded to lower EFS in both cohorts (HR, 1.448; 95% CI 0.980–2.139); (HR, 1.486; 95% CI 1.055–2.093), according to descriptive p-values. At baseline, median MTV was found to be 231.07 mL (range, 0.04–16669.3) overall and was comparable in both the axi cel and SOC cohorts, but it did not associate with PK or PD values, and the benefit in the EFS of axi cel versus SOC was demonstrated in both the low- and high-MTV subgroups. The study authors concluded that MTV serves as a better prognostic and predictive indicator than the sum of the product of perpendicular diameters (SPD) for assessing tumor burden because the method FDG PET-CT allows for the discrimination of necrotic lesions from viable tumors [4].

9.3.2 *Tisagenlecleucel*

Tisagenlecleucel (tisa cel) is a CD19 targeted with a CD3ζ/4-1BB costimulatory domain. CAR is manufactured after T-cell selection by using a lentivirus vector. The phase 3 BELINDA clinical trial showed that second-line tisa cel was not improved after SOC in aggressive B-cell lymphoma as second-line treatment, as reported by Bishop et al. in 2021 in *NEJM* (median EFS in both groups being 3 months). On the basis of the phase1/2 ELIANA trial, tisa cel received FDA approval for the pediatric and young adult R/R B-ALL patient population up to age 25 and for adults with R/R LBCL. In this pediatric and young adult patient population, an OS of 76% and an EFS of 50% were demonstrated after infusion at 12 months. Adverse events (AEs) included CRS at 77% and neurological disease at 40%. Overall, 77% of patients had CRS, whereas 40% of patients experienced neurological toxicities. For third- or subsequent-line therapy for DLBCL, the phase 2 JULIET trial first showed data featuring an ORR of 52% (95% CI = 41–62; 93 patients infused) and a CR of 40%. CRS of any grade was 58%, that of grade 3 was 23%, and grade 3+ ICANS were 11% and considered infrequent [3].

9.3.3 *Lisocabtagene Maraleucel*

Lisocabtagene maraleucel (liso cel) is CD19 targeted, having a CD3ζ/4-1BB costimulatory region CAR that is uniquely manufactured with a lentivirus in a 1:1 CD4+/CD8+ T-cell ratio that showed superior CAR T-cell performance in preclinical studies; however, this is unknown in clinical settings. It is the third CAR T-cell therapy approved for R/R LBCL after two previous lines of systemic treatment and is also approved for follicular lymphoma grade 3B as a result of its inclusion in the trial (Table 9.2).

9.3.4 *TRANSCEND, TRANSFORM, and PILOT Studies*

The TRANSCEND trial ($n = 344$; $n = 269$ received infusion) enrolled patients who underwent leukapheresis, and it demonstrated an ORR of 73% (95% CI 66.8–78.0) ($n = 256$ evaluable patients), with 53% maintaining a CR at 18.8 months. The OR was 53% (95% CI 56.8–59.4) for liso cel in third- or subsequent-lines of LBCL treatment. In TRANSCEND, evaluating liso cel in third and subsequent lines, patients experiencing renal dysfunction, cardiac dysfunction, and secondary CNS involvement were included, and when compared to ZUMA-1 and JULIET, where 41% of patients were 65 or older (median age of 63), 58 and 24%, in ZUMA-1 and 56 and 23%, in JULIET [3].

Table 9.2 Background information on lisocabtagene maraleucel

Structure	CD19-directed, genetically modified autologous T-cell immunotherapy administered as a defined composition of $CD8^+$and $CD4^+$ T cells (1:1). The CAR is composed of an FMC63 mAb-derived single-chain variable fragment (scFv), IgG4 hinge region, CD28 transmembrane domain, 4-1BB (CD137) costimulatory domain, and CD3 zeta activation domain. CD3 zeta signaling is critical for initiating activation and antitumor activity, whereas 4-1BB (CD137) signaling enhances CAR T-cell expansion and persistence
Mechanism of action	CAR binding to CD19 expressed on the cell surface of tumors and normal B cells induces the activation and proliferation of CAR T cells, the release of proinflammatory cytokines, and the cytotoxic killing of target cells
Pharmacokinetics in LBCL	Following infusion, lisocabtagene maraleucel exhibited an initial expansion, with a median time of maximal expansion of 10–12 days, followed by a bi-exponential decline. Presence was detected in peripheral blood over an estimated median of 12.1 months
FDA-approved indications	The treatment of adult patients with LBCL, including DLBCL not otherwise specified (including DLBCL arising from indolent lymphoma), high-grade B-cell lymphoma, primary mediastinal large B-cell lymphoma, and follicular lymphoma grade 3B who have either refractory disease to first-line chemoimmunotherapy or relapse within 12 months of first-line chemoimmunotherapy (June 2022); refractory disease to first-line chemoimmunotherapy or relapse after first-line chemoimmunotherapy and who are not eligible for HSCT due to comorbidities or age (June 2022); or relapsed or refractory disease after two or more lines of systemic therapy (February 2021) Limitations of use: It is not indicated for the treatment of patients with central nervous system lymphoma

Source: US Prescribing Information. (Adapted from Elmacken et al. [5])
Abbreviations: *LBCL* large B-cell lymphoma and *DLBCL* diffuse large B-cell lymphoma

The safety and efficacy profiles for liso cel in the second-line setting for R/R LBCL were shown in the TRANSFORM study, as reported by Kamdar et al. *Lancet* in 2022 featured an FDA approval summary provided by Elmacken et al. in clinical complete response (CCR), with additional data on the PILOT study.

Liso cel versus SOC (CT followed by ASCT) was investigated in the interim, open-label, randomized phase 3 trial TRANSFORM across 47 sites in primary R/R early (under 12 months) LBCL patients. EFS was assessed through independent review committee (IRC) was the primary endpoint, which found improvement with the administration of liso cel, (10.1 months (95% CI 6.1–not reached) vs. SOC (2.3 months); (stratified HR 0.35; 95% CI 0.23–0.53)), with a statistically significant higher CR rate (66% vs. 39%) and an improved median DoR (not reached vs. 14.5 months) versus the SOC arm. Liso cel was also associated with a superior CR rate (61 of 92 patients (66%); 95% CI 56–76) vs. SOC (36 of 92 patients (39%); 95% CI 29–50), with the treatment group having a longer mDoR versus the SOC group (median not reached (95% CI 6.8–not reached) vs. 14.5 months (4.7–not reached)). ORR was reported as 86% in the liso cel group (79 patients; 95% CI 77–92%) and 48% (44 patients; 37–59%) in the SOC group. There were 28 progression-free survival (PFS) events in the liso cel group, with a fourfold increase in median EFS (10.1 months (95% CI 16.1–NR) vs. 2–3 months (95% CI 2.2–4.3)), and 43 PFS events in the SOC group were also observed.

A 27% higher CR (83% vs. 50%) was demonstrated, and an ORR of 65% vs. 32% at a median follow-up 24.9 months was also shown, along with a more than 2.5-fold increase in mPFS (14.8 months (95% CI 6.6–NR) versus 5.7 months (95% CI 3.9–9.4)) when compared to SOC. The results demonstrate superior clinical outcomes, with favorable safety outcomes associated with liso cel versus SOC in early R/R LBCL. The common AEs were grade 3 neutropenia, reported in 74 of 92 patients (80%) in the liso cel arm and 46 of 91 patients (51%) in the SOC arm; thrombocytopenia, anemia, and prolonged cytopenia were observed 45 (49%) vs. 58 (64%); 45 (49%) vs. 45 (49%); 40 (43%) vs. 3 (3%), respectively). CRS and neurological events occurred in one and four of 92 patients (1% and 4%, respectively) in the liso cel group, respectively, with no grade 4 or 5 AEs reported. According to the authors, no safety signals arose in second-line settings given that no patients discontinued therapy or had dose modifications due to toxicity, and bridging therapy was associated with consistent benefit.

The study authors concluded that liso cel in the second-line setting is an effective therapy for early R/R LBCL according to the phase 3 TRANSFORM trial results, representing a clinically meaningful option over SOC because it was effective in a minority of patients and supporting a change in clinical practice from other recent phase 3 studies. It also had implications for other autologous CD19 targets and for other settings, including 12 months after treatment in the first-line settings, aligning with the latest results in therapy [6].

The single-arm phase 2 trial PILOT, conducted on 61 patients who were ineligible for transplant but fit to undergo therapy, also evaluated liso cel in second-line management, and the IRC-CR rate was reported as 54% (95% CI 41–67), with a 68% continued response rate. CRS was reported in 45% of patients, and grade 3 events occurred in 1.3% of patients, where neurotoxicities were observed in 27% of patients (7%) with grade 3 events. ORR was 80% (95% CI 68–89), and "the median time to first CR or PR was 1.0 month (range, 0.8 to 3.0 months), and the median time to first CR was also 1.0 month (range, 0.8 to 6.9 months)."

9.3.5 Key Results

- CR ($n = 33$)
  - 6 months: 83% (95% CI 64–93)
  - 12 months: 68% (95% CI 45–83); mDOR not reached
- PR: mDOR was 2.1 months (95% CI 1.4–2.3).
- CRS, fever, and fatigue were shown (39%, 38%, and 44%, respectively).
- Common grade 3 AEs were infections and musculoskeletal pain (3.3% and 4.9%, respectively).
- Neutropenia, lymphopenia, thrombocytopenia, anemia, and alpha-1 antitrypsin deficiency (AAT) increase were grade 3–4 laboratory abnormalities occurring in $\geq$ 30% of patients.

The authors note that patient fitness is required for lymphodepletion (LD), and a safety label for liso cel describes risk-mitigation strategies for CRS and neurotoxicity. The authors conclude that TRANSFORM and PILOT provide substantial evidence for clinical efficacy and favorable safety profiles of liso cel for R/R LBCL patients as second-line treatment with a magnitude of clinical benefit and an overall favorable benefit–risk profile.

9.3.6 Brexucabtagene Autoleucel

Brexucabtagene autoleucel (brexu cel) is CD19 directed, having a CD3ζ/CD28 costimulatory domain utilizing a T-cell selection step in its manufacturing process, with the analogous CAR construct as axi cel, which has approval for R/R MCL, as shown by the ZUMA-2 trial, where this patient population was included. The treatment showed clinical efficacy and a manageable safety profile, especially in patients between ages 65-75 years old and high-risk patients. Pretreatment included anti-CD20 antibodies, and PFS values were 77% (6 months) and 51% (12 months) after infusion, respectively, whereas OS values were 83% (6 months) and 61% (12 months) after infusion.

A real-world study was performed by Trando et al. [7] on R/R DLBCL patients (n = 66) receiving tisa cel (11%) and axi cel (89%). Extranodal disease (HR 2.22, 95% CI 1.15–4.31; p = 0.018) and Eastern Cooperative Oncology Group (ECOG) status (HR 2.65, 95% CI 1.30–5.41) were shown as the best predictors of response in the cohort with a median age of 59.5, where 21% were over 70 years old. Due to adverse toxicity profiles (CRS and ICANS) and the poor prognosis for nonresponders, constituting half of the patient population, a study was conducted by DiBiasi et al. evaluating post–CAR T-cell therapy patients who were also nonresponsive, PFS and OS were a dismal 2.8 and 5.2 months, respectively, meriting a study revealing clearly defined prognostic and predictive biomarkers. Salvage therapy included targeted treatment, bispecific antibodies, and hematopoietic stem-cell transplantation (HSCT) (allogeneic). The UCSD study included data on CRS and neurotoxicity and on factors associated with disease relapse and clinical response after CAR T-cell therapy relapse.

9.3.7 Key Results

- CRS: n = 58 (68%), grade 1–2 (57, or 86%)
- ICANS: n = 37 (56%), grade 1–2 (20, or 30%)
- Anemia: n = 66 (100%), grade 1–2 (21, or 32%) and grade 3–4 (45, or 68%)
- Neutropenia: n = 66 (100%); grade 3–4 (66, or 100%)
- ORR at median follow-up of 16.3 months, 67%; CR (53%) or 35 of 66 with three relapses, and among the remainder of 31 patients, nine (14%) had PR and 17 (26%) SD or PD

- mPFS 10.3 months (95% CI 3.3–NR); for patients experiencing CR, PR, or SD/PD, mPFS was NR, 3.65 months (95% CI 2.04 to NR), 1.38 months (95% CI 1.22–3.29) (HR 7.77, 95% CI 4.15–14.56, statistically significant)
- mOS 28.4 months (95% CI 12.4–NR); CR, PR, SD/PD, mOS = NR (95% CI 34.95–NR); 7.99 months (95% CI 3.29–NR and 6.48 months (95% CI 3.52–NR) (HR 3.00, 95% CI 1.93–4.68; $p < 0.001$)
- Stratified according to age
  - mPFS < 70 years: 7.45 months (95% CI 3.29–NR)
  - mPFS > 70 years: 28.37 months (95% CI 4.24–NR)
  - (HR 0.79, 95% CI 0.35–1.8, not significant)
  - mOS < 70 years 21.5 months (95% CI 10.26–NR)
  - mOS > 70 years: 28.37 months (95% CI 28.37–NR), (HR 0.70, 95% CI 0.27–1.84, not significant)
- Stratified according to ECOG
  - mPFS ECOG of 0–1: 28.37 months (95% CI 4.11–NR)
  - mPFS ECOG 2–4 3.22 (95% CI 1.12–NR)
  - Patients with ECOG of 0–1 reported a significantly longer PFS in comparison with patients with an ECOG of 2–4 (HR 2.49, 95% CI 1.23–5.05)
  - mOS ECOG 0–1: 34.95 months (95% CI 18.51–NR)
  - mOS ECOG 2–4: 5.29 months (95% CI 2.36–NR)
  - ECOG of 0–1 reported a significantly longer OS in comparison with ECOG of 2–4
- CR
  - < 70 years: 27/52 patients (52%)
  - > 70 years: CRR: 30/53 patients (57%)

The authors discussed how their results compare with the ZUMA and JULIET trials and noted that their results are comparable. They concluded that biomarkers for therapy urgently need to be uncovered and determined that no consensus has been reached on which biological, clinical, or imaging biomarkers would predict therapy outcomes [7].

9.3.8 Idecabtagene Vicleucel

Idecabtagene vicleucel (ide cel) is BCMA directed, with a CD3ζ/4-1BB costimulatory domain (lentiviral vector), for CAR T-cell therapy, approved for relapsed/refractory multiple myeloma (RRMM) after four or more prior lines of treatment, including a proteasome inhibitor, an immunomodulatory agent, and an anti-CD38, according to the results of the phase 2 KarMMa study for heavily pretreated patients (median six prior lines of treatment), with patients undergoing bridging therapy

(88%), undergoing apheresis ($n = 140$), and receiving the agent ($n = 128$) [1]. In the open-label, international phase 3 KarMMa-3 study, Rodriguez-Otero et al. evaluated ide cel in comparison with SOC for triple-class exposed R/R multiple myeloma (MM), as reported in the *NEJM*, with random assignment to ide cel ($n = 254$) and the standard regimen ($n = 132$). In that study, 254 patients were randomly assigned to ide cel and 132 to the standard regimen. In the standard regimen group, patients received daratumumab, pomalidomide, and dexamethasone ($n = 30$); carfilzomib and dexamethasone ($n = 43$); elotuzumab, pomalidomide, and dexamethasone ($n = 30$); ixazomib, lenalidomide, and dexamethasone ($n = 22$); and daratumumab, bortezomib, and dexamethasone ($n = 7$).

In the intention-to-treat (ITT) population, PFS was 13.3 months (95% CI 11.8–16.1) versus 4.4 months for the SOC group (HR 0.49, 95% CI 0.38–0.65), indicating remarkable results, and the PFS clinical benefit was seen across all subgroups, even those with high-risk profiles (high tumor burden, refractory status after triple-class exposure, and cytogenetic abnormalities). The ide cel group also saw a greater percentage of patients with PR (71% (181 of 254; 95% CI 66–77) versus 42% (55 of 132, 95% CI 33–50)) and complete response (39% vs. 5%). Median DOR was 14.8 months (95% CI 12.0–18.6) and 9.7 months (95% CI 5.4–16.3) in the ide cel and the SOC group, respectively. The ide cel group showed a higher minimal residual disease (MRD)-negative status, which was confirmed in 51 patients versus one patient in the SOC group. The investigators also performed an exploratory analysis on cellular kinetics, showing that the expansion of ide cel was also associated with longer PFS, whereas bone marrow tumors cells indicating BCMA expression were seen in six evaluable biopsies. AEs were reported in 248 patients (99%) and 123 patients (98%) in the ide cel and SOC cohorts, respectively, with 233 and 94 in each cohort, respectively, experiencing grade 5 events. The most common AEs were hematologic in nature, being neutropenia (78% vs. 44%), anemia (66% vs. 36%), and thrombocytopenia (54% vs. 29%). Grade 3 or 4 infection occurred in 61 days (24%) or 23 days (18%), respectively, the most common being upper respiratory tract infections. Grade 5 TRAEs occurred in 3% of ide cel patients. CRS occurred in 197 out of 225 patients (88%), mostly grade 1 or 2 in the ide cel cohort, and investigator-defined neurotoxicity occurred in 34 of the 225 ide cel patients, mostly grade 1 or 2, and were managed with glucocorticoids in 15 patients. The study authors concluded that in this hard-to-treat patient population in which a lack of established SOC, particularly in triple-class exposed disease, ide cel makes for an attractive therapeutic option because the therapy is associated with a significantly longer PFS than the standard of care, deeper and more-durable responses, and a 51% lower risk of death. Even though a significant proportion of patients in the ide cel arm experienced CRS, along with higher incidences of hematologic toxicity and infections, it is consistent with observations in other KarMMa trials. The authors also noted that these benefits were derived from a single infusion and that ide cel may prove to be fruitful in hard-to-treat triple-class exposed relapsed/refractory multiple myeloma (RRMM) with these prolonged PFS results across subgroups with typically poor survival outcomes [8].

9.4 Ciltacabtagene Autoleucel

CARTITUDE-4 showed that ciltacabtagene autoleucel (cilta cel), also a BCMA-targeting CAR, has robust responses in earlier lines of therapy in refractory MM patients with prior treatment featuring lenalidomide versus SOC, which was reported in the *NEJM*. They found that in MM patients refractory to lenalidomide, a single infusion of cilta cel led to a lower risk of both disease progression and death as the primary endpoint when compared to Daratumumab-Pomalidomide (DP) (median follow-up 15.9 months). PFS was reported as 75.9% for cilta cel versus 48.6% for SOC. Patients receiving cilta cel also experienced deeper, more-durable responses, had higher measures of MRD negativity (60.6% versus 15.6%, RR of 2.2; (95% CI 1.8–2.6)), and had an OR of 8.7 (95% CI 5.4–13.9). However, the authors also note that two triplet regimens have been shown to have high clinical efficacy, and isatuximab, carfilzomib, and dexamethasone and daratumumab, carfilzomib, and dexamethasone did not undergo evaluation and have since entered clinical practice. In this trial, 419 patients were randomized to receive either cilta cel (n = 208) or SOC (physician's choice, n = 211). Median PFS was not reached in the cilta cel cohort and was 11.8 months in the SOC cohort (HR, 0.26; 95% CI 0.18–0.38).

9.4.1 Key Results

- Cilta cel: PFS (12 months) 75.9% (95% CI 69.4 to 81.1); greater OR 84.6%; CR 73.1%; absence of MRD 60.6%
- Standard of care: PFS (12 months) 48.6% (95% CI 41.5 to 55.3); OR 67.3%; CR 21.8%; absence of MRD 15.6%
- Death from any cause: 39 patients and 46 patients (HR: 0.78; 95% CI 0.5 to 1.2); RR 2.9 (95% CI 2.3 to 3.7); OR 10.3 (95% CI 6.5 to 16.4)
- Serious adverse events
  - Cilta cel: 92 (44.2%)
  - Standard of care: 81 (38.9)
- Second primary malignancies
  - Cilta cel: Nine (4.3%)
  - Standard-of-care group (most common): 14 (6.7%)—hematologic events and cutaneous or noninvasive cancers
- CRS
  - Cilta cel: 134/176 (76.1%) (grade 1 or 2: 132; grade 3: 2)
- Neurotoxic events: 36 patients (20.5%) (grade 1 or 2: 31; grade 3 or 4: five). ICANS: Eight (4.5%; grade 1 or 2); median of 9.5 days (range, 6 to 15)

With this favorable benefit–risk profile, the authors concluded that a strong PFS benefit and durable outcomes demonstrate the great promise of cilta cel as an established treatment option for relapsed MM [9].

Swan et al. reviewed CAR T-cell therapy for MM and described two approved BCMA-directed treatments (ide cel and cilta cel). Ide cel was evaluated in the phase 2 KarMMA trial in 54 patients receiving a high CAR T-cell dose, where the ORR was reported as 81%, the CR rate was at least 39%, and PFS was 12.1 months. Of patients with CR, MRD showed a level of 10(−5), and 59% had sustained MRD negativity after 12 months according to next-generation sequencing (NGS). CRS and neurotoxicity occurred in 84% and 18% of patients, respectively. Ide cel was approved in RRMM after four prior lines of therapy, with similar results with PD within 18 months of induction therapy, ASCT, and lenalidomide maintenance. At a median follow-up of 21.5 months, ORR was reported as 83.8% and CR rate as 45.9%, and MRD negativity was achieved in 11 of 13 evaluable patients (10(−5)). Median PFS was demonstrated as 11.4 months, whereas mOS was not reached. Patients who were triple-class exposed were evaluated in the phase 3 KarMMA-3 trial comparing ide cel with this SOC, with significant improvement in mPFS being shown in the ide cel arm, where an mPFS of 13.8 compared to 4.4 months and a 51% reduced risk of death or PD, with an ORR of 71% vs. 42% and an CR of 44% versus 5%, were reported. CRS occurred in 88% and neurotoxicity in 15%. Cilta cel was evaluated in the CARTITUDE studies, with CARTITUDE-1 enrolling 97 RRMM patients, 87% being triple refractory and 42% being pentarefractory. ORR was 98%, CR was 80%, and MRD negativity at a level of 10(−5) was achieved in 92% of evaluable patients. The FDA has reported CRS developing in 95% of patients and neurotoxicity in 23%, with movement and neurocognitive TRAEs in 6%. Median PFS was 34.9 months, and the estimated OS of 63% occurred at 36 months. CARTITUDE-2 evaluated RRMM patients after one to three prior lines of therapy, comparing cilta cel with pomalidomide; bortezomib and dexamethasone; or daratumumab, pomalidomide, and dexamethasone with an enrollment of 419 patients and 208 randomized to receive cilta cel; 176 received an infusion of cilta cel. MRD negative was significantly higher in the cilta cel arm, with ORR reported at 85% versus 67% and a CR rate of 73% vs. 22%; mPFS was not reached vs. 11.8 months in SOC. 12-month PFS was shown to be 76% in the cilta cel arm versus 49% in the control arm. CRS occurred in 76% of patients, and 4.5% of patients had ICANS and cranial nerve palsy. Problems arising with CAR T-cell administration in MM patients include a loss of BCMA expression, an immunosuppressive MM microenvironment, and suboptimal CAR T-cell function and manufacturing tissues. This can be alleviated by using a fully human BCMA-binding domain, with a fully humanized anti-BCMA being designed in zevorcabtagene autoleucel (zevor cel). Additionally, 18 RRMM patients were infused with fully humanized anti-BCMA CAR T CT103A in a phase 1 study, where ORR was 100% and CR was 78% at a median of 41 months. Seven patients remained MRD negative at data cutoff. Also, mPFS and mOS were 23 and 42 months, respectively, with a 419 median CAR T persistence, significant given that in CARTITUDE-1 most patients did not show considerable transgene persistence at 6 months. Equecabtagene autoleucel (eque cel) was shown in the FUMANBA-1 study evaluating 103 RRMM patients with prior P1 to have an ORR of 96%, a CR of 74%, and a 12-month PFS of 79%. The treatment could still be detected in 40% of patients, and of the 88 patients who were MRD negative, 78% remained as such over 6 months and 74% over 12 months. In terms of approaches to BMCA loss, BCMA expression decreased and subsequently recovered, with BCMA being cleaved from the MM cell surface by gamma secretase, resulting in increased BCMA serum levels and reduced cellular expression, which is an adverse prognostic factor. Trogocytosis leads to increased BCMA secretion as well. Dual antigen targeting also reduces the likelihood of BCMA loss, with the CAR T-cell construct incorporated in the truncated form of APRIL enabling a dual targeting of BCMA and TACL with its antigen binding domain. When evaluated in a phase 1 study, it showed an ORR of 43% ($n = 11$), and a bispecific BCMA/CD38 CAR T-cell construct evaluated in RRMM patients ($n = 16$) in a single-center phase 1 study showed an ORR of 87.5%; PFS was 69%, and OS was 75%. The upregulation of proinflammatory cytokine genes, NKFB-signaling genes, and apoptotic genes overcame an immunosuppressive TME. High levels of PD-L1 have also been shown to contribute to an immunosuppressive environment and have been associated with inferior results with in vitro MM cell lysis after cilta cel treatment. A novel BCMA CAR T agent—namely CART-ddBCMA anitocabtagene autoleucel (anito cel)—with a completely synthetic d-domain-based antigen binding site was tested in a phase 1 trial ($n = 13$) and demonstrated an ORR of 100% and an 89% MRD negative rate. Another BCMA-directed CAR T agent, the allogeneic ALLO-715, is a disrupted CD52 expression and was shown in the phase 1 UNIVERSAL trial ($n = 43$) to have an ORR of 71% and a CR of 25%. Three out of 43 patients who underwent infusion died as a result of grade 5 infections. Other systems using the piggyBac nonviral integration-based one, such as P-BCMA-ALLO1, also an allogeneic BCMA CAR T, have less-complex manufacturing processes and are less costly than viral vector-based approaches, regarded as more traditional [10].

Nasari et al. [11] also discuss some of the problems with the administration of ide cel and cilta cel, with response durations of 8.6 months and 34.9 months, respectively, with patients frequently facing relapse. Limitations occurring endemically with T-cell availability and persistence and with modifications in aspects of the T cell while patients are being treated are seen as mitigating factors. The shedding of myeloma antigen expression in the context of an immunosuppressive TME and the inherent complexities in CAR T-cell penetration in tissues are also posited as factors that need to be addressed. A solution has been proposed for developing engineered allogeneic T cells serving as a universal source for CARs expression and the utilization of CAR expression on other immune cells (NK cells). Research is being conducted on the adoption of dual-specific or multispecific antigen targeting receptors that integrate a diverse set of costimulatory domains with designing genes to coexpress cytokines through genetic alterations. When it became apparent that the persistence of CAR T cells and success of CAR T-cell approaches did not correspond with the absolute number of infused cells, efforts were made to optimize persistence and functionality, leading to enhancements in the design of CAR constructs and CAR T-cell production. Stimulating CAR T-cell cultures with recombinant cytokines such as IL-5, IL-7, IL-8, and IL-12 as well as IL-21 and IL-23 has been found to enhance persistence and promote memory cell formation when compared to effector cells, and fourth-generation CAR T-cell-generating BCMA expressing CCL19 and IL-17 has as shown to be superior to second-generation CAR T cells, considered to be traditional in the context of migration and cytotoxicity. Other constructs, such as Bb21217, that use a PI3K inhibitor were added ex vivo to stimulate memory and T-cell production and showed an ORR of 55%, which encouraged its development and completion. GC012F is a dual BCMA/CD19 that targets a CAR T product that is undergoing investigation in a phase I study across multiple centers for MM patients in China. BMS-986354 and PHE885 are other constructs undergoing investigation, with the former undergoing the NEX-T approach to lessen the time for manufacturing and the latter being a fully humanized BCMA CAR T-cell product, with the T-Charge platform undergoing evaluation in a phase I study. Innovations are taking place in the development of allogeneic CAR T cells for enhancements in safety for an off-the-shelf solution that can be readily accessible for R/R patients as well. UCARTCS1A is an allogeneic CAR T-cell therapy undergoing clinical development for MM that has the T-cell receptor (TCR) utilizing TALEN and as well as ALLO-715 and ALLO-605 that are modified allogeneic anti-BCMA CAR T cells and utilize TALEN technology, allowing for the deactivation of the TCR alpha constant gene and CD52; when combined with ALLO-647, an anti-CD52 monoclonal antibody, they allow for temporary but selective lymphodepletion prior to CAR T-cell administration. As the authors state, T cells that are double negative for CD4+ and CD8+ receptors are suppressive of GvHD independent of limitations in MHC with nonspecific antigen recognition, and they have been recognized as having potential in the allogeneic setting with demonstrated clinical efficacy through tumor growth inhibition, as observed in preclinical models. Antigen heterogeneity interfering with T-cell recognition has also been shown to be an issue that leads to a reduction in efficacy and to trogocytosis, as shown by BCMA cleaved by gamma secretase, as alluded to earlier, which leads to release for cleaved BCMA into circulation and T-cell fratricide. Also, resistance mechanisms have emerged through BCMA escape through the downregulation of BMCA as a result of nontruncating mutations and an in-frame deletion in the EXC domain of BCMA. In the BCMA locus of the chr16p region, a heterozygous deletion along with a nonsense mutation of the other allele results in biallelic BCMA suppression. To overcome heterogeneity and BCMA evasion, the repertoire of antigens has been expanded to include signaling lymphocyte activation molecule family-7, found in the immunosuppressive component of CAFs, promoting MM cell production, with autologous targets to CAR T cells and allogeneic targeting Carta and BCMA/SLAM:

- SLAMF-7—expression in 95% MM
- CD138—expression in 90–100% MM
- CD38—expression in 80–100% MM
- CD56—expression in 70–90% MM

- Kappa (κ) light chain—expression in 35% MM
- Overexpressed antigens—natural-killer group 2 member D (NKG2D)

Stress-induced ligands with MHC-1 chain–related proteins, and diverse, structurally unique, long 16-binding proteins 1 to 6 are upregulated in MM and bind to receptors on NK and T cells, forming a hexameric structure consisting of an adaptor protein DAP1 functional for eliminating tumor cells. GPCR class C group 5 member D (GPRC5D, a largely myeloma-specific orphan receptor), CD44v6, CD74, TnMUC1, integrin-Beta7, MMG49, NY-ESO-1, and proteins are marked by abnormal glycosylation accompanied by tumor overexpression. The CAR TnMUC1 is incorporated into the transmembrane CD8 alpha region in addition to two intracellular signaling domains: CD2 (the signaling of which led to prolonged T-cell persistence and reduced exhaustion in the TME, as shown in a phase 1 study) and CD3ζ. APRIL and TACI B-cell activating factor contribute to MM resistance through the binding of BAFF-R and the transmembrane activation of TAC1 receptors, triggering the expressing of PD-L1 and promoting T-cell exhaustion. These findings led to the construction of an APRIL-CAR, relying on a natural ligand rather than an scFV-derived antibody containing TAC1 and BCMA-based CAR T targets and relying on a natural ligand as opposed to an antibody-derived scFv with TAC1 and BCMA targeting both BCMA/TAC1 simultaneously to address heterogeneous antigens and CD19. Integrin Beta7 is also highly expressed by MM, contributing to migration, adhesion, invasion, and drug resistance. Nirogacestat inhibits Notch signaling with a small molecule gamma secretase inhibitor and enhances the efficacy of BCMA-targeted therapies. The Notch signal regulates the CXCR4 chemokine system, promoting MM cell proliferation via cyclin D1 upregulation, and HEY1, the hairy enhancer of split-1 and the hairy enhancer of a split-related receptor with YRPW motif protein. In terms of the immunosuppressive TME environment, disrupting checkpoint genes through genome-editing technologies improves CAR outcomes by leading to the growth of CAR T cells and their cytotoxicity within the TME, retaining the ability of the T cell to eliminate the cancer cells [11].

Reddy et al. performed an additional review of CAR T-cell therapies for MM, describing the targets specific for MM, early- and late-line setting treatments, the determinants of response and resistance, and tumor factors such as target antigen and pretreatment burden, tumor microenvironment factors such as CAR T-cell trafficking to the tumor site and the immunosuppressive environment, and clinical factors such as using MRD to predict outcomes. The ideal target should be uniformly expressed on malignant cells with very little expression on normal cells, with BCMA and GPR5CD being examples. In MM, BCMA, a member of the tumor necrosis factor (TNF) receptor family, promotes MM cell survival, growth, and proliferation. As described earlier, targets such as GPRC5D and SLAMF7, expressed on malignant MM cells but not on hematopoietic cells, are undergoing preclinical and clinical development. T-cell factors, such as T-cells' phenotype in memory and effector cells, the latter of which have the CD45RA phenotype, have more prevalence in patients with chronic infection and with MM for several years. CD4+ and CD8+ T cells have been shown to improve the expansion of CD8+ T cells and lead to intrinsic cytotoxic killing. BCMA expression varies between patients, prior therapy impacts BCMA expression, and no studies have confirmed the threshold for BCMA expression; however, studies have shown that a loss of BCMA expression by genomic deletion and protein downregulation can be detected, whereby genetic homozygous loss may resolve and protein downregulation may allow for retreatment with BCMA-targeting therapy. In patients whose tumors no longer express antigen, BCMA-directed therapy leads to resistance. In terms of tumor burden, no universal biomarker is yet available for assessing MM [12].

To address the limitations of allogeneic BCMA-directed CAR T-cell therapy, limitations that include a time-consuming manufacturing process (4–5 weeks at 1.5% and 18% rates in the KarMMa and CARTITUDE trials, respectively) and a risk of contamination by pathogens, scientists have been attempting to create an allogeneic approach for CAR-based immune cell treatment (Figs. 9.3 and 9.4). The procedures consist of beginning with a collection of healthy donor blood, isolating the relevant and specific immune cells, genetically modifying them, and expanding them in vitro for further quality control testing and in vitro expansion, with the advantage being to apply them "off the shelf." The examples described by Du et al. are gene-edited alpha-beta T cells, gamma-delta T cells, and NK cells. ALLO-715, as described earlier, is a BCMA T cell that has been genetically modified and uses TALEN technology for disrupting the TCR to reduce GvHD, which has been tested in a phase I study. An interim report showed that 53% had grade I and 2 CRS and that 14% experienced neurotoxicity. ORR in the 320 × 10(6) cohort was 71%. ALLO-605 is an alternative allogeneic cellular BCMA treatment that was given the FDA fast track designation in 2021 and the orphan drug designation in 2022. Having a constitutively active chimeric antigen receptor (CACCR), it regulates T-cell exhaustion and improves T-cell potency and functioning. Gamma-delta T cells make up a minor CD3+ T-cell population that expresses a V-delta chain that recognizes antigens in a human leukocyte antigen (HLA)–independent fashion, being able to recognize endogenous isopentenyl pyrophosphate that is overexpressed in

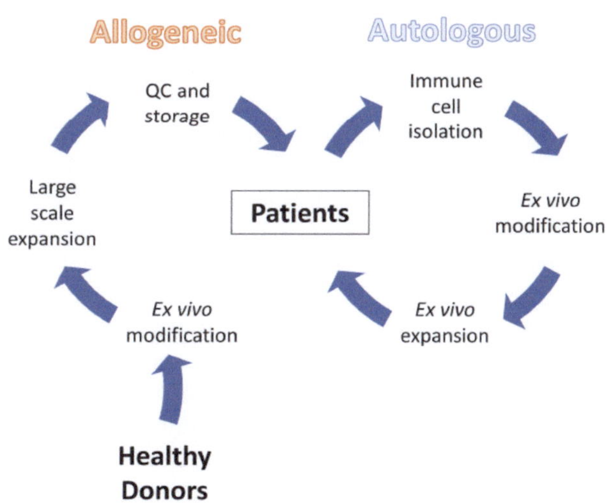

Fig. 9.3 The allogeneic and autologous adoptive transfer of CAR-based immune cells. (Adapted from Du [13])

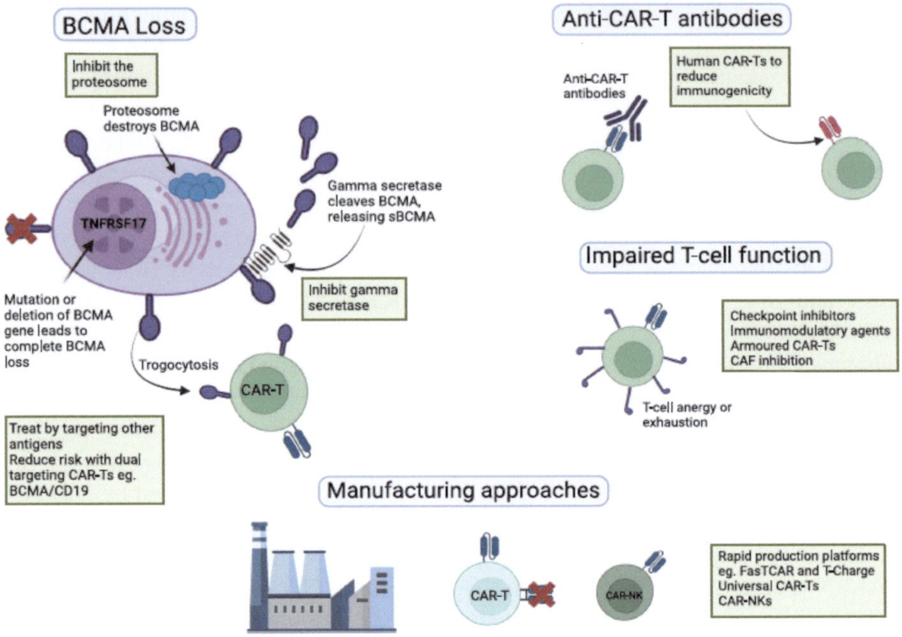

Fig. 9.4 An approach to improving CAR T efficacy in multiple myeloma. (Adapted from Swan [10])

tumor cells. However, because of low T-cell abundance and T cells' innate yet precise regulatory functions, problems emerge in effector and efficiency functions in gene editing and in vitro expansion capacity, with expansion protocols utilizing Il-2 and IL-15 in development to alleviate these issues. NK cells have no need from antigen presentation through the HLA recognition mechanism and possess natural cytotoxicity with allogeneic applications. Their adoptive transfer has been allogeneically shown to have tolerability in several clinical trials in treating MM; however, anti-BCMA CAR NK cells are less prevalent, with no data yet released by three clinical trials that chose CB, NK-92, and iPSCs as the origins of NK cells. Upon the activation of MM cells, anti-BCMA CAR NK cells transferred with mRNA display have shown superior in vitro cytotoxicity through degranulation and the release of interferon-gamma (IFN-gamma) when compared to control NK cells. When compared to the NK-92 cell line transduced by a lentivirus anti-BCMA CAR, a second-generation agent, superior cytotoxicity was shown against K562, XG-1, and U2266. Challenges remain in transducing primary NK cells using lentivirus and retrovirus; therefore, a better option for NK cell genetic modification may be through nonviral transfection systems. CAR-NK cells have innate potential through their in vivo activity. Also, enhanced NK receptor expression could be achieved through in vitro manipulation, leading to the downregulation of the homing receptors on NK cells. The authors also found that CXCR4 significantly improved migration and homing capacities, with coexpression showing further tumor-eradicating effects in an MM xenograft model. Without cytokine support, NK cells have limited existence in peripheral blood; however, mitigation through IL-2 injection has been conducted [13].

Ravi et al. performed a phase I clinical study on the autologous BCMA CAR T that was manufactured as a NEX-T CAR T-cell therapy (BMS-986354) in triple-class exposed RRMM ($n = 65$); 39% were cytogenetic high risk, 91% were triple-class refractory, and 43% have extramedullary disease. Part A served as the dose-escalation phase, whereas part B served as the dose-expansion phase. RP2D was found to be 40 × 10^6 CAR T cells. CRS occurred in 82%, neurotoxicity in 8%, and infections in 32% of participants. Compared to the CAR T-cell therapy orvacabtagene autoleucel, the same CAR construct, the investigational treatment had a higher proportion of Tcm cells, with proliferative abilities and improved potency. The authors note that bridging therapy leads to 10% attrition between infusion and apheresis and that CRS is life-threatening in certain situations with ide cel and cilta cel, with prolonged cytopenias that require intensive management. Given the necessity of improving the manufacturing process and the safety and efficacy of autologous BCMA-targeted therapy, the necessity for developing novel CAR T-cell constructs arises. In this study, 25 patients (39%) had myeloma with high-risk chromosomal abnormalities (17p13 deletion, 17p del, t4;14, or t14;16), with 28 patients (43%) having extramedullary plasmacytomas and 59 patients (91%) being triple-class exposure. DLTs were prolonged neutropenia and thrombocytopenia and decreased fibrinogen; at all three dose levels, they were considered tolerable, whereas tocilizumab and dexamethasone for CRS were also shown to be tolerable. Moreover, 8% of participants had neurological toxicity, including four grade 1 and one grade 2 ICANS. TEAEs consisted of grades 3 and 4 neutropenia and thrombocytopenia in 48 (74%) and 25 (39%) of all participants, respectively. Three patients developed myelodysplastic syndrome (MDS), with one case after 1 month showing a newly demonstrated loss of chromosome 5q. An NGS panel revealed TP53 mutations. Deep and fast responses were observed at all dose levels, with PR at 87 (99%) and very good partial response (VGPR) at 30 (46%) (95% CI 34%–59%). In total, 47 patients were treated at RP2D, with 44 (94%, 95% CI 82%–99%) having PR or better and 18 (38%, 95% CI 25%–54%) having CR/sCR. The value of 1 month (range 0.9–4.0) served as the median time to response. Also observed was long-term disease control due to persistence, with the percentage of Tmem cells correlating with better antitumor activity and better and longer-term disease control. Effector cells, on the other hand, were short-lived and yet responsible for early immune response while correlating with toxicity and a lack of sustained response, which is significant given that the progressive differentiation that CAR T cells undergo leads to a loss of the ability to proliferate after infusion. As the authors conclude, "BMS-986354, with a higher percentage of memory phenotype, offers a potentially efficacious CAR T manufacturing platform" with manageable safety, with similar CRS events as those seen in CARTITUDE trials [14].

Du et al. reported updates on an open-label phase I study on BCMA/CD19 dual target CAR T cell construct GC012F for RRMM. GCO12F is a dual targeting construct with both CD19 and BCMA dual target developed on the FasTCAR-T platform that requires only 22–36 h of manufacturing. In this study, 29 patients were evaluated for CR and VGPR, yielding 82.8% (n = 24) and 89.7% (n = 26), respectively. PFS was 38.0 months, with CRS reported in 25 patients (86.2%), of which most CRS cases were grade 2. MRD negative rate levels also showed a deep and durable response with potential for further clinically evaluating GC012F for RRMM to confirm efficacy [15].

9.5 Recent Clinical Trials (Figs. 9.5 and 9.6)

Gagelmann et al. developed and validated a prediction model outcome after BCMA-targeting CAR T-cell therapy in RRMM. The international study, composed of a European cohort and a US cohort (n = 136; n = 133), aimed to develop models with the ability to predict outcomes, identifying patients who may benefit from ide cel (n = 171) and cilta cel (n = 38). Academically produced BCMA CAR T was also evaluated (n = 60). Safety results included a grade > 2 of CRS in 10 patients (7%) in the European cohort and 7 patients (5%) in the US cohort. ORR was 87%, and when evaluating OS at 12 months, no significant difference was observed between the cohorts (Europe 79% (95% CI 71 to 87) vs. the United States 65% (95% CI 54 to 75)). Risk factors for failure with early treatment within 5 months of infusion included high-risk cytogenetics such as, the presence of del (17p), sex, age and lenalidomide-refractoriness-adjusted ferritin levels before lymphodepletion. Each risk factor had a score that contributed to the MyCARe model. Scores ranged from

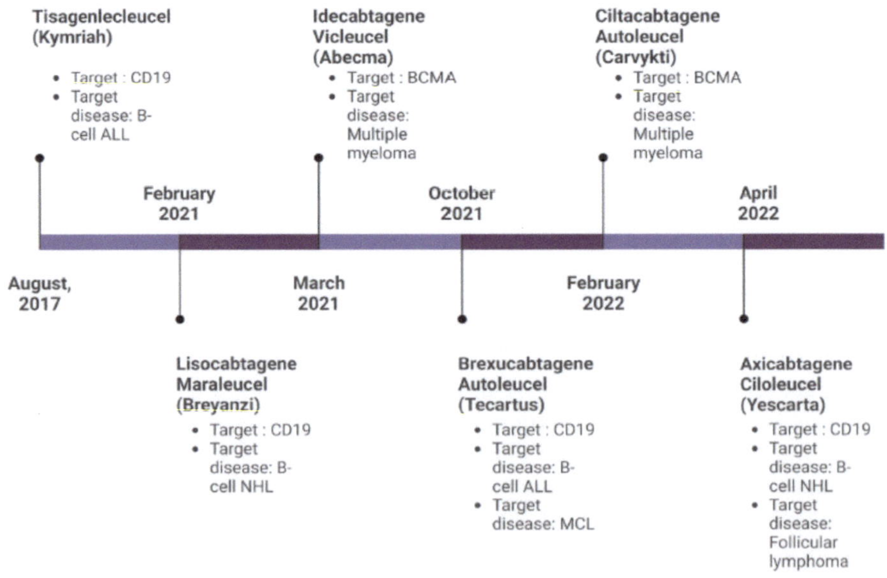

Fig. 9.5 FDA-approved CAR T-cell therapies. (Adapted from Huang et al. [16])

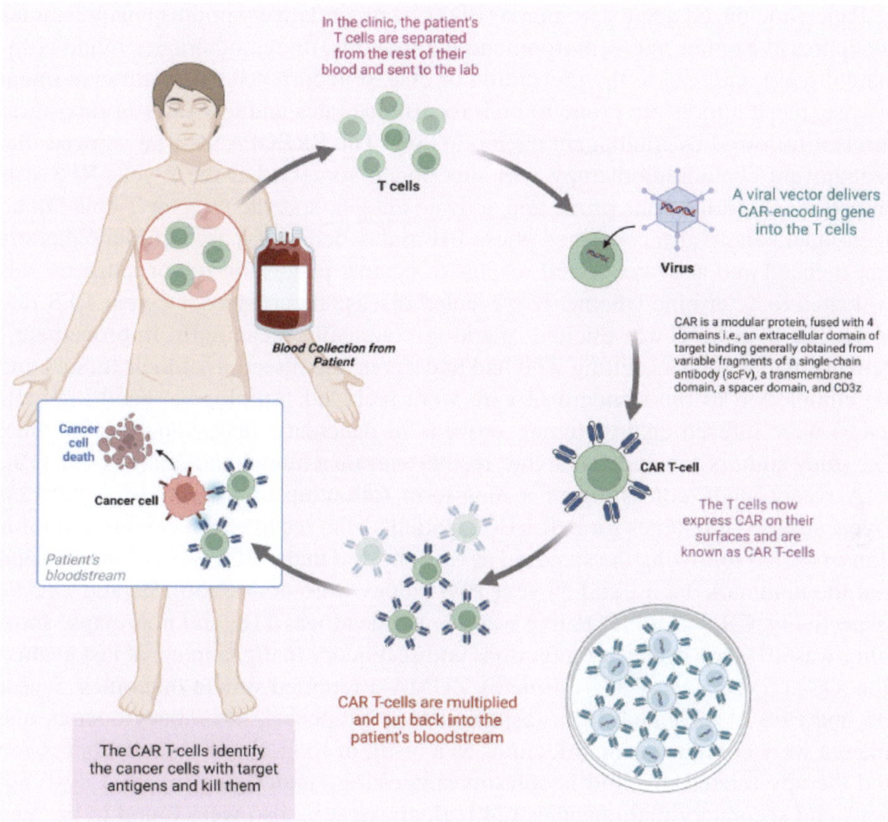

Fig. 9.6 Recent clinical trials. (Adapted from Huang et al. [16])

0 to 4, with scores of 0 to 1 being low, scores of 2 to 3 being intermediate, and a score of 4 being high risk. The study authors showed that the MyCAR model also had prognostic utility for patients based on an age of 65 years or 65 years or older [17].

In a pooled analysis of two early-phase studies, the safety and efficacy of the CAR-modified T-cell therapy CT041 targeting Claudin 18.2 in solid tumors were shown in previously treated pancreatic cancer ($n = 24$ patients). Five patients previously had one at one line of therapy, with 19 receiving more than one line. Objective response rate (ORR) was 16.7%, and disease control rate (DCR) was 70.8%. CRS and gastrointestinal (GI) disorders were the most common AEs. Median PFS was 3.3 months after infusion (95% CI 5.5 to 17.6). Median DoR was reported as 9.5 months (95% CI 2.6 to not reached). All patients had extensive metastasis at enrollment. CRS was reported in 21 patients (87.5%), where CRS cases were grade 1 and 2. Tocilizumab was administered after enrollment. Swimmer plots displayed the decreasing size of target lesions, with decreases in tumor load [18].

Pancreatic ductal adenocarcinoma (PDAC) has a relatively nonresponsive immunosuppressive tumor microenvironment; without this, immunotherapies might eliminate disease and lead to the prevention of disease recurrence. After curative intent disease, these tumors are prone to high recurrence rates and low rates of long-term survival followed by multiagent chemotherapy. The PREOPANC trial showed that neoadjuvant chemoradiotherapy was superior to surgery, but the 2-year RFS was only 40%. Dendritic cells prime and activate antigen-specific effector T cells. In an open-label, single-arm combined phase I/II trial, a dendritic-based immune therapy that induced and activated T-cell responses against pancreatic tumor antigens was evaluated to determine whether it prevented disease recurrence. A 2-year RFS rate of greater than 60% was elicited, marking "clinically meaningful improvement." Patients in the adjuvant setting who had undergone the resection of their tumors and the completion of the standard of care were included. Autologous dendritic cells (DCs) were infused against tumor antigens in pancreatic ductal adenocarcinoma. The study authors concluded that the "results warrant a future randomized trial" [19].

A recent study consisting of a long-term follow-up of patients (n = 275) on 5-year survival outcomes for R/R LBCL patients who received axi cel through infusion (n = 275) following the standard of care showed that mPFS was 8.7 months and that the landmark 1-, 3-, and 5- year PFS values were 47.3%, 36.1%, and 28.5%, respectively. CR was 84; PD/alive was 33; PD/dead was 118; and nonrelapse mortality was 40 (16% driven by infections and secondary malignancies) at last evaluation. OS at 5 years was 40% (estimate). ZUMA-1 reported similar outcomes: 5-year OS and PFS of 43% and 32%, respecteively. Cytopenias, thrombocytopenia, and anemia were common. Late infections as a result of long-term immunosuppression and therapy-related myeloid neoplasms suggesting "underlying myeloid dysfunction" and secondary malignancies (24 patients, or 9%) also were found to be "key survivorship issues" and reduced long-term survival after CAR T therapy, especially in patients 65 to 75 years old. patients, who after CAR T-cell therapy have a lower risk of relapse but a higher risk of late no-relapse mortality (NRM) [20].

An algorithm was created to stratify risk and quantify tumor-infiltrating lymphocytes on the basis of H&E-stained whole slide images (WSIs). The study authors retrospectively explored the relationships between survival outcomes and tumor-infiltrating lymphocyte (TIL) density in colorectal cancer (CRC) patients by using the Cancer Genome Atlas (TCGA) and the molecular and cellular oncology international cohort. They created LinkNet17, an automated deep-learning network, "to develop a cellular-level TIL detector." They found a risk of disease progression and a nonlinear relationship between TIL abundance on one hand and OS and PFS on the other in the TCGA cohort. In a univariate Cox proportional hazard (beyond the scope of this book), the TIL(Link) score was associated with improved PFS and OS in CRC.

9.5.1 Key Results

- "The TIL-high group (> 0.252%) showed a significantly longer time to PFS. (HR, 0.259; 95% CI 0.163 to 0.412) than the TIL-low group (< 0.252%) in the TCGA cohort with similar, significant trends in favor of the TIL-high group also observed for OS in both TCGA (HR, 0.464; 95% CI 0.274 to 0.784) and MCO patients (HR, 0.708; 95% CI 0.568 to 0.882)."

- "The TIL-high patients had an approximately 70% reduction in the risk of disease progression compared with the TIL-low patients (HR, 0.272; 95% CI 0.118 to 0.624)."

The prognostic association with TIL(Link) score is independent of other clinicopathological factors in multivariate analysis (beyond the scope of the book). This study remains significant because given that TILs are prognostic, therapeutic decision-making could be better informed about tumors harboring high TIL densities that may benefit from ICI therapies [21].

Ciltacabtagene autoleucel was also shown to be safe and clinically effective for RRMM patients "who have previously received three or more lines of therapy or whose cancer was not responsive to a proteasome inhibitor, an immunomodulatory drug, or an anti-CD38 antibody ($n = 97$)," and at a median follow-up of 18 months, ORR was a very favorable 98%, with a CR of 80.4% and a PR of 94.8%. Response rates were in the range of 95% to 100% for prior lines of treatment and cytogenetic risk (https://dailynews.ascopubs.org/do/early-data-suggest-investigational-car-t-cell-therapy-provides-deep-durable-responses).

9.6 Allogeneic CAR T-Cell Strategies

With remarkably efficacy in hematological malignancies such as lymphoma and multiple myeloma, CAR T cells combine mAbs with the cytotoxic effects of T cells to kill tumor cells by using CD19 and BCMA targets. They have less efficacy in solid tumors, however, due to an immunosuppressive TME and tumor heterogeneity. Studies have been performed to evaluate CAR T-cell therapy, including second-generation and third-generation constructs that lead to cytotoxic T-cell activity in tumors such as melanoma and GBM despite the challenges posed by solid tumors.

One study on multiple solid tumors that evaluated tandem CAR T cells directed against both CD70 and B7-H3 demonstrated potency in preclinical models, showing that despite relapse after initial CAR T-cell therapy as a result of heterogenous expression and antigen variants, the combinatorial targeting of TAAs enhance antitumor targeting. A target-antigen binding moiety was designed with two CD70 targeted CARs consisting of a distinct antigen binding domain, a shortened CD27- and CD70-specific scFv, and bivalent tandem CAR, with target expression on multiple solid tumors, such as breast, kidney, and melanoma, showing high activity on CD70 tumor cells [22].

Pal et al. conducted both preclinical and clinical studies on an allogeneic CD70-directed CAR T-cell therapy developed for advanced or refractory clear cell renal cell carcinoma (ccRCC). They report that the agent, CTX130, showed favorable cytotoxicity profiles and preclinical proliferation with the complete regression of RCC tumors in xenograft models. Also, 16 R/R ccRCC patients were enrolled in a phase I study that evaluated CTX130 in which no patients experienced DLT, and a

DCR of 81.3% was reported. A durable complete response of 3 years was observed in one patient. These results are significant because the standard of care for ccRCC is targeted vascular endothelial growth factor (VEGF) therapy in combination with ICIs, yet only a minority of patients show CR, with mPFS in the range of 5 to 8 months and ORR between 28% and 43%. The target for this agent is CD70, a member of the costimulatory tumor necrosis factor (TNF) family of molecules, transiently expressed on dendritic cells (DCs) and antigen-presenting cells (APCs) in the GI tract and activated lymphocytes. It is constructed by an anti-cD70 expression case into the T-cell receptor alpha constant (TRAC) locus that disrupted beta macroglobulin, eliminating the surface expression of MHC class I molecules and disrupting CD70 expression. According to the authors, current evidence may suggest that signaling through CD70 is a possibility, promoting tumor growth by limiting the expansion of T cells and driving immune-suppressive Treg cell proliferation, which enables further immune evasion. Immunohistochemistry (IHC) samples showed that CD70 was evident in 43% of solid tumor samples and is considered a biomarker for ccRCC, with its expression regulated by hypoxia-inducible factor (HIF) mutations in the von Hippel-Lindau (VHL) gene, leading to CD70 activation and targets located downstream, leading to the possibility of anti-CD70 targeting for CD70-expressing tumor types such as ccRCC, of which CTX130 is an example, being an investigational CD70-directed allogeneic CAR T-cell therapy. CTX130 was shown through in vitro studies and in vivo efficacy studies to demonstrate specificity for CD70 and completely inhibit tumor growth in all five mice, and it showed that a PD-1 knockout reduced CAR T potency. CTX130 was also shown in an open-label phase I study investigating the efficacy, safety, and PD of CTX130 in R/R ccRCC to have favorable safety profiles, with no grade 3 CRS events reported, no patients experiencing ICANS, and no instances of hemophagocytic lymphohistiocytosis (HLH) and secondary malignancies, where 13 patients (81%) achieved DCR with CR (one, or 6%), PR, and SD (12, or 73%). Also, mPFS and mOS were 2.9 months (95% CI 1.7–6.0) and 2.9 months (95% CI 14.3 to not available (NA)), respectively. In terms of PK analysis, rapid expansion with peak concentration took place from approximately day 7 to day 15, with CTX130 cells declining by day 28. IHC analysis displayed "high CD70 tumoral expression with a median and mean tumor CD70 positivity of 100% and 75.7%, respectively." The authors conclude on the significance of CTX130 in this heavily pretreated patient population with an excellent safety profile and clinically meaningful results that overcome many of the limitations of CAR T-cell therapy in solid tumors, such as tumor antigen heterogeneity and a suppressive TME. They also conclude that their findings represent proof-of-concept evidence for additional studies on CD70-engaging CAR T cells in ccRCC and other CD70 malignancies and illustrate that these studies evaluated other improved CD70 CAR T-cell constructs relevant for allogeneic CAR T products beyond those for ccRCC [23].

Zhang et al. detail a list of studies on CAR T-cell therapies for urologic tumors. One study for RCC showed that CAR T cells directed against the human carbonic anhydrase IX can secrete human anti-PD-L1 antibodies in a humanized preclinical model of RCC exhibiting tumor suppression as evidence of post-treatment with these antibodies. A panel of anti-CD70 scFv-based CAR T-cells showed potent antitumor activity in RCC cell lines as well. C-Met may also be used as a therapeutic target for RCC through the creation of antihuman c-Met-directed CAR T cells and may be used in the study of the antitumor effects in xenograft models with the ability to infiltrate cancer tissues and thus lead to tumor growth inhibition. These types of treatments could be combined with axitinib to synergistically enhance antitumor CAR T-cell responses. Prostate cancer treatment through CAR T cells is also detailed in that ICIs have less efficacy against them. Prostate-Specific Membrane Antigen (PMSA) and Prostate Stem Cell Antigen (PSCA) can serve as CAR T-cell therapy targets, with one study investigating the efficacy and tolerability of autologous PSMA-specific CAR T cells against refractory castration resistant prostate cancer (CRPC). PSMA targets are also enhanced through the expression of a dominant-negative TGF-βRII (dnTGF-βRII) for further enhanced cytokine secretion and lymphocyte proliferation, with a phase I study ($n = 18$) underway for the treatment of TGFbeta resistance CAR T cells. The combination of CAR T-cell PSMA targets with low-dose CT such as docetaxel led to controlled tumor growth, as did the combination of CAR T-cell PSMA targets with IL-23 Ab. The inclusion of a 4-1BB costimulatory domain proved superior to a CD28 domain in improving the tumor killing of PSCA-CAR-containing cells. A STEAP can also be utilized as a target antigen for PCa treatment and has shown reactivity at a low antigen density for antitumor activity. The authors posit that the existence of Treg cells, myelodysplastic stem cells (MDSCs) tumor associated macrophages (TAMs) and other immunosuppressive cells in solid tumors lead to multiple protumorigenic effects in urological tumors [2].

A recent study designed a CAR T-cell therapy for rare types of melanoma by utilizing the "surface expression of TYRP1 [as] a relevant target for CAR T-cell therapy for patients with melanoma." TYRP1 is a tyrosinase-related protein and a transmembrane glycoprotein involved in melanin synthesis, and it forms a novel and useful target given that the protein is expressed on both malignant cells and normal cells; however, its expression on skin is limited to retinal pigment epithelium. An mAb targeting TRYP1 was evaluated in a clinical study in R/R melanoma with a DCR of 41%, with no adverse events occurring, confirmed through scRNA sequencing and IHC. According to the study authors, melanoma cells expressing TYRP1 were targeted by a TYRP1 CAR T-cell therapy that was designed for the optimal detection of low-level TYRP1 expression on cell surfaces, with the transmembrane, signaling, and costimulatory domains and CD3zeta T-cell coreceptor constructed for IFN-gamma release and targeted cell killing. The authors found that CD28 and 4-1BB were more likely costimulatory signals leading to antitumor activity. Moreover, 20D7SL-28ζ and 20D7SL-BBζ CAR T cells recognize TYRP1 with high specificity, and 20D7SL-28ζ CAR T cells exert strong tumor control, accompanied by low toxicity in the immunocompetent B16 melanoma model's 20D7SL-28ζ–treated tumors, with increases in T-cell infiltration. CRS and systemic inflammation were the most common toxicities. With the high expression of TRYP1 in uveal and acral melanoma, the CAR T construct could have clinical efficacy [24].

The feasibility and safety of GD2-iCAR-PBT was evaluated in metastatic melanoma. The expression of CAR T cells was observed with a specific protocol that leads to a naive-like phenotype with the expression of memory T stem cells through manufacturing that promoted a naive-like CD45RA + CCR7+ CD95+ CD45RO. No

DLTs were reported, with no determination of MTD. In a study, 12 patients were enrolled, with one patient experiencing an AE. Fever, diarrhea, and anorexia at 33% each were the most common AEs, with rash at 50%. PR plus BRAF inhibitor and MEK inhibitor administration was achieved with a concurrent infusion of GD2-CAR-PBT (5/12), whereas V600 BRAF-mutant metastatic melanoma patients receiving concurrent dabrafenib and trametinib as the standard treatment for their V600 BRAF-mutant metastatic melanoma demonstrated low-grade AEs at 59%. A tumor biopsy showed CAR T-cell infiltration, identifying tumor-infiltrating GD2-CAR T cells in three of six formalin-fixed, paraffin-embedded (FFPE) tumor biopsies [25].

Many functional challenges exist in the administration of CAR T-cell therapies that implicate T-cell differentiation and exhaustion. CAR T-cell therapies associated with shorter responses possess deficient proliferative properties that are reflective of the exhausted state and terminal differentiation. The early T-cell differentiation of T cells demonstrates therapy effectiveness through the proliferative capacity of cells. T memory cells promote efficacy, whereas many transcriptional and epigenetic factors prolong the T-cell exhaustion state. After antigen exposure, the increased population of T effector cells leads to the proliferation and persistence of memory T cells, also with high development and proliferative capacity, which circulate and can persist with cytokine proliferation, whereas effector cells lose their proliferative ability but still possess cytotoxic activity. However, chronic antigen exposure leads to the accumulation of the T exhaustive cells that are promoted by LAG-3, PD-L1, and CTLA-4, with a diminished ability to carry out cytokine production. The transcription factor activity of TOX, BATT, IKT4, and NFAT also extend this exhausted state. The authors also point out a distinct epigenetic landscape with T mem characterized by an open chromatin structure where the T box transcription factor and basic leucine zipper are enriched for binding sites. Exhausted T (Tex) cells are uniquely enriched for NFAT and NR4A cytokine effector genes that show high levels of DNA methylation and are epigenetically locked in a Tex state. During late dysfunction, traditional effector properties producing IL-2, TNF, and IFN-gamma fade away. According to Buillard et al., transcriptional and epigenetic signatures are associated with genetic contributions to memory and with the effector and dysfunctional states of T cells. One such example is an approach to defining the memory state by determining the association between CD62L and CCR7 that has remained elusive, with few studies available to determine correlations between clinical outcomes and these traditional homing markers. Studies affecting these markers have yet to find a correlation between less-differentiated products and improved persistence. Further alterations in generating longer-lasting memory cells with less enrichment of these markers has not led to the mitigation of the T-cell-differentiated state, leading to a better manufacturing processes and better clinical outcomes. The authors postulate that CD27 may be a better predictive marker. RUNX3, T-BET, and BLIMP-1, together with IRF4, upregulate IL-12 and downstream differentiation, whereas BATF is induced by IL-12 and IL-21 in CD8+ T cells to regulate chromatin accessibility, regulating transcription factor expression. BATF also has the function of propagating inflammatory signals, whereas RUNX3, another basic leucine zipper

ATF-like transcription factor (BATF-induced TF), governs chromatin acceptability, upregulates BLIMP-1 and IRF4, and downregulates BACH2 and TCF-1. IL-12 further leads to direct differentiation by inducing BLIMP-1 and BET-T expression and downregulating TCF-1 and IL-7RA, thus promoting the effector molecule expression of granzymes and repressing the memory state of TCF-1, IL-7RA, and CD62L. The control of CD8 T-cell differentiation is further enhanced by the Type I interferon induced expression of the Notch, IL-2R, and mTOR. The transcriptional and epigenetic exhaustion program is further driven by the balance between AP-1 and NFAT cells, a balance that directs chronic TCR stimulation and hyporesponsiveness versus physiological differentiation. Furthermore, BLIMP-1 antagonizes memory formation and is highest in the differentiated exhausted state. The NR4A family of neuronal transcription factors further leads to T-cell exhaustion by inhibiting AP-1 function, upregulating PD-1 expression, and repressing effector gene function, thus orchestrating a genome-wide exhaustion linked to the CAR T-cell transcriptional and epigenetic landscape. The authors elaborate on using cell engineering to control CAR T-cell differentiation in which a memory cells are stably engineered to retain their characteristics after infusion through a regulatory network and engineering strategies, stably reprogramming CAR T-cell differentiation and the exhaustion state by involving the constitutive expression of BCL-6 for CD4+ T-cell differentiation and the repression of BLIMP-1 and cJUN overexpression; also, BATF deletion improves the antitumor immunity conferred by CAR T cells. The inducible constitutive activation of FOXO1 also leads to an increased persistence of CAR T cells, as does the enforced expressing of BACH2 and RUNX3. The suppression of the T exhausted state is another approach featuring the deletion of DNMT3A, increasing TCF-1 expression and LEF-1 and CCR7- sustained cytokine secretion, resulting in cytolytic activity evident even when facing persistent and repetitive antigenic challenge [26].

Resistance mechanisms for CAR T-cell therapies are often responsible for treatment failures such as CAR T-cell dysfunction, generalized immune dysfunction, and intrinsic tumor resistance. CAR T-cell dysfunction is exemplified by T-cell dysfunction that occurs with the repetitive antigenic stimulation of T cells, leading to exhaustion markers, with intratumoral T cells demonstrating high levels of T-cell exhaustion at baseline, corroborated by clinical studies delineating the impact of T-cell exhaustion (Fig. 9.7). Using ICIs in combination and increasing the stimulation of costimulatory pathways are some of the ways to overcome T-cell exhaustion. Differentiation states of T cells are also factors that highlight the early lineage of T memory that when used as starting material result in better antitumor activity in murine models when compared to late-lineage cells such as T effector or effector memory cells. Early-lineage T cells have better clinical outcomes and expansion kinetics. When compared to ALL, non-Hodgkin lymphoma (NHL) is less likely to feature the enrichment of early-lineage T cells, which may explain the expansion difference whereby the depletion of early-lineage T-cell fractions took place, and this depletion suggests that the differentiation of early- and late-lineage T cells is affected by cytotoxic treatment. Prior treatment also skews the T-cell compartment, and less-differentiated products are associated with lower levels of systemic

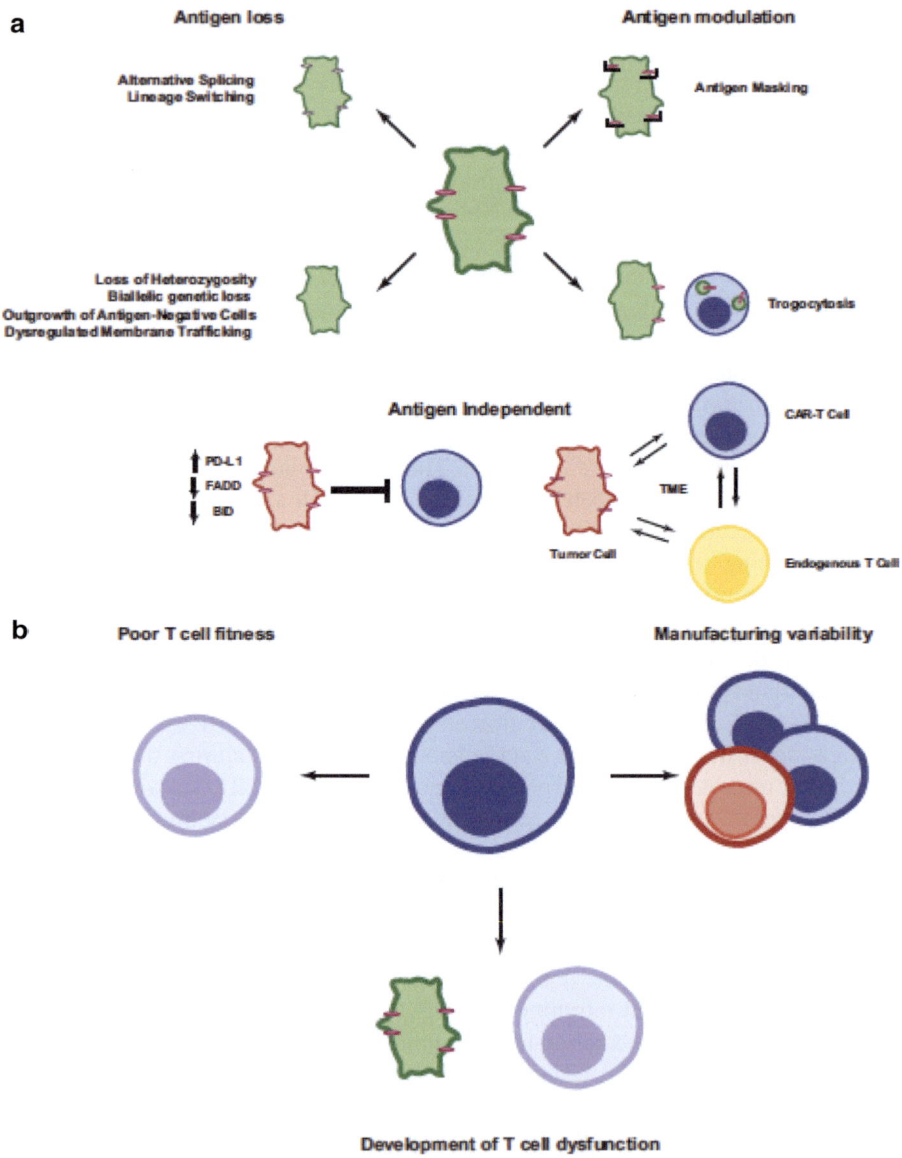

Fig. 9.7 Mechanisms of resistance and relapse: (**a**) tumor-dependent and (**b**) T cell-dependent mechanisms that lead to CAR T failure

proinflammatory cells and improved EFS. As shown through RNA sequencing, CR correlated with CD8 T-cell memory signature, whereas poor molecular response was associated with CD8 T-cell exhaustion signatures. In a study comparing tisa cel and axi cel infusion in NHL patients, axi cel treatment showed enrichment for the CD8 Tem and Tn phenotype, and tisa cel treatment showed enrichment for the CD4

Tcm and Teff phenotype. Higher postinfusion expansion was also associated with higher enrichment for Tcm. In light of this, allogeneic CAR T cells are being tested in early-phase studies, which have the advantage of being manufactured from a less-differentiated state. The role of IL-17 and IL-15 in the differentiation of Tn and Tscm cells is being studied in a clinical trial using these cytokines during the manufacturing of TCR-engineered T cells and led to an increased frequency of early-lineage T cells, such as Tscm frequency, increased antitumor cytotoxicity, and improved apoptotic resistance after repetitive antigen exposure. Improved proliferation and a decreased expression of exhaustion markers also resulted. Modulating intracellular pathways is also stipulated as a potential way of improving antitumor activity, such as by inhibiting AKT signaling during manufacturing, which increases Tcm percentage in preclinical modes that regulates FOXO1, whose overexpression increases the memory phenotype. Generalized immune dysregulation is also a factor, with tumor burden and associated systemic inflammation markers such as IL-6, IL-15, and TNF-alpha correlating with poor outcomes, where the presence of MDSC is evident in the blood of axi cel–treated LBCL patients. The intrinsic resistance of the tumor cell and target antigen loss are also factors with mechanisms in the expression of splice variants, acquired mutations, and trogocytosis. Target antigen transfer occurs from tumor cells to CAR T cells, promoting CAR T-cell fratricide, which has been mitigated by the administration of pharmacological agent and multiantigen targeted CAR T cells. An FIH study evaluating CD20/CD19 CAR T cells showed that 19 patients with NHL had an ORR at day 28 was 82% and a CR of 64%, a PFS of 44%, and OS of 69% at 2 years. Intrinsic resistance occurs through the BCL2 family of signaling in the mitochondria and the extrinsic pathways of the TNF and FAS families. FAS expression had predictive value for outcomes in ZUMA-1, and in cfDNA samples, FAS was associated with poor PFS following CD19 targeted CAR T cells in LBCL patients. BCL2 tumor cell expression was associated with poor outcomes in NHL patients treated with axi cel and tisa cel. In this context, venetoclax treatment after administration has improved cytotoxicity with direct antilymphoma affects. TP53 and APOBEC have also been implicated in immune cell dysregulation [27].

A recent study reported in *Cellular Oncology* found that rituximab in combination with CAR T-cell therapy improves overall clinical outcomes in B-ALL by "sensitizing leukemia cells to CAR T-mediated cytotoxicity and reducing CAR T exhaustion." The methodology of the study compared patients receiving rituximab prior to CAR T infusion with control patients who had comparable features and underwent CAR T-cell therapy without rituximab. Rituximab conferred a favorable prognosis, and the 2-year OS and LFS rates in the rituximab arm were longer, and that group exhibited greater increases in IFN-gamma, TNF-alpha, and IL-2, with a decreased expression of exhaustion factors LAG-3, PD-1, and TIM-3. This study remained significant in the context of high cases of refractory and relapse in B-ALL patients receiving CAR T after treatment, a high risk of recurrence, and disease burden. The authors noted that "mitigating pre-CAR disease burden and CAR T -cell exhaustion" could be factors promoting long-term clinical response. However, few studies have shown that rituximab can lead to these outcomes, and the authors investigated the efficacy and safety of administering rituximab prior to CAR T-cell treatment in R/R B-ALL, and they determined whether any acidity was in the in vitro B-ALL cells. CR was defined as no extramedullary sites of disease, remission as less than 5% bone marrow blasts, and MRD negativity as defined by less than 0.01% bone marrow blasts. Relapse was determined by the reappearance of blasts in blood and bone marrow. CRS and ICANS were also assessed. Clinical response was shown by MRD negativity achieved at a median time of 5.03 months; at analysis, 8/10 (80%) remained alive in the rituximab arm, whereas 3/10 (30%) remained alive in the control arm. Six proceeded to allo-HSCT, with 5/6 achieving CR and surviving. In the control group, eight patients underwent HSCT, and only 3/8 patients were alive, demonstrating a CR. Immune-modulating cytokines such as IL-2, IL-6, IFN-gamma, and TNF-alpha were also evident in the rituximab group, and OS and LFS were higher in the rituximab group (90% vs. 26.7% and 41.7% vs. 25%, respectively), which also improved for relapsed patients (88.9% vs. 25% and 87.5% vs. 15%, respectively) with a long-term prognosis in the rituximab arm, being superior to that in the control group. When evaluated, the killing ability of rituximab showed the expansion and killing of CD19/CD22 CAR T cells, which rapidly proliferated upon challenge, with Nalm-6 reaching on day 5 a peak level of expansion and with CD20 binding to the cell surface, leading to the inhibition of tumor cell proliferation, the induction of apoptosis, and the sensitization of tumor cells to CT. The authors found that unlike the control, rituximab in combination with CAR -T repeatedly eliminated tumor cells. They concluded that when tumor cells were pretreated with rituximab, CD19/CD22 expansion efficiently occurred in vitro, leading to a reduction in tumor burden, promoting the killing efficiency of CAR T, and improving LFS in patients failing multiple lines of therapy—leading to the implication that rituximab shows effectivity and may serve as an option in relapsed patients [28].

9.7 Adverse Events and Toxicity Profiles Associated with CAR T-Cell Therapy

A remarkable review article was written by Hughes et al. (Figs. 9.8 and 9.9), providing detailed summaries of the main AEs associated with CAR T-cell therapy, their symptoms, and their management: CRS, ICANS, and HLH-like syndrome or immune effector cell–associated HLH-like syndrome (IEC-HS). Many of these toxicities are unique and life-threatening, whose biology and risk factors need to be understood and assessed for targeted approaches. As the authors state, hyperinflammation and cytokine storm characterize these events; however, the relevant cytokines and immune cells driving pathophysiology differ. The first patient experiencing CRS had high-spiking fevers progressing to CV and respiratory failure with numerous cytokine elevations (IL-6, IL-10, and IFN-gamma), which led to dramatic improvement after receiving tocilizumab. The biology and pathophysiology of the

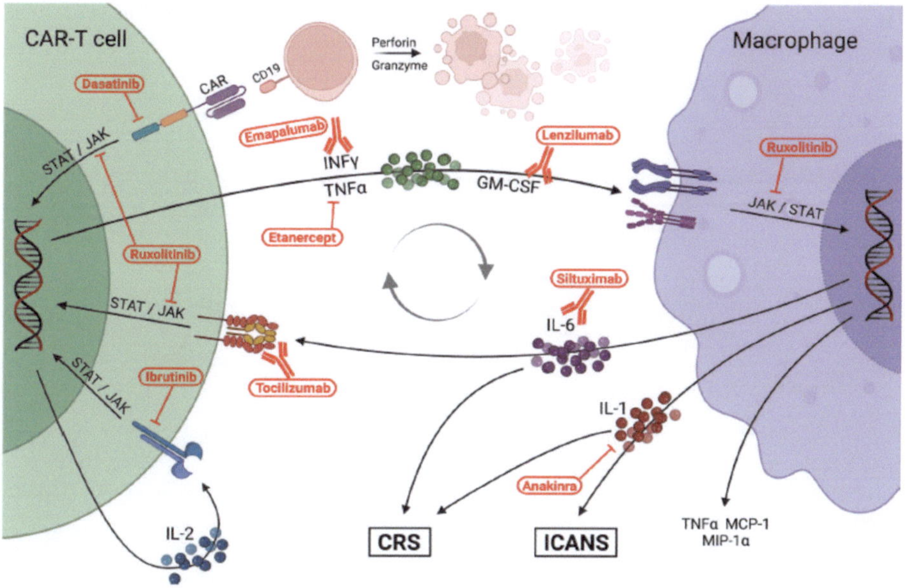

Fig. 9.8 A schematic detailing the current understanding of the pathophysiology of CRS and ICANS caused by cross-talk between CAR T cells and macrophages, where several of the current and emerging therapies for CRS and ICANS are shown in their mechanism of action. (Created with biorender.com and adapted from Hughes et al. [30])

inflammation result in capillary leak and fever, leading to hypoxia and hypotension. ICANS is marked by seizure, ataxia, and cranial nerve palsy; IEC-HS is characterized by high ferritin levels, cytopenias, coagulopathy, and multiorgan failure. ZUMA-1 showed that 93% of patients had CRS, 13% of whom had severe ones. CRS is marked by the relevance of IL-6 in its origin, along with the macrophage release of CXCL9, MIG, CXCL10, IFN-alpha, and MIP1a and MIP1b. However, notably, toxicity does not correlate with clinical response, because patients treated with axi cel and tisa cel who developed CRS had no difference in PFS or OS. Disease burden is correlated with the severity of toxicity and is associated with worse symptoms but did not have predictive value. "For example, manipulating the structure of the CD8α domain of the CAR while keeping the 4-1BB/CD28 and CD3ζ signaling domains unchanged was found to preserve anti-tumor efficacy in patients with B-cell lymphoma while significantly reducing the incidence CRS and neurotoxicity." Tocilizumab is considered the main management agent and is also preventive. Corticosteroids are administered as second-line therapy, also found to be preventive in the ZUMA-1 trial. Other agents are being developed, such as the IL-1 receptor antagonist anakira and the IFN-gamma blocking antibody emapalumab. The symptomology of ICANS is delirium motor dysfunction including ataxia, dysphagia, seizures, and encephalopathy. Encephalopathy is further graded by immune effector cell–associated encephalopathy. ICANS is more prevalent in patients treated with CAR T CD28 products and tends to occur later in the treatment process, after

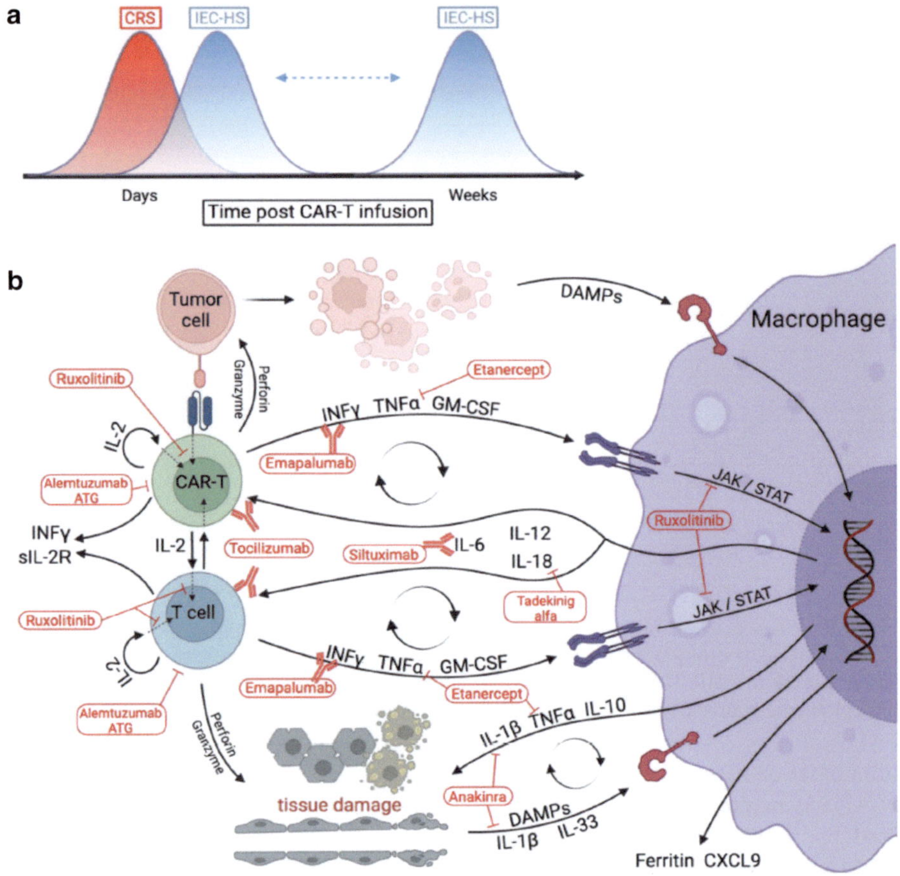

Fig. 9.9 IEC-HS timing is distinct from that of CRS in that it occurs as CRS is resolving or later, after CRS has resolved. The general concept is that CAR T activation creates feed-forward loops with macrophages and endogenous T cells, activated by and resulting in cytokine secretion and tissue damage. Schematic detailing the current understanding of the pathophysiology of IEC-HS, inferred from lines of evidence in secondary HLH, (**a**) and the mechanisms of action of several proposed therapies for IEC-HS, which are incorporated into the schematic to illustrate how they may work to ameliorate this pathology (**b**). (Created with biorender.com)

CRS. The serum levels of cytokines IL-6, IL-18, IFN-gamma, IL-8, and Il-10 are associated with ICANS, with elevated levels of glutamate in the cerebrospinal fluid (CSF). Givng corticosteroids is the primary therapy because they are able to cross the blood–brain barrier (BBB), unlike tocilizumab; however, higher doses have led to metabolic derangements, hypertension, and infection. Anakira is being considered as a prophylactic agent. Shah et al. reported rapid and sustained resolution with intrathecal (IT) administration of hydrocortisone end methotextrate. Immune effector cell–associated HLH-like syndrome (IEC-HS) is characterized by a state of hyperinflammation with hyperferritinemia, cytopenias, and multiorgan dysfunction;

is recognized as clinically and biochemically similar to HLH with organ failure, hepatosplenomegaly, neurologic toxicities, cytopenia, and hyperferritinemia; is caused by immune activation due to dysregulated interaction between T cells, NK cells, and macrophages; is more common in patients with 4-1BB costimulatory domain; and is distinguished by ferritin levels of 10,000 ng/mL and higher. The biology is presupposed to feature the macrophage activation of CAR T via IFN-gamma signaling, leading to tissue damage with high levels of ferritin, IL-1B, and TNF-alpha secretion that mediates this tissue damage and immune cell activation. IFN-gamma blockade with emaplalumab has been approved for primary HLH. Hemodynamic instability, worsening cytopenias, coagulopathy, and hypertriglyceridemia were associated with the administration of tocilizumab, further showing the efficacy of emapalumab. CXCL9 is found to be a useful biomarker. Ruxolitinib is now being increasingly used as frontline therapy. Both severe CRS and later IEC-HS have clinically, biologically, and pathophysiologically overlapping features with HLS and high ferritin, and multiorgan failure and cytopenias with elevated IL-6, IL-10, and IFN-gamma portend worse prognosis. As the authors conclude, the assessment of CAR T–associated toxicities is evolving with refining definitions of CRS and management along with the poorly understood biology of ICANS and the newly recognized IEC-HS, which is now highlighted by timing [29, 30].

Ghilardi et al. reported on a case of T-cell lymphoma after commercial CAR T-cell therapy with a JAK3 variant that exhibited a CD8+ phenotype for NHL. The study investigators assessed the risk of secondary primary malignancy after CAR T-cell therapy, analyzed 449 patients, and found that 16 patients had a secondary primary malignancy at a median onset time of 26.4 and 9.7 months for solid tumors and hematologic malignancies and a projected 5-year cumulative incidence of 15.2% and 2.3% for solid tumors and hematologic malignancies, respectively, with one case of T-cell lymphoma (TCL). The study was in the context of the FDA warning about BCMA therapy, titled "Serious Risk of T Cell Malignancy Following BCMA-Directed or CD19-Directed Autologous Chimeric Antigen Receptor (CAR) T Cell Immunotherapies," where this risk was declared when cases of secondary malignancy were reported in patients with a prior diagnosis of hematologic malignancy (HM). NHL patients have a fivefold higher incidence of secondary TCL and a relative risk of an 11–17-fold higher incidence, with DNA damaging agents and radiotherapy increasing the risk through genomic alterations. MDS and AML also lead to poor prognosis, characterized by a complex karyotype. Secondary malignancies are reported in 15% of patients, with HMs such as MDS, MM, and nonmelanoma skin cancers resulting. In an analysis of patients with NHL receiving tisa cel, 16% developed a secondary malignancy at a 5-year follow-up period. Lung cancer, AML, MDS, prostate cancer, and melanoma were the most frequently characterized secondary malignancies. One case arose because the CAR transgene was inadvertently introduced into CAR T manufacturing. Other patient case studies were reported, with one appearing following an infusion of the piggy-Bac transposon engineered CD19-directed CAR T, showing a CAR expressing CD4+ TCL with high transgene and point mutations and altered copy numbers, which resulted in death. A chronic lymphocytic leukemia (CLL) patient also experienced CAR T expansion that included 94% T-cell clonality. Genetic mutations such as CAR+ TCL (TET2, NFKB) and JAK3 and "CAR insertion in PBX2 represented [possible contributors] to TCL development." The case described by the authors is a patient receiving axi cel with a diagnosis of B-cell lymphoma, with a gray zone lymphoma (GZL) that had no relevant mutations, as shown via NGS, with MAF loss, as revealed via fluorescence in situ hybridization (FISH). After receiving chemoimmunotherapy (CIT) and pembrolizumab, a PR was observed but was complicated by grade 4 autoimmune cells. After receiving brentuzumab vedotin as a bridging therapy to third-line axi cel therapy, one patient's clinical course was followed. The case study is as follows:

> Before CART-19, he received lymphodepletion with fludarabine/cyclophosphamide (dose reduced by 25%; day −5 to −3) and was then infused with 2 × 106 CAR T cells per kg on day 0. The time from apheresis to CAR T infusion was 28 days. He tolerated the treatment well with mild toxicity, including grade 1 cytokine-release syndrome and neurotoxicity. Of note, the infused axi-cel CAR+ cells expanded to high levels (44,261.06 CAR copies per μg of gDNA) at day 7 after infusion compared to other patients with large B cell lymphoma (LBCL) treated with commercial CART-19; however, at day 14, CAR T cells were already decreasing (3,542.52 CAR copies per μg of gDNA), as expected. Completed metabolic remission was seen at the GZL, but after three lymph nodes lesions resulting, a peripheral TCL arose CD79a and CD138 highlighted scattered plasma cells that seem polytypic by kappa and lambda staining. Immunohistochemistry analysis showed large, atypical cells that were CD45+, CD30+, CD2+, CD3+, CD5 (partial weak)+, CD4 (partial weak)+, CD8+ and perforin+. The presence of the JAK+ variant was also detected. The TCL was therefore diagnosed as a CD8+ peripheral TCL, NOS with a cytotoxic phenotype, with a clonal TRG rearrangement identified. qPCR also showed the possession of very low levels of CAR transgene. It was also determined that the T cell population from which the neoplastic T cell population clone arose was circulating at the time of apheresis at day 28. The possession of a high levels of CAR T transgene with the relevant timing showed an uncommon cytotoxic immunophenotype suggesting the contribution of T cel activation during CAR T manufacturing post CAR T inflammation. [31]

9.8 Focusing on Treatment for Solid Tumors with CAR T-Cell Therapy

Ai et al. and Chen et al. have written extensive reviews on CAR T-cell therapy for solid tumors, which cover strategies for employing individual CAR T-cell subsets, combinatorial treatments, optimizing CAR T structure design, modification and production, targeting appropriate tumor-specific antigens, combating an immunosuppressive tumor microenvironment in solid tumors, and mitigating side effects and toxicities. As they state, the effectiveness of CAR T-cell therapies in solid tumors is limited due to a variety of factors, such as a lack of tumor-specific target antigens, the immunosuppressive TME, restricted T-cell proliferation and invasion, and s risk of severe toxicity. For solid tumors, CAR T cells face challenges in finding the appropriate TSAs, the heterogeneity of tumor target antigen, and the immunosuppressive environment, which can be overcome by using combination therapies and the results from ongoing clinical studies. Conventional targets in solid tumors such as EGFR, HER2, and MSLN are tumor-associated antigens that exist in normal tissue as well and a lack the specificity of tumor-specific antigens that are associated with off-target effects that lead to serious negative events. Tumor escape is also an issue because of the limited ability of CAR T cells to recognize only a single surface marker, raising the risk of tumor recurrence. The problems raised by tumor heterogeneity and escape are mitigated by a number of strategies, including pooled CAR T-cell therapy, entailing the sequential and concurrent use of multiple CAR T-cell types designed for targeting a specific antigen; bispecific CAR T cells expressing two CARs simultaneously; a tandem CAR combining two TAA-specific scFvs alone, forming a unified CAR with an intracellular signaling component on the cell surface; the use of the Notch signaling pathway through the construction of SynNotch to induce CAR expression in T cells; and on-switch CAR separating the coregulatory domain from the signal domain, promoting the assembly of the two CAR fragments through small molecule heterodimerization, leading to T-cell activation. According to studies, in "pooled CAR T cell therapy, the capacity of CAR T cells to identify and attach to corresponding tumor cells is enhanced, reducing the likelihood of tumor resistance." Two examples are the use of cholangiocarcinoma to target EFGR and CD33 and the coapplication of PSCA-targeting antigen and MUC1-directed CAR T cells to eradicate tumor cells. Bispecific CAR T cells coexpress IL13Rα2 and HER2 CAR molecules and demonstrate reduced tumor escape and stronger antitumor ability; "dual CAR T-cells employ an AND-logic-gated strategy to effectively target dual TAA positive cancer cells," which has shown safety and effectiveness against PCa cells expressing CEA and MSLN. The SynNotch receptor contains a synthetic extracellular (EXC) recognition domain, a core regulatory domain from Notch, and a synthetic intracellular transcription domain. Upon antigen binding, transmembrane cleavage is induced, releasing transcription factors and thus activating the expression of target genes. SynNotch induces the expression of CAR in T cells, whereupon T-cell activation ensues as the CAR binds to antigen on target cells, and more significantly, the activation of T cells occurs only when tumor cells express two specific surface antigens, effectively minimizing off-target toxicity given that cells expressing one antigen are unaffected. ROR1 CAR T cells were modified to express this receptor with specificity for EpCAM and B7-H3. On-switch CAR separates the coregulatory domain from the signal domain activating T cells by promoting the assembly of two CAR fragments by introducing heterodimerized small molecules. The enabled precision leads to the regulation of T-cell time, location, and activity; activation dose-reducing off-tumor toxicity; and first-pass toxicity, with benefits extending to the activity of CAR T cells in solid tumors through its dose dependency and dose titration. Overcoming the immunosuppressive TME, including TAMs and MDSCs, involves creating a proinflammatory stimulatory environment through a number of mechanisms. A second-generation CAR targeting the macrophage marker F4/80 "demonstrated that F4.CAR T cells could selectively kill F4/80+ macrophages and locally release" IFN-gamma and TNF. Reducing M2 macrophages while promoting the M1 phenotype is another effective strategy, as shown by the construction of the folate-targeted Toll-like receptor 7 agonist to bind endosomal TLR7 and initiate signaling pathways for reprogramming both TAMs and MDSCs into proinflammatory M1-myeloid-like cells while repolarizing the M2-like anti-inflammatory phenotype to an M1-like proinflammatory phenotype. CAR T cells and endogenous T-cell activation and accumulation are thus promoted. MDSCs are other mediators of poor response in solid tumors, and TGFbeta serves as a crucial mediator of immune suppression. MDSCs induce the production of Tregs and the release of IL-10 and TGFbeta and produce MMP-9, which remodels the extracellular membrane (ECM), leading to angiogenesis and tumor aggression and spread. TGFbeta also promotes the production of Tregs and restrains T-cell activity by attaching TGFbetaR1 and TGFbetaRII receptors, resulting in mitigated cytotoxic capability and in decreased proliferation with approaches under investigation to counteract this TGFβ-mediated immune suppression through the development of a TGFβ-switch receptor (TGFβ SwR) with the combination of both "transmembrane and intracellular domains of IL-2/IL-15 receptor β and γ chains and the EXC domains of TGFβ receptor I and II, with the ability to transmit activating signals for T cells when triggered by TGFβ." As the authors state, they "co-expressed the TGFβ SwR with CARs, allowing for CAR T cells to maintain effective and persistent function in TGFβ-rich environments." Physical barriers also impose limitations, such as a dense ECM and aberrant vasculature. Disrupting the chemokine-receptor network is also a strategy that was shown by the CAR T cells overexpressing the IL-8 receptors CXCR1 and CXCR2 for improved antitumor effects through tumor infiltration [32].

9.8.1 Selecting T-Cell Subsets and Modifying the CAR T-Cell Structure

Alternative sources of CAR T-cell generation are being actively explored, such as CD4+ T cells, CD8 + CD161+ CAR T cells that release perforin and granzyme, CAR-γδT cells that secrete chemokines and cytokines, and CAR-TN/SCM cells that increase persistence and eliminate exhaustion and the memory phenotype. A clinical study with patients receiving CD4+ and CD8+ CAR T cells in a 1:1 ratio led to enhanced antitumor efficacy, as shown by liso cel achieving high response rates at specific CD4+ and CD8+ doses. CD161 distinguish various T-cell subsets, such as CD8 alpha-beta T cells for enhanced cytotoxic and memory characteristics. CD8 + CD161+ T cells transduced with CAR showed an increased expression of perforin and granzyme B as well as innate-like receptors that show enhanced antitumor survival. Substituting γδ T cells with αβ T cells lowers the risk of GvHD and employs unique MHC-independent mechanisms. These cells can target multiple tumor types, enhance chemokine and cytokine production, and act as APCs for αβT-cell activation. In metastatic CRPC, they were "found to activate CAR-γδT cells independently of CAR, and the endogenous Vγ9Vδ2 T cell receptor enhances γδT cell function." CAR-γδT cells are being further refined by "engineering Vδ1 T cells, a γδT cell subset with a 4-1BB/CD3ζ and GPC-3 CAR" for boosting their naive memory phenotype, leading to cytokine production, increased proliferation, and cytotoxic activity against in vitro hepatocellular carcinoma (HCC). Other strategies being actively investigated are natural killer T (NKT) cells that have increased cytotoxicity, lower GvHD incidence, and more-favorable safety profiles and that can be stimulated through lipid antigens present on CD1d. They also activate apoptosis pathways through the release of perforin and granzyme. CAR T structure modification involves a three-pronged strategy of designing novel targets (CLDN6, B7-H3, CD123/CLL1, and CD19/CD22), costimulatory modification (IL12 integration, 4-1BB, and optimized CD28 stimulation), and using a PD1/CD28 chimeric-switch receptor, thus overcoming the immunosuppressive TME, causing IFN-gamma expression, blocking PD-1/PD-L1, using BiTEs, secreting anti-CD40 antibodies, and leading to IL15 and IL21 costimulation. Claudin 6 is more expressed in extracellular (EC) and nearly absent in healthy tumors, and elevated levels upregulate pathways for tumor proliferation, cell-cycle progression, and receptor ECM interaction. In the phase 1/2 BNT211–01 trial, CLDN6 CAR T cells in R/R CLDN6-positive solid tumors demonstrated significant efficacy, particularly in germ cell tumors, which was evident at even high doses, showing the highest ORR from treatment with CLDN6-specific CAR T cells while maintaining tolerable safety profiles. Other targets include angiogenic pathways such as EphA2-specific CAR T cells, which showed antitumor effects in a xenograft model of EphA2-positive NSCLC, with a decreasing correlative trend of increased IFN-gamma expression. B7-H3, present on solid tumor cells and associated blood vessels, was employed as a target in the construction of TOP CAR cells with a unique mAb. Bispecific and tandem CARs, as alluded to earlier, that target CD123/CLL-1 and CD19/CD22 outperform single targets, showing greater efficacy against B-cell malignancies and eliminating leukemic cells via cytokine release. A flexible design of dual target CAR T cells enhances their targeting accuracy toward tumor cells and reduces off-target toxicity, with extended survival times through the targeting of both PRDM1 and NR4A3. CD28 stimulation has been associated with exhaustion and reduced persistence, and modifying it can reduce these effects. A mutant CD28 was developed for a CD19-specific CAR T cell that also included 4-1BB. The optimized CD28-enhanced CAR T cell showed antitumor activity and improved the memory phenotype, boosting proliferation and increasing lymphocyte-specific protein TK to the tumor site. CD27 expressed on immunogenic cells, and its ligand CD70 was found on APCs and DCs, and macrophages activating NF-kappaB led to "T-cell activation differentiation and clonal expansion." CD27 CAR T cells have an effective antigen-stimulated effector function with increased survival in ovarian cancer (OC) mouse models. HVEM and GITR have also been incorporated into CAR T-cell constructs. HVEM is expressed on B cells and T cells and has been incorporated into CAR T-cell constructs; interaction with its ligand LIGHT leads to T-cell activation and proliferation; and its binding to BTLA inhibits T-cell activation. In one report, HVEM G2 CAR T cells showed increased production of inflammatory cytokines and higher antitumor effects when compared to CD28 or 4-1BB G2 CAR T cells [33].

An approach to modifying CAR T cells by targeting genes and regulating the gene expression involved in cellular proliferation, exhaustion, and cytokine production is an area of active investigation utilizing pharmacological agents to inhibit or activate signaling molecules. One example is to increase the expression of FOXO1 to enhance T cells' cytotoxicity and persistence. When expressed in solid tumors, high levels of FOXO1 exhibit superior cytotoxicity and improved efficacy. When combined with elevated levels of IL-15, CAR T cells have increased longevity and lead to tumor suppression, as shown through in vivo models featuring genetically modified CAR T cells, reducing tumor size by 30% and increasing the survival rate by 50% with the dual regulation approach. In addition, introducing loss-of-function mutations into PIK3CD and its regulatory subunits (LCK, SOS1, AKT1, RHOA) into CAR T cells increases IL-2 production and enhances AP-1 and NK-KappaB, improving the tumor elimination efficacy of in vitro assays and in vivo models. Other strategies aiming to modulate the TME include the engineering of CAR T cells to concurrently release a bispecific trap protein targeting PD-1 and TGFbeta, reducing inhibitory T-cell signaling. The development of CD40L expressing CAR T cells to transiently express CD40L on T cells after TCR stimulation activates dendritic cells and cytotoxic T cells and induces apoptosis in CD40+ expressing cells and the development of a meso3-CD40 CAR T cell targeting MSLN that secretes anti-CD40 CAR T cells, showing IFN-gamma secretion and potent cytotoxicity in target cells [33].

A pivotal preclinical study of a Claudin 18.2 CAR T-cell target was conducted by Barrett et al. on multiple solid tumors, including gastric, pancreatic, and esophageal cancers. The target, AZD6422, is an autologous CAR-T that "incorporates defensive dnTGFβRII armoring and an optimized, shortened manufacturing process" and was evaluated for preclinical efficacy and safety in xenograft tumor models, which further supported the clinical development of this armored CAR T product. According to the study authors, "Claudin 18 (CLDN18) is a well-characterized four-transmembrane protein and one of a family of at least 27 CLDNs that regulate cell–cell adhesion, cell permeability, and cell polarity in epithelial cells in a tissue restricted manner." The study proved significant in the design of a construct that could combat the immunosuppressive TME of solid tumors. Its experimental design included a scFv, enhanced CD28 and CD3z costimulatory and signaling domains, and TGFbeta armoring that allowed for a shortened manufacturing process. Cytotoxicity was shown both in vitro and in vivo and also had greater persistence, further supporting its clinical development. Chen et al. describe the clinical trial evaluating the novel CAR T construct, in which 37 patients with CLDN18.2 positive GI cancer received three doses, with a 94.6% rate of grade 1 or 2 CRS, no serious AEs, an ORR of 57.1%, and a DCR of 75% and with a survival rate of 81.2% at 6 months [34].

In short, CAR T-cell therapy is considered the standard of care in hematologic malignancies with ongoing evaluation in solid tumors. It constitutes an innovative treatment with many FDA approvals and an increasing number of clinical studies, with their role as a mainstay as a cancer immunotherapy being established [35].

References

1. Berger TR, Boardman A, Brentjens R, and Maus MV. Biology of CAR-T Cells. in Gene and Cellular Immunotherapy of Cancer. A. Ghobadi, J. F. DiPersio (eds.) Springer Nature Switzerland AG 2022
2. Zhang G, Wang Y, Lu S, Ding F, Wang X, Zhu C, et al. Molecular understanding and clinical outcomes of CAR T cell therapy in the treatment of urological tumors. Cell Death Dis. 2024;15(5):359.
3. Boardman AP, Salles G. CAR T-cell therapy in large B cell lymphoma. Hematol Oncol. 2023;41(Suppl 1):112–8.
4. Locke FL, Oluwole OO, Kuruvilla J, Thieblemont C, Morschhauser F, Salles G, et al. Axicabtagene ciloleucel vs standard of care in second-line large B-cell lymphoma: outcomes by metabolic tumor volume. Blood. 2024;143(24):2464–73.
5. Elmacken M, Peredo-Pinto H, Wang C, Xu Z, Tegenge M, Jaigirdar AA, et al. FDA approval summary: Lisocabtagene Maraleucel for second-line treatment of large B-cell lymphoma. Clin Cancer Res. 2024;30(11):2309–16.
6. Kamdar M, Solomon SR, Arnason J, Johnston PB, Glass B, Bachanova V, et al. Lisocabtagene maraleucel versus standard of care with salvage chemotherapy followed by autologous stem cell transplantation as second-line treatment in patients with relapsed or refractory large B-cell lymphoma (TRANSFORM): results from an interim analysis of an open-label, randomised, phase 3 trial. Lancet. 2022;399(10343):2294–308.
7. Trando A, Ter-Zakarian A, Yeung P, Goodman AM, Hamdan A, Hurley M, et al. Outcomes of chimeric antigen receptor (CAR) T-cell therapy in patients with large B-cell lymphoma (LBCL): a single-institution experience. Cancers (Basel). 2023;15(18)
8. Rodriguez-Otero P, Ailawadhi S, Arnulf B, Patel K, Cavo M, Nooka AK, et al. Ide cel or standard regimens in relapsed and refractory multiple myeloma. N Engl J Med. 2023;388(11):1002–14.
9. San-Miguel J, Dhakal B, Yong K, Spencer A, Anguille S, Mateos MV, et al. Cilta cel or standard care in lenalidomide-refractory multiple myeloma. N Engl J Med. 2023;389(4):335–47.
10. Swan D, Madduri D, Hocking J. CAR-T cell therapy in multiple myeloma: current status and future challenges. Blood Cancer J. 2024;14(1):206.
11. Nasiri F, Asaadi Y, Mirzadeh F, Abdolahi S, Molaei S, Gavgani SP, et al. Updates on CAR T cell therapy in multiple myeloma. Biomark Res. 2024;12(1):102.
12. Reddy ST, Hosoya H, Mikkilineni L. CAR T-cell therapy to treat multiple myeloma: current state and future directions. Cancer Metastasis Rev. 2024;44(1):14.
13. Du Z, Zhu S, Zhang X, Gong Z, Wang S. Non-conventional allogeneic anti-BCMA chimeric antigen receptor-based immune cell therapies for multiple myeloma treatment. Cancers (Basel). 2023;15(3)
14. Ravi G, Richard S, Kumar S, Atrash S, Liedtke M, Kaur G, et al. Phase 1 clinical trial of B-cell maturation antigen (BCMA) NEX-T(R) chimeric antigen receptor (CAR) T cell therapy CC-98633/BMS-986354 in participants with triple-class exposed multiple myeloma. Leukemia. 2025;39(4):816–26.
15. Du J, Fu W-J, Jiang H, Dong B, Gao L et al. Updated results of a phase I, open-label study of BCMA/CD19 dual-targeting fast CAR-T GC012F for patients with relapsed/refractory multiple myeloma (RRMM). Abstract. American Society of Clinical Oncology. 2023.
16. Huang Z, Chavda VP, Bezbaruah R, Dhamne H, Yang DH, Zhao HB. CAR T-cell therapy for the management of mantle cell lymphoma. Mol Cancer. 2023;22(1):67.
17. Gagelmann N, Dima D, Merz M, Hashmi H, Ahmed N, Tovar N, et al. Development and Validation of a Prediction Model of Outcome After B-Cell Maturation Antigen-Directed Chimeric Antigen Receptor T-Cell Therapy in Relapsed/Refractory Multiple Myeloma. J Clin Oncol. 2024;42(14):1665–75.
18. Qi C, Zhang P, Liu C, Zhang J, Zhou J, Yuan J, et al. Safety and Efficacy of CT041 in Patients With Refractory Metastatic Pancreatic Cancer: A Pooled Analysis of Two Early-Phase Trials. J Clin Oncol. 2024;42(21):2565–77.

19. van't Land FR, Willemsen M, Bezemer K, van der Burg SH, van den Bosch TPP, Doukas M, et al. Dendritic cell-based immunotherapy in patients with resected pancreatic cancer. J Clin Oncol. 2024;42(26):3083–93.
20. Jain MD, Spiegel JY, Nastoupil LJ, Tamaresis J, Ghobadi A, Lin Y, et al. Five-year follow-up of standard-of-care axicabtagene ciloleucel for large B-cell lymphoma: results from the US lymphoma CAR T consortium. J Clin Oncol. 2024;42(30):3581–92.
21. Liu A, Li X, Wu H, Guo B, Jonnagaddala J, Zhang H, et al. Prognostic significance of tumor-infiltrating lymphocytes determined using LinkNet on colorectal cancer pathology images. JCO Precis Oncol. 2023;7:e2200522.
22. Yang M, Tang X, Zhang Z, Gu L, Wei H, Zhao S, et al. Tandem CAR-T cells targeting CD70 and B7-H3 exhibit potent preclinical activity against multiple solid tumors. Theranostics. 2020;10(17):7622–34.
23. Pal SK, Tran B, Haanen J, Hurwitz ME, Sacher A, Tannir NM, et al. CD70-targeted allogeneic CAR T-cell therapy for advanced clear cell renal cell carcinoma. Cancer Discov. 2024;14(7):1176–89.
24. Jilani S, Saco JD, Mugarza E, Pujol-Morcillo A, Chokry J, Ng C, et al. CAR-T cell therapy targeting surface expression of TYRP1 to treat cutaneous and rare melanoma subtypes. Nat Commun. 2024;15(1):1244.
25. Gargett T, Truong NTH, Gardam B, Yu W, Ebert LM, Johnson A, et al. Safety and biological outcomes following a phase 1 trial of GD2-specific CAR-T cells in patients with GD2-positive metastatic melanoma and other solid cancers. J Immunother Cancer. 2024;12(5).
26. Bulliard Y, Andersson BS, Baysal MA, Damiano J, Tsimberidou AM. Reprogramming T cell differentiation and exhaustion in CAR-T cell therapy. J Hematol Oncol. 2023;16(1):108.
27. Kearl TJ, Furqan F, Shah NN. CAR T-cell therapy for B-cell lymphomas: outcomes and resistance mechanisms. Cancer Metastasis Rev. 2024;44(1):12.
28. Li Y, Cui Q, Liu S, Liu L, Li M, Gao J, et al. Rituximab potentially improves clinical outcomes of CAR-T therapy for r/r B-ALL via sensitizing leukemia cells to CAR-T-mediated cytotoxicity and reducing CAR-T exhaustion. Cell Oncol (Dordr). 2024;47(5):1649–61.
29. Hayden PJ, Roddie C, Bader P, Basak GW, Bonig H, Bonini C, et al. Management of adults and children receiving CAR T-cell therapy: 2021 best practice recommendations of the European Society for Blood and Marrow Transplantation (EBMT) and the Joint Accreditation Committee of ISCT and EBMT (JACIE) and the European Haematology Association (EHA). Ann Oncol. 2022;33(3):259–75.
30. Hughes AD, Teachey DT, Diorio C. Riding the storm: managing cytokine-related toxicities in CAR-T cell therapy. Semin Immunopathol. 2024;46(3–4):5.
31. Ghilardi G, Fraietta JA, Gerson JN, Van Deerlin VM, Morrissette JJD, Caponetti GC, et al. T cell lymphoma and secondary primary malignancy risk after commercial CAR T cell therapy. Nat Med. 2024;30(4):984 9.
32. Chen T, Wang M, Chen Y, Liu Y. Current challenges and therapeutic advances of CAR-T cell therapy for solid tumors. Cancer Cell Int. 2024;24(1):133.
33. Ai K, Liu B, Chen X, Huang C, Yang L, Zhang W, et al. Optimizing CAR-T cell therapy for solid tumors: current challenges and potential strategies. J Hematol Oncol. 2024;17(1):105.
34. Barrett AM, Britton ZT, Carrasco RA, Breen S, Broggi MAS, Hatke AL, et al. Preclinical evaluation of AZD6422, an armored chimeric antigen receptor T cell targeting CLDN18.2 in gastric, pancreatic, and esophageal cancers. Clin Cancer Res. 2024;30(23):5413–29.
35. Joy R, Phair K, O'Hara R, Brady D. Recent advances and current challenges in CAR-T cell therapy. Biotechnol Lett. 2024;46(1):115–26.

Chapter 10
Artificial Intelligence in Precision Oncology

A basic framework for artificial intelligence (AI) in precision oncology or personalized medicine in oncology applies big data to detect patterns in radiological images and histological slides and to process the vast streams of data from next-generation sequencing (NGS) advancements in whole-genome sequencing (WGS), whole transcriptome sequencing (WTS), and whole-exome sequencing (WES), along with proteomic, metabolomic, and epigenomic data. The foundation relies partly on the necessity for accurate diagnosis in oncology and the use of artificial intelligence (AI) tools to analyze high-throughput data to advance cancer genomics. The value of AI in prognosis and predictability in oncology is an emerging field made possible by these vast streams of omics for analysis. AI, machine learning (ML), and deep learning, a subset of ML, can find patterns in data well beyond human detection and can considerably enhance the accuracy, sensitivity, and specificity of radiological and pathology diagnosis, which has been astutely characterized as a phenomenon underscoring the multimodal aspect of data analysis inherent in oncological decision-making with the primacy of evidence-based care. Other accounts have articulated the ability of AI and ML to process large-scale and heterogenous data to reveal patterns with clinical relevance, such as the process of detecting abnormal features in histologic slides to aid in diagnosis by using automated methods with little human input for risk prediction. Large language models (LLMs) can extract data from electronic health records (EHRs) to optimize clinical decision-making [1, 2].

AI can be applied to many of the main features of precision oncology that have been described in the previous chapters, such as molecular profiling, clinically actionable alterations, targeted therapies for solid tumors and hematologic malignancies, the development of immunotherapies and tumor-agnostic therapies and conducting adaptive clinical trials. AI in precision oncology can go "beyond patient stratification" and applications in pattern recognition through the supervised classification of imaging datasets and omics data [3]. Chang et al. describe the ten hallmarks of AI in precision oncology, grouped into cancer screening asymptomatic

P. Hays, *Personalized Medicine in Oncology*,
https://doi.org/10.1007/978-3-032-14437-9_10

patients, detection following symptoms and profiling diagnosed cancers, patient outcome prediction, treatment planning, and identifying effective treatments and drug design. ML models, including support vector machines and decision trees, use neural networks such as convolutional neural networks (CNNs) and artificial neural networks (ANNs). While AI implications run the gamut of imaging modalities, clinical data, molecular profiling, omics analysis, and prognostic and predictive outcomes with efficacy by developing response biomarkers are also areas of application for AI tools. AI has improved the efficiency and accuracy of screening, such as with the development of a smartphone camera photo input to a CNN model. Early detection can dramatically decrease mortality rates through radiologic imaging, histology, tissue biopsy, and liquid biopsy, an example being the ML-based targeted methylation analysis of cfDNA. A CNN model was developed for cancer classification trained on 130,000 digital images of skin lesions with comparable competence to that of dermatologists. AI can lead to the prediction of tissue origin for unknown cancers and is increasingly relying on molecular characteristics, with its tools being able to conduct this type of characterization with greater accuracy by identifying driver alterations, tumor mutational burden (TMB), and PD-L1 expression. Estimating survival and recurrence rates is also amenable to a random forest algorithm, which generated a 22-gene genomic expression signature for prostate cancer prognosis. A DL model trained and validated on 2072 whole slide images (WSIs) and tumor-stage data predicted disease recurrence risk in endometrial cancer (EC) [4].

Large-scale cancer line data have been used to predict drug synergy through AI tools such as LLM Cancer GPT by using synergy datasets from rare tissues converting tabular data into free text and yielding synergy prediction (Chang). When applying algorithms to tissue types with various histologic features, the spatial distribution of the cancer and neighborhood cells can lead to prognostic and predictive algorithms when applied with other data. For instance, imaging mass cytometry when applied to a tissue sample from 416 NSCLC patients demonstrated that the CNN-based spatial analysis identified five markers (CD14, CD16, CD94, CD117, and alpha-SMA) from immune lineages [5].

10.1 Machine Learning Models and Deep Learning Methods

A fascinating study on deep-learning methods determined prognostic information for CD3 and CD8 in colorectal cancer (CRC) receiving adjuvant chemotherapy. Tumor tissue was derived from the dataset of the QUASAR study, which enrolled 3239 patients with CRC. For prognostic analysis, relapse free survival (RFS) served as the primary outcome, and immunohistochemistry (IHC) and VENTANA scanner along with the deep learning (DL) classification system was used to image algorithms of CD3 and CD8 densities. The results show an association of outcomes with cell-density measures. The optimal cell-density cut points were CD3 (290 (69%) high-risk patients) and CD8 (246 (58%) in the high-risk group). The training set featured an RR of a high risk rate that was twice that of the low risk rate for all measures: CD3-CT 2.00 RR, and CD8-CT 2.17 RR. The training and validation sets were among proportions of tumors with high-risk CD3 and CD8. "QUASAR chemotherapy reduced 2-year recurrence by 42% in all risk groups. The number of patient needed to treat with adjuvant chemotherapy was for first 2 years: 11 high risk; 21: intermediate risk group; 36 for low risk group." The authors concluded that "from the QUASAR trial, high CD3 and CD8 [tumor-infiltrating lymphocyte (TIL)] densities both CT and IM were strongly associated with reduced tumor recurrence postsurgery." However, "CD3 and CD8 densities did not predict chemotherapy sensitivity" [6].

A recent study analyzed hematoxylin and eosin slides through a deep-learning model for predicting homologous recombination deficiency (HRD) and homologous recombination proficiency (HRP). Breast cancer (BC, $n = 1008$) and ovarian cancer (OC, $n = 459$) from the Cancer Genome Atlas (TCGA), malignancies amenable to platinum chemotherapy approaches, and PARP inhibitors underwent analysis by a weakly convolutional neural network architecture. Representing an advancement over molecular profiling through traditional pathologic analysis, DeepHRD does not involve a CLIA-certified genomic test, which costs up to USD 3000 and a 4–6 week waiting period, precluding application and clinical studies. DeepHRD predicted HRD from whole-slide images, and the results showed that the model was able to detect complete response (CR) and progression-free survival (PFS) specific to platinum chemotherapy. Trained breast cancer models were subject to adjusting training parameters and final model testing. According to the study investigators, DeepHRD predicts whether a cancer is HRD or HRP, allowing for subsequent histopathologic investigations, and when applied to an external platinum-treated metastatic BC arm ($n = 77$), a 3.7-fold increase in median progression-free survival (mPRS) occurred (14.4 vs. 3.9 for HRD patients and HRP patients, respectively). A flash-frozen ovarian cancer model was also performed, and the overall survival (OS) of patients predicted to be HRD and HRP were 4.6 and 3.2 years (HR, 0.46 (95% CI 0.23 to 0.93)), respectively. The DeepHRD model indicated that a "deep-learning framework is applicable to routinely sectioned tissue blocks" across cancer types [7].

One study relates how AI has impacted molecular tumor boards, citing an example of a virtual molecular tumor board. The characteristics of this virtual molecular tumor board (VMTB) are as follows:

- It is a cloud-based board that includes a scoring model, a rules engine of > 51,000 rules, and a knowledge and a reporting tool with a virtual chat room. The VMTB led to reductions in time period from data receipt to the delivery of the report. Biomarker-driven trials were found for patients to develop personalized treatment plans through the VTMB rather than solely through commercial lab results.

One caveat that was mentioned was duration response variability to targeted therapy, which could be mitigated by taking into consideration intrapatient tumor heterogeneity.

A noteworthy study on the economic impact and life years gained (LYG) for NGS testing for actionable driver oncogenes (ADOs) reported that "[e]ach incremental 10% increase in NGS testing produces an average of 2,627.4 additional LYG, with an average cost savings per LYG of USD 75." ADOs included EGFR, ALK, ROS1, BRAF, RET, MET, and NTRK, with "an average additional 21,096 LYG and a reduced cost per LYG by an average of USD 599," gained by replacing single-gene testing with NGS. The conclusion of the authors was that the total average cost of LYG would be close to USD 17,000 if 100% of eligible patients were identified with matched treatment after NGS evaluation and testing, where its widespread adoption would yield clinically relevant gains in survival accompanied by non-negligible reductions in costs. The study (which used a statistical model) focused on non–small cell lung cancer (NSCLC) because single-gene testing for a few genomic alterations still exists for this cancer despite comprehensive genomic profiling (CGP) recommendations [8].

A similar study on the cost-effectiveness of NGS versus single gene testing (SgT) was also conducted in the setting of a Spanish reference center. In this study, 9734 NSCLC patients were estimated in the target population.

Key Results

- NGS could lead to the detection of 1873 more alterations versus SgT, with 82 more patients enrolling in clinical trials, accentuated by using NGS for providing 1188 additional quality-adjusted life years (QALYs) in the target population when compared with SgT.
- However, "the incremental cost of NGS versus SgT in the target population was €21,048,580 for a lifetime horizon (€1,333,288 for the diagnosis phase only).
- The obtained incremental cost–utility ratios were €25,895 per QALY gained, below the standard cost-effectiveness thresholds, leading to NGS being a cost-effective strategy."

Using a decision tree model that covered the diagnostic phase after treatment was assigned, partitioned survival models were developed and used to determine health consequences and long-term costs. The authors concluded that implementing NGS in Spanish reference centers would lead to clear benefits, with LYs gained (1,188.08 LY, 812.84 QALYs) because more candidates would receive optimate treatment according to genetic testing, which outweighs the costs of targeted therapies given that the "ICURs obtained are below usual cost-effective thresholds" [9].

10.2 Computationally based and Network Analysis Applications

A computationally based analysis for predicting drug combinations was reported in a review by Flanary et al., showing that a number of computational models, including networks, regression-based machine learning, classifier machine-learning models, and deep-learning approaches, can predict the efficacy of cancer therapies and identify novel compounds. The review focused on studies published over the past 10 years. Network-based methods show relationships between genes, proteins, and pathways and lead to designing combinatorial therapies, whereas regression-based methods are machine-learning models that predict sensitivity (missing dose-response values) for "synergy calculations." Classifier-based machine-learning models also use synergy calculations and drug targets to predict novel drug combinations. Deep-learning methods tackle complex data to devise combination approaches.

Networks include drug–disease, drug–target, drug–drug, and protein–protein interaction networks to identify drug-repurposing candidates. Regression-based methods, on one hand, lead to the prediction of outcomes on relationships between independent variables and dependent variables, a linear relationship being an example. Classifier-based approaches, on the other hand, classify observations according specific mathematical boundaries and classify the drug interactions as either additive, synergistic, or antagonistic. Deep learning handles (involving artificial neural networks) large amounts of data that can be used to "discern significant biological relationships" to make predictions. Deep learning also outperforms other machine-learning methods in predicting several pharmacodynamic properties for the purposes of drug discovery, such as drug toxicity and activity, and it outperforms other ML methods for these tasks. Not only has deep learning been used to predict several pharmacodynamic properties for drug discovery purposes, such as drug activity and toxicity, but it has also been shown to outperform other machine-learning methods for these tasks—DeepSynergy and CCSynergy being two examples. The review authors conclude that comprehensive models using these computational methods can lead to improvements in implementing patient multi-omics data with pharmacodynamic considerations to predict the ability of effective drug regimens for cancer, reducing drug development costs and time and leading to better patient outcomes [10].

An integrated Clinical and Genomic Information System (CGIS) was presented in one report as a way to aid precision oncology by providing systematic interpretations of genomic alterations from NGS data. The methodology involves a web-based CGIS that processes NGS data, annotates variants, and integrates clinical information to recommend therapies and support patient cohort exploration. Key findings include the ability of the system to identify actionable genomic targets, stratify patients on the basis of molecular data, and provide interactive tools for variant exploration and survival analysis. The conclusion emphasizes that the CGIS software is designed for both clinicians and medical scientists, integrating diverse genomic resources to facilitate biomarker development and clinical decision-making. Potential implications include improved precision medicine through an enhanced understanding of genomic data, patient stratification, and targeted therapy options. The integration workflow is shown Fig. 10.1. Like prior similar studies, the development of the CGIS was an early example of establishing the importance of NGS for oncology and the processing of clinical information for determining effective therapies through actionable genomic targets [11–13]. In Fig. 10.1, information flow among various components is indicated in arrows. BioDataBank is the central knowledgebase of information for genes, variants, drugs, curated records, cohort population data, etc.

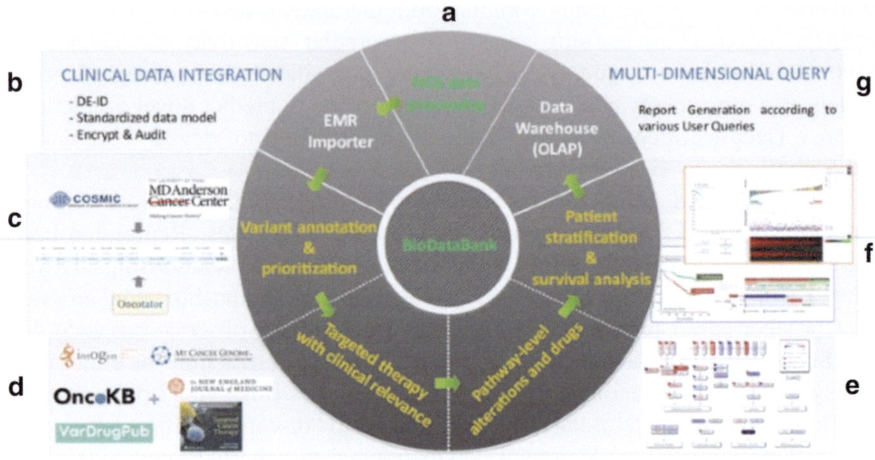

Fig. 10.1 System architecture of our CGIS software, where the labels beside component panels (**a**–**g**) correspond to description markers in the section featuring the implementation/overview of the system and its features

10.3 Multi-Omics

A fascinating study on multi-omics and three-dimensional (3D) tumor models was conducted by Jose et al., which, in light of drug discovery and precision medicine, integrated 3D tumor models such as patient-derived tumor organoids with pan-omics technologies, including genomic NGS, microarrays, and transcriptomics, comprising RNA-seq, scRNA-seq, and epigenomics, including ChIP-seq and ATAC-seq, leading to the development to novel drug targets and the differentiation of drug sensitivity (Figs 10.1 and 10.2). This report highlighted that the application of 3D tumor models would be advantageous over conventional yet valuable two-dimensional (2D) cultures. In one study, the prognostic ability of PARP inhibitors was enhanced, where those who benefited could be identified through HRR analysis through X-ray exposure to patient derived organdies (PDOs). Transcriptomic analysis of PDOs derived from metastatic liver samples from CRC patients showed drug sensitivity to EGFR, RAS, and TP53 after drug-sensitivity testing. Another cited study used ChIP-seq and RNA-seq data analysis, which led to the identification of epigenomic and transcriptomic reprogramming in prostatic epithelial cells, confirming the role of Myc and "significant, androgen dependent alteration" in transcriptional and histone methylation patterns in N-Myc by using in vivo, in vitro, and PDO models. As the review authors highlight, 3D tumor modeling is highly effective in assessing cancer therapy through its ability to "recapitulate the complexities of in vivo tumors with better prediction of therapy sensitivity," including the cells of the tumor microenvironment and extracellular matrix (ECM) modeling [14].

In another quantitative study, whole transcriptome and DNA sequencing results were analyzed from a database and matched with Kaplan–Meier estimates to

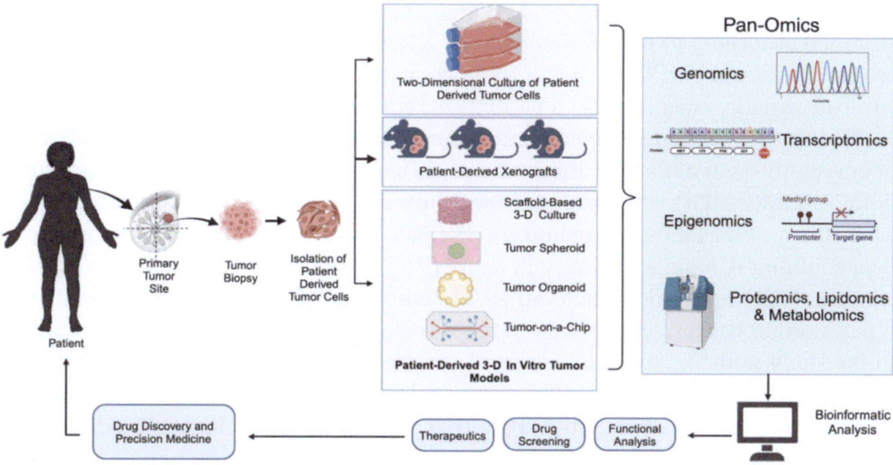

Fig. 10.2 Graphical abstract

differentiate between young-onset pancreatic cancer (YOPC) clinical outcomes and adult-onset pancreatic cancer (AOPC) clinical outcomes.

Key Results

- Higher proportions of MMR/MSI-H, BRCA2-mutant, and PALB2-mutant tumors were among YOPC patients than among AOPC patients, and the former had fewer CDKN2A-, RNF43-, SMAD4-, and SF3B1-mutant tumors.
- A lower incidence of KRAS mutation was shown among YOPC patients in comparison to AOPC patients (81.3% vs. 90.9%). YOPC tumors in the KRASWT subtype (n = 227) demonstrated fewer TP53 mutations and were driven mainly by NRG1 and MET fusions, whereas among AOPC patients, BRAF fusions were exclusively observed.
- A significant enrichment of NK cells, monocytes, M2 macrophages, and CD8+T cells was also observed in YOPC patients relative to AOPC patients, corresponding to lower rates of HLA-DPA1 homozygosity.
- Improved OS was associated with KRAS-WT tumors among YOPC patients when compared with AOPC patients who were also KRASWT status (16.2 vs. 10.6), but this was not evident in KRAS-mutant tumors (12.9 vs. 10.0 months).

The study authors concluded that age-stratified molecular differences in pancreatic ductal adenocarcinoma (PDAC) in this real-world, large multi-omics study showed that YOPC is associated with differentially regulated signaling pathways of the tumor transcriptome that has prognostic and therapeutic implications and a distinct molecular landscape that could lead to targeted options because YOPC harbored an increased incidence of BRCA2 and PALB2 but lower rates of KRAS, which demonstrated better overall survival (OS) in the wild-type form. Immune cell subsets were also enriched in this real-world YOPC cohort when compared to AOPC. Differential expression was observed among a relatively narrow number of genes when comparing YOPC and AOPC, and evidence showed that OS could be stratified according to KRAS mutated and KRASWT, suggesting "that survival differences between YOPC and AOPC patients in the overall cohorts may be driven by survival variation specifically in patients harboring KRASWT tumors" [15].

A recent AI study developed regulated cell death, a sequential form of cell death operating through molecular mechanisms, as a biomarker to predict immune checkpoint inhibitor (ICI) response, and the study authors conducted a comprehensive assessment of its status and features at the pan-cancer level to reveal emerging evidence linking ICI and regulated cell death (RCD) efficacy, such as OS, in malignant cancers. RCD levels determine an RCD score and RCD landscape across cancer types, normal tissues, and cells from large-scale 82 scRNA-Seq datasets. According to the study authors, an RCD signature was developed from seven ML algorithms and 18 ICI cohorts to predict ICI response. In total, 18 RCD genes were collected from previous studies, revealing TP53, BCL2, and BAX, which suggested common nodes and hubs between RCD modalities. Collected transcriptomic data showed that RCD levels between cell lines of different cancer origins varied considerably. The association between RCD levels on one hand and functional signaling pathways and genomic variations on the other at the pan-cancer level showed that RCD scores had negative associations with cell-cycle signaling and DNA repair but had positive associations with inflammation and metastasis, showing that failures in DNA repair and "abnormal assembly of oncogenic signaling hubs trigger cell death." RCD score correlation with TMB, copy number variation (CNV), and intra-tumor heterogeneity showed that the RCD levels were negatively associated with CNV score and positively associated with TMB in colon cancer and breast cancer (OCAD and BRCA). Therefore, the RCD level may serve as a relevant biomarker for ICI treatment, being an effective complement to TMB and intra-tumor heterogeneity (ITH). RCD heterogeneity levels in various tumors may impact clinical outcomes and serve as a robust and feasible predictor for prognosis. The expression of immune checkpoints may have a positive correlation with RCD scores. Additionally, 29 signatures categorized into pro-TME, anti-TME, fibrosis, angiogenesis, and malignant cell proprieties demonstrate a positive relation between signature and RCD level, with several steps in the cancer-immunity cycle being related to RCD levels in individual cancer types. When the study authors considered 1793 immune-related genes, the majority of genes were signals associated with RCD levels in almost all solid cancer types. A positive correlation was also shown with objective response rate (ORR), and TMB immune cell infiltration showed that high-RCD subgroups and low-RCD subgroups were related to high-ITH and low-ITH subgroups. High RCD scores were shown in nonresponder subgroups, and the proportion of cells was higher, as shown with scRNA-Seq data. A predictive model for ICI response was based on the RCD signature as constructed with comparable assessments. Furthermore, 18 bulk-level transcriptomic cohorts treated with ICI revealed an area under the curve (AUC) of 0.56 to 0.72 in a validation dataset. The patients in the high-risk group had worse OS than those in the low-risk group (HR 7.54). The testing of individual cohorts revealed an AUC ranging from 0.58 to 0.85, indicating the robustness of the predictive model through the optimally predictive model, with

13 published signatures, in which the RCD-Sig-based model demonstrated high predictive effectiveness, and consistently, ICI response based on RCD signature also had predictive value, "demonstrating remarkable robustness and superiority compared to previously published signatures." Solid tumors had an RCD that positively correlated with ICI effectiveness and was prevalent across a wide range of cancer types and pan-cancer RCD signatures, showing that RCD-Sig-containing genes demonstrated a correlation with RCD. An RCD-Sig pan-cancer survival signature showed that oncology patients across multiple independent datasets had strong associations with prognosis and prediction [16].

A study on an AI-based image analysis of the IHC assessment of PD-L1 expression in diffuse large B-cell lymphoma (DLBCL) also displayed similar results of presenting as a prognostic and predictive biomarker for the malignancy. In contrast to solid tumors, where tumor regions can differentially identify PD-L1 expression, tumor B cells, and nonmalignancy, immune cells can coexpress PD-L1 in the TME. In the study, a PD-L1 scoring framework for lymphoma was accurately quantified for tumor proportion score (TPS). Tumor cells were digitally screened for DLBCL in IHC slides, and primary and validation cohorts were constructed with large-scale available annotations. Three senior pathologists scored TPS in 220 PD-L1 and WSIs in a double-blind manner for correlation measurement. The correlation between AI algorithm outcomes and pathology results along with results in PD-L1 scoring demonstrated that the algorithm consistently provided stable quantitative findings that were closely aligned with pathologists' findings.

Key Results

- The concordance between surgical specimens and intra-pathologist scores was 0.91 (95% CI 0.87 to 0.94).
- The intraclass correlation coefficient (ICC) between the mean scores of pathologists and the algorithm's results was 0.95 (95% CI 0.93 to 0.97).
- The concordance between the median scores of pathologists and the algorithm's results was 0.96 (95% CI 0.94 to 0.98).
- Fine needle biopsy on the IPC was 0.96 (95% CI 0.94 to 0.97).
- The ICC between the mean scores of pathologists and the algorithm's results was 0.96 (95% CI 0.95 to 0.97).
- The ICC between the median scores of pathologists and the algorithm's results was 0.95 (95% CI 0.93 to 0.97).

These results support strong agreement between pathologists and the algorithm's assessment. According to the authors, a new PD-L1 quantification rule for DLBCL was used to address the difficulty of tumor cell identification in expression quantitation with an objective and interpretable tool for quantifying and analyzing PD-L1 expression in DLBLC patients. These AI-based models can be sued for determining quantifiable results. This would help pathologists face limitations in accurate cell counting and calculations, avoid misclassifying patients as positive or negative, potentially deprive patients of the advantages of receiving immunotherapy, and avoid potentially harmful treatments, with the authors' analytics indicating stable and consistent performance. They show that their two-stage cell segmentation model streamlines qualitative discrimination in DLBCL, yielding quantitative results closely aligning with and complementing pathologists' assessment through an integrative pipeline of cell detection and segmentation. The authors' hypothesis was that tumor cells exhibit larger morphologies, and this would lead to distinguishing membrane positive cancer cells and provide an "intelligence-assisted framework" for accurately quantifying PD-L1 expression in a digital manner with objectivity and interpretability thanks to the AI-based models being optimized for DLBCL patient analysis, ensuring a high level of concordance between pathologists' evaluations and AI-generated results. The authors conclude that, taken together, their "findings show that pathologists of different levels of experience can potentially benefit from the AI-assisted model to enhance the immunotherapy decision making for DLBCL patients" [17].

Challenges exist in the implementation of AI for personalized medicine in oncology, including insufficient data, the interpretability of the data, and dealing with multiple data modalities. ML applications are developed to automate the process of different levels of data integration, including combinations of data from different inputs, such as omics data, with difficulties in extracting predictive patterns in patient outcomes concomitant with this challenge. Access to massive high-quality datasets is also an issue due to the relative lack of reference datasets for molecularly characterized tumors. Furthermore, the machine learning (ML) system's ability to make predictions must be understandable and interpretable to humans, with higher-complexity models posing interpretability challenges, such as in detailed depictions of evidence relationships behind individual predictions [3].

As this chapter on the exciting field of AI in precision oncology comes to a close, this book finds its conclusion in the vast enterprise of personalized medicine in oncology, with points made, concepts and ideas outlined, and innovations and technologies detailed. With the graphic representation of the cancer-immunity cycle leading to a deep understanding of immunology in developing cancer immunotherapies, the discovery of signaling pathways and genomic alterations paving the way for targeted therapies, and improvements in diagnosis through liquid biopsy, the paradigm could be considered established and fully implemented in mainstream medicine. Medicine may have been profoundly affected and considerably advanced.

References

1. Ballester PJ, Carmona J. Artificial intelligence for the next generation of precision oncology. NPJ Precis Oncol. 2021;5(1):79.
2. Ballester PJ, Carmona J. Artificial intelligence for the next generation of precision oncology. npj Precis Oncol. 2021;5:79.
3. Azuaje F. Artifiical intelligence for precision oncology: beyond patient stratification. Npj Precision Oncol. 2019;3:6.
4. Chang T-G, Park S, Schaffer AA, Jiang P, Ruppin E. Hallmarks of artificial intelligence contributions to precision oncology. Nature Cancer. 2025;6:417.

5. Fountzilas E, Pearce T, Baysal MA, Chakraborty A, Tsimberidou AM. Convergence of evolving artificial intelligence and machine learning techniques in precision oncology. Npj Digital Med. 2025;8:75.
6. Williams CJM, Gray R, Hills RK, Shires M, Zhang L, Zhao Z, et al. Evaluation of CD3 and CD8 T-Cell Immunohistochemistry for Prognostication and Prediction of Benefit From Adjuvant Chemotherapy in Early-Stage Colorectal Cancer Within the QUASAR Trial. Journal of Clinical Oncology. 2024;42(29):3430–42.
7. Bergstrom EN, Abbasi A, Díaz-Gay M, Galland L, Ladoire S, Lippman SM, et al. Deep Learning Artificial Intelligence Predicts Homologous Recombination Deficiency and Platinum Response From Histologic Slides. Journal of Clinical Oncology. 2024;42(30):3550–60
8. Lemmon CA, Zhou J, Hobbs B, Pennell NA. Modeling Costs and Life-Years Gained by Population-Wide Next-Generation Sequencing or Single-Gene Testing in Nonsquamous Non-Small-Cell Lung Cancer in the United States. JCO Precis Oncol. 2023;7:e2200294.
9. Arriola E, Bernabe R, Campelo RG, Biscuola M, Enguita AB, Lopez-Rios F, et al. Cost-Effectiveness of Next-Generation Sequencing Versus Single-Gene Testing for the Molecular Diagnosis of Patients With Metastatic Non-Small-Cell Lung Cancer From the Perspective of Spanish Reference Centers. JCO Precis Oncol. 2023;7:e2200546.
10. Flanary VL, Fisher JL, Wilk EJ, Howton TC, Lasseigne BN. Computational Advancements in Cancer Combination Therapy Prediction. JCO Precis Oncol. 2023;7:e2300261.
11. Stuart T, Butler A, Hoffman P, Hafemeister C, Papalexi E, Mauck WM, 3rd, et al. Comprehensive Integration of Single-Cell Data. Cell. 2019;177(7):1888–902 e21.
12. Xing XW, Zhang JT, Ma YB, He MW, Yao GE, Wang W, et al. Metagenomic Next-Generation Sequencing for Diagnosis of Infectious Encephalitis and Meningitis: A Large, Prospective Case Series of 213 Patients. Front Cell Infect Microbiol. 2020;10:88.
13. Jang Y, et al. An integrated clinical and genomic information system for cancer precision medicine. BMC Med Genomics. 2018;11(Suppl 2):34.
14. Jose A, et al. Integration of pan-omics technologies and three-dimensional in vitro tumor models: an approach toward drug discovery and precision medicine. Mol Cancer. 2024;23(1):50.
15. Ogobuiro I, Baca Y, Ribeiro JR, Walker P, Wilson GC, Gulhati P, et al. Multiomic Characterization Reveals a Distinct Molecular Landscape in Young-Onset Pancreatic Cancer. JCO Precis Oncol. 2023;7:e2300152.
16. Zhang. Pan-cancer evaluation of regulated cell death to predict overall survival and immune checkpoint inhibitor response. NPJ Precis Oncol. 2024;8(1):77.
17. Yan F. Artificial intelligence-based assessment of PD-L1 expression in diffuse large B cell lymphoma. NPJ Precis Oncol. 2024;8

Index

P. Hays, *Personalized Medicine in Oncology*,
https://doi.org/10.1007/978-3-032-14437-9

T

U

MIX
Papier aus verantwortungsvollen Quellen
Paper from responsible sources
FSC® C105338

If you have any concerns about our products,
you can contact us on
ProductSafety@springernature.com

In case Publisher is established outside the EU,
the EU authorized representative is:
Springer Nature Customer Service Center GmbH
Europaplatz 3, 69115 Heidelberg, Germany

Printed by Libri Plureos GmbH
in Hamburg, Germany